D1158344

GENE–ENVIRONMENT INTERACTIONS IN DEVELOPMENTAL PSYCHOPATHOLOGY

Duke Series in Child Development and Public Policy

Kenneth A. Dodge and Martha Putallaz, *Editors*

GRACE LIBRARY CARLOW UNIVERSITY
PITTSBURGH PA 15213

Gene–Environment Interactions in Developmental Psychopathology

RJ
499
G385
2011

Edited by
KENNETH A. DODGE
MICHAEL RUTTER

THE GUILFORD PRESS
NEW YORK   LONDON

CATALOGUED

© 2011 The Guilford Press
A Division of Guilford Publications, Inc.
72 Spring Street, New York, NY 10012
www.guilford.com

All rights reserved

No part of this book may be reproduced, translated, stored in a retrieval
system, or transmitted, in any form or by any means, electronic, mechanical,
photocopying, microfilming, recording, or otherwise, without written
permission from the publisher.

Printed in the United States of America

This book is printed on acid-free paper.

Last digit is print number: 9   8   7   6   5   4   3   2   1

Library of Congress Cataloging-in-Publication Data
Gene–environment interactions in developmental psychopathology / edited by
Kenneth A. Dodge, Michael Rutter.
    p. ; cm.—(Duke series in child development and public policy)
  Includes bibliographical references and index.
  ISBN 978-1-60623-518-8 (hardcover: alk. paper)
  1. Child psychopathology—Genetic aspects.   2. Child psychopathology—
Environmental aspects.   3. Nature and nurture.   I. Dodge, Kenneth A.
II. Rutter, Michael, 1933–   III. Series: Duke series in child development
and public policy.
  [DNLM: 1. Child Behavior Disorders—genetics.   2. Behavioral
Symptoms.   3. Child Development Disorders, Pervasive—genetics.
4. Child.   5. Environment.   6. Genetic Predisposition to Disease.
7. Health Policy.   WS 350.6]
  RJ499.G385 2011
  618.92′89—dc22

                                                        2010040309

About the Editors

Kenneth A. Dodge, PhD, is William McDougall Professor of Public Policy, Professor of Psychology and Neuroscience, and Director of the Center for Child and Family Policy at Duke University. His research focuses on how genes and environments interact to produce chronic antisocial behavior. He has used his research findings to create, implement, and evaluate preventive interventions for children and parents, and is currently interested in designing policies for communities to prevent violence. Dr. Dodge is a recipient of the Distinguished Scientific Contribution Award from the American Psychological Association and the Senior Scientist Award from the National Institutes of Health.

Michael Rutter, MD, FRS, is Professor of Developmental Psychopathology at the Institute of Psychiatry, Kings College, London, United Kingdom. He has long been interested in gene–environment interdependence, has undertaken numerous studies of environmental influences on psychopathology, and has been involved in both behavioral genetic and molecular genetic studies of mental disorders. Throughout his research and clinical career, he has focused on research–clinical interplay and the policy implications of research findings. Dr. Rutter was knighted in 1992 and is an honorary member of the British Academy, a Fellow of the Royal Society, and founding Fellow of the Academia Europaea and the Academy of Medical Sciences.

Contributors

Avshalom Caspi, PhD, Department of Psychology and Neuroscience, Duke University, Durham, North Carolina

Robert Cook-Deegan, MD, Center for Genome Ethics, Law, and Policy, Institute for Genome Sciences and Policy, Duke University, Durham, North Carolina

E. Jane Costello, PhD, Department of Psychology and Behavioral Sciences, Duke University School of Medicine, Durham, North Carolina

Kenneth A. Dodge, PhD, Center for Child and Family Policy, Sanford School of Public Policy, Duke University, Durham, North Carolina

Guang Guo, PhD, Department of Sociology, University of North Carolina at Chapel Hill, Chapel Hill, North Carolina

Ahmad R. Hariri, PhD, Department of Psychology and Neuroscience and Institute for Genome Sciences and Policy, Duke University, Durham, North Carolina

Andrew Holmes, PhD, National Institute on Alcohol Abuse and Alcoholism, National Institutes of Health, Rockville, Maryland

Joan Kaufman, PhD, Department of Psychiatry, Yale University, New Haven, Connecticut

Andreas Meyer-Lindenberg, MD, Central Institute of Mental Health, Mannheim, Germany; Department of Psychiatry and Psychotherapy, University of Heidelberg, Heidelberg, Germany

Terrie E. Moffitt, PhD, Department of Social, Genetic, and Developmental Psychiatry, Institute of Psychiatry, Kings College London, London, United Kingdom

Stephen J. Morse, JD, PhD, Law School and Department of Psychiatry, University of Pennsylvania, Philadelphia, Pennsylvania

Jenae M. Neiderhiser, PhD, Department of Psychology, The Pennsylvania State University, University Park, Pennsylvania

Francheska Perepletchikova, PhD, Department of Psychiatry, Yale University School of Medicine, New Haven, Connecticut

David Reiss, PhD, Child Study Center, Yale University, New Haven, Connecticut

Michael Rutter, MD, FRS, Department of Social, Genetic, and Developmental Psychiatry, Institute of Psychiatry, Kings College London, London, United Kingdom

Rudolf Uher, PhD, MRCPsych, Department of Social, Genetic, and Developmental Psychiatry, Institute of Psychiatry, Kings College London, London, United Kingdom

Series Editors' Note

Perhaps the most important concept to emerge in the field of child development over the past several decades has been the notion of gene–environment interplay, specifically, the interaction effect. Michael Rutter first articulated the basic hypothesis years ago, namely, that the impact of genes on human development depends on the particular environment in which the child is reared and the impact of the environment depends on one's genes. Only in the past decade, however, has this hypothesis been subjected to rigorous empirical testing in hundreds of studies. We now know, for example, that early life stressors lead to depressive disorder only in a subgroup of children who have a polymorphism in the serotonin transporter gene, and that genetic risk for this disorder does not lead to inevitable outcomes that are unaltered by life experiences. The body of these empirical findings ends the nature–nurture war by declaring that behavioral development is the product of nature with nurture.

Several factors conspired to bring about this revolution in science. Ongoing longitudinal studies of cohorts of children who have been followed from early life through adulthood afforded rich data about qualities of early environments and ready access to these participants for new collection of DNA. Technological advances enabled genotyping of individuals' DNA at reasonable cost. New empirical research in other species offered hypotheses about candidate genes and processes in development. And vibrant multidisciplinary intellectual climates at places such as the Institute of Psychiatry in London nurtured scientific interest in these questions for developmental psychopathology. The result has been an unprecedented set of replicated empirical findings across multiple genes, environments, and psychiatric disorders.

The scientific field has paid attention. The journal *Science* declared the gene–environment interaction effect to be the most important discovery in all of science for the year 2003. Early pivotal articles by Avshalom Caspi and colleagues have been cited thousands of times, and attempted replications now reach triple digits.

Far less clear is the meaning of this body of research for future scientific inquiry, clinical practice, and public policy. Empirical research on gene–environment interactions has progressed so rapidly that many important implications have not yet even been identified. At the same time, some observers have prematurely answered other questions, declaring, for example, that the day of personalized psychiatric medicine is here and the blueprint for genetic engineering of behavior is at hand.

This volume addresses these questions for developmental psychopathology, clinical practice, and public policy. The first part of the volume on scientific understanding, offers concise statements and reviews of research by the leading scientists who have contributed to the revolution. Michael Rutter lays out scientific issues and challenges for conducting this science. Avshalom Caspi and colleagues review the case of the serotonin transporter gene and life stress as co-factors in the development of depression. Ahmad R. Hariri describes how these same gene–environment interactions operate on the development of psychiatric disorders by biasing the neurobiological processing of threat information. Andreas Meyer-Lindenberg goes a step further by describing the neural mechanisms through which gene–environment interactions operate. Finally, Rutter and Kenneth A. Dodge appraise the state of this collective science, note the implications for the future conduct of science in this field, and highlight the challenges that remain.

The second part of the volume addresses clinical practice and policy. David Reiss and Jenae M. Neiderhiser summarize their findings on gene–environment interactions in marital dynamics and the implications of this work for family interventions. Guang Guo reviews findings on gene–environment interactions in adolescent delinquency and asserts implications for prevention of delinquent behavior. Rudolf Uher addresses the potential for personalized pharmacological treatments for depression based on genetic risk; his review is both exciting in its promise and sobering in its acknowledgment of the many steps that remain before the practice of personalized psychiatric medicine is realized. Joan Kaufman and Francheska Perepletchikova tell a fascinating but worrisome story of how politics can intrude on research in gene–environment interaction effects in maltreated children. E. Jane Costello steps back and takes a broader view of how environments affect secular trends in broad behavioral characteristics such as intelligence and psychopathology. Stephen J. Morse moves the discussion to the justice domain by asking whether findings in gene–environment interactions should alter legal definitions of criminal responsibility. Robert Cook-Deegan reflects on how science has been used maliciously in calls for eugenics, and he raises new questions given the context of gene–environment discoveries. Finally, Dodge and Rutter integrate these issues with a statement of how science can and should inform practice and policy, but at an appropriate pace.

The goal of the Duke Series in Child Development and Public Policy is to bring cutting-edge research in the vibrant field of child development to bear on important problems facing children and families in contemporary society. The current volume, *Gene–Environment Interactions in Developmental Psychopathology*, is ideally suited to this task.

Each volume in the series has grown out of a national conference held at the Center for Child and Family Policy at Duke University. The conference held for this volume was particularly multidisciplinary. Participants across conferences have included nationally renowned scholars from multiple disciplines, officials in public service who are charged with improving the lives of families and children, and students who are learning how to integrate scholarship with service.

Reflecting the goal of intersecting basic behavioral science with public policy, the series is a partnership between the Duke University Department of Psychology and Neuroscience and the Duke Center for Child and Family Policy, with Series Editors Martha Putallaz and Kenneth A. Dodge anchoring these two groups, respectively. Each volume in the series also follows the model of an editorial partnership between a scholar at Duke University and a leading scholar at another university. As Series Editors, we owe a great debt to Professor Sir Michael Rutter, of the Institute of Psychiatry at Kings College in London, for his collaboration.

Like previous volumes, the current volume has benefited from financial support provided by the Duke Provost's Office. We are grateful to Duke Provost Peter Lange, PhD, and Duke Vice Provost Susan Roth, PhD. We acknowledge and appreciate the important contributions of conference organizer Erika Layko and Center for Child and Family Policy Associate Director Barbara Pollock. We also thank Zoë Dodge for graphic design and editing.

KENNETH A. DODGE, PhD
MARTHA PUTALLAZ, PhD

Contents

GENE–ENVIRONMENT INTERACTIONS
IN DEVELOPMENTAL PSYCHOPATHOLOGY

PART I

SCIENTIFIC UNDERSTANDING

CHAPTER I

Gene–Environment Interplay

Scientific Issues and Challenges

Michael Rutter

The focus of this book is on gene–environment interactions (G × E) in developmental psychopathology. The discovery of G × E effects in depression and conduct disorder has been met with both excitement and skepticism. In order to appreciate the contributions of these discoveries for understanding the mechanisms of psychopathology, it is crucial to appreciate that the G × E interaction is only one out of several forms of gene–environment interplay, and therefore we will have to consider how G × E fit into this overall pattern and how other forms of gene–environment interplay need to influence how we study G × E. Similarly, although the chapters in this volume deal with a limited number of mental disorders, a quite small number of identified genes, and a narrow range of measured environments, in considering the scientific issues and the challenges they provide, the background considerations must be examined more broadly. In addition, because the study of G × E involves a variety of statistical issues and several key methodological hazards, these too need to be discussed.

BACKGROUND CONSIDERATIONS REGARDING DISORDERS

Most mental disorders are *multifactorial*, meaning that their causation involves multiple genes and multiple environmental factors. Also, most disorders both operate dimensionally and involve dimensional risk factors

(Rutter, 2003). In addition, many disorders involve a spectrum. It should be added that the operation of a spectrum applies to several Mendelian disorders as well as to multifactorial ones (e.g., the range of manifestations in tuberous sclerosis is extremely wide). With respect to multifactorial disorders, a spectrum is apparent, for example, with respect to autism, schizophrenia, Tourette syndrome, and affective disorders (see relevant chapters in Rutter et al., 2008). Most mental disorders involve overlapping disorders or symptom patterns. Thus, anxiety, inattention, and agitation all appear as key features in several different disorders. This plays a part in bringing about high levels of supposed comorbidity, much of which is likely to be artifactual. Often, too, there are developmental changes in symptom patterns, making continuity in diagnostic criteria across the lifespan quite problematic (Rutter, Kim-Cohen, & Maughan, 2006). Neurodevelopmental impairment in childhood is important for some disorders (such as autism, schizophrenia, and attention-deficit/hyperactivity disorder [ADHD]), but not for others (such as bipolar disorder or depression/ anxiety). Finally, the heritability of mental disorders is quite variable. For example, heritability is very high for autism, schizophrenia, and ADHD, but only moderate for many other disorders (Plomin, De Fries, McClearn, & McGuffin, 2008).

BACKGROUND CONSIDERATIONS REGARDING GENES

Each single gene that codes for proteins actually involves multiple DNA elements affecting transcription and expression (Rutter, 2006; Thapar & Rutter, 2008). Most identified susceptibility genes are *pleiotropic*, meaning that they have multiple effects. This is obvious, for example, from the effects of the *ApoE4* gene in relation to both Alzheimer's disease and ageing, on the one hand, and cholesterol metabolism, on the other. Similarly, the *COMT* gene has a substantial range of effects (Caspi et al., 2008). These varied effects may reflect different chemical pathways or they may reflect the diverse consequences of differences in functioning within a single pathway. Genes often affect biological pathways relevant for multiple disorders and for variation in individuals without disorder. The latter feature has been strikingly shown in the experimental studies of G × E (Meyer-Lindenberg et al., 2006). Genetic effects are crucially dependent on gene expression (which is subject to environmental influences, chance variation, and background genetic effects). Most known genetic effects involve probabilistic risks associated with common allelic variations rather than with major pathological mutations, although opinions vary on the frequency of operation of rare and of common variants. Genetic effects may depend on interacting patterns of genes, although good evidence on this assertion in relation to mental disorders is largely lacking at the moment.

Both schizophrenia and autism are associated with reduced fecundity, and it remains a puzzle why this feature has not resulted in both conditions being eliminated from the population over time (Keller & Miller, 2006). The implication is that the genetic mechanisms associated with schizophrenia and autism are likely to differ from disorders (such as depression) where there is no reduced fecundity.

Some genetic effects operate within disorders. For example, a replicated finding has emerged that *COMT* affects antisocial behavior within ADHD, unaccompanied by main effects of *COMT* on either antisocial behavior in the absence of ADHD or on ADHD in the absence of antisocial behavior (Caspi et al., 2008). Some genetic effects involve genomic imprinting. For example, the genes on the long arm of chromosome 15 lead to either Prader–Willi syndrome or Angelman syndrome, according to whether they derive from the father or the mother (Skuse & Seigal, 2008). Some genetic effects also involve transgenerational change through the mechanism of trinucleotide repeats expansion, such as fragile X anomaly and Huntington's disease (Skuse & Seigal, 2008). These complex effects imply that some genetic transmission is neither straightforwardly Mendelian nor polygenic/multifactorial. Also, genetic effects on liability to mental disorders may operate via the neuroendocrine system or immunity mechanisms rather than via neurotransmitters. Some genetic effects operate via quantitative trait loci (QTLs) rather than categorical differences (Bishop, 2009). Finally, it is important to appreciate that it is misleading to view genes as providing only *susceptibility* to disease. Genes also provide *protection* from disease. Cancer genetics clearly shows the separate operation of both oncogenic genes and tumor-suppressant genes (Tobias & Black, 2002).

A key puzzle is why the individual susceptibility genes that have been identified so far have such tiny effects. Twin studies have demonstrated in a convincing fashion that the overall effect of genes on psychiatric disorders accounts for some 30–90% of the variance (Rutter, 2006). Despite this large effect, however, the odds ratios for individual genes are rarely above 1.2 or 1.3 (Kendler, 2005; Maher, 2008). The traditional answer has been that the small effects are a function of hundreds of different genes being involved and a huge genetic heterogeneity. While both of these effects are likely to apply in many instances, they constitute a restricted answer that fails to attend to other considerations. As is implicit in what has already been said, small effects may arise because genetic influences operate on behaviors that are within diagnostic categories, because genetic influences differ between the sexes, and because genetic influences operate on dimensions that are only indirectly associated with psychopathology. In addition, as we shall see, single-gene main-effect studies ignore the importance of epigenetic effects, the role of copy number variations (CNVs), and the importance of both gene–environment correlations (rGE) and G × E.

SOME BACKGROUND CONSIDERATIONS REGARDING ENVIRONMENTAL AND STOCHASTIC EFFECTS

Evidence supports strong environmental causes of disease, including mental disorder (Academy of Medical Sciences, 2007). Nevertheless, many claims on environmental causes are unsound because they fail to consider genetic mediation, reverse causation, and unmeasured confounders. The causal inference can be tested through the use of "natural experiments," of which there is a considerable range (Rutter, 2007). None of these natural experiments provides the perfect strategy but, taken together, they can do much to confirm or refute the causal inference.

Nongenetic effects may involve developmental perturbations brought about through stochastic effects rather than specific environmental hazards (Molenaar, Boomsma, & Dolan, 1993). For example, the higher risk for Down syndrome in babies born to older mothers clearly operates in this way. Environmental influences may be prenatal and not just postnatal, as is shown, for example, by the effects of both maternal smoking and maternal consumption of alcohol during pregnancy. Taking these two points together, it may be concluded that there are strong reasons for expecting developmental perturbations to be common and also reasons for supposing that they may be involved in risk effects for psychopathology. Brain development is essentially probabilistic. That is, neuronal overproduction is followed by neuronal pruning in order to correct initial errors (Bourgeois, Goldman-Rakic, & Rakic, 1999). Minor errors in development are very common (as shown by congenital anomalies and CNVs) and there is the reality of parental age effects such as those on autism (Reichenberg et al., 2006). The research implication is that it is crucial to determine the origins for developmental perturbations as well as their effects. Why, for example, are chromosome anomalies, congenital anomalies, minor congenital anomalies, and CNVs so frequent in autism?

It is also crucial to appreciate the need to consider the effects of environments on biology. That is, how do environments get "under the skin" when they bring about lasting changes that persist way after the environmental hazards have ceased to be present or to be operative? Possible ways in which this enduring effect occurs may be through biological programming, effects on the hypothalamus–pituitary–adrenal (HPA) axis, or changes in mental models. As already indicated, some nongenetic effects (such as high parental age) may operate through effects on mutations.

SOME STATISTICAL CONSIDERATIONS IN RELATION TO G × E

During the second half of the last century there was a famous dispute between Ronald Fisher with his biometric concept of G × E as a purely statistical feature and Lancelot Hogben with his biological concept (Tabery, 2007, 2008). For Fisher, G × E was simply a "nuisance" term that needed to be removed in order to proceed with the serious business of partitioning the variance into genetic and environmental components. Thus, organisms are biologically programmed to adapt to the environmental conditions prevailing at key sensitive periods of development (see Bateson et al., 2004). The Hubel and Wiesel (2005) findings on the role of visual input on the development of the visual cortex is perhaps the best-known example, but it is clear that experience–adaptive programming also operates with respect to variations within the normal range (see Kuhl et al., 1997; Maye, Werker, & Gerken, 2002; Werker, 2003). There is an abundance of evidence that both acute stressors and chronic adversities have effects on neuroendocrine functions (Gunnar & Vázquez, 2006), but do they serve as mediators of psychological sequelae? There is also much evidence that, from infancy onward, children think about and process their experiences—thereby developing mental models of these experiences and of their own role in them. It is plausible that individual differences in the details of such models might mediate differences in psychological outcomes, but do they? By contrast, Hogben (see Tabery, 2007) argued for a developmental and biological notion of G × E that needed to be tackled more broadly through developmental biology rather than just mathematical manipulations. For Hogben, G × E was not something to be removed by scaling modifications nor was it an answer in its own right. Rather, the finding of G × E pointed to a phenomenon that required a biological understanding. On the other hand, Hogben, as a mathematician, certainly accepted the important points that Fisher made about the problem of variations in scaling creating artifactual interactions and also the importance of taking rGE into account when dealing with interactions. As Tabery (2007) argued, most people have come nowadays to accept that Hogben was right in his plea that it is the biology on which we must focus, although it is also the case that the statistical issues must be taken seriously.

All too often the debate about G × E narrows to the presence or absence of a statistically significant interaction effect. Rutter and Pickles (1991) argued that this criterion is almost never appropriate. There should be a continuing interplay among theory, postulated mechanisms, the purpose of the investigation, and the apparently abstract statistical technicalities. Among other things, they noted the need to appreciate that the usual focus on multiplicative interactions requires a logarithmic mode of measurement, but that synergistic interactions may also operate through scales that are not logarithmic. The choice between additive interactions and multiplicative interactions has to be decided on conceptual grounds rather than statistical ones. The effect, however, is that $G \times E$ may be apparent on one model and not on the other. Even that solution oversimplifies the breadth of possibilities in that, as Rutter and Pickles pointed out, there is a broader range of link functions. An interaction term is just one element in an overall statistical model of the data and cannot be understood without reference to the rest of that model. Rutter and Pickles also discussed the differences of opinion between the regression school, which performs forward selection requiring identification of main effects, before proceeding to examine interactions, and the analysis of variance (ANOVA) school, which performs backward selection. The ANOVA school argues that main effects cannot be interpreted if they are also involved in interactions and so starts with all interactions present, removing only those that are nonsignificant. There is not an unambiguous universal answer as to which approach is "best" because each approach involves a rather different set of assumptions and a different set of advantages and limitations.

MULTIPLE VARIETIES
OF GENETIC–NONGENETIC INTERPLAY

There are three main varieties of such interplay: nongenetic effects on gene actions, genetic effects on environmental risk exposure; and gene–environment co-action or synergistic interaction.

There are positive reasons for expecting that epigenetics will play a key role not only in $G \times E$, but also with its operation in relation to causal influences on susceptibility to disease and disorder (Jirtle & Skinner, 2007; Meaney, 2010; Mill & Petronis, 2007). Numerous animal studies have demonstrated the reality and importance of epigenetic effects. The rat studies by Meaney's (2010) group on the effects of archback nursing would be one example and Jirtle's studies of genomic imprinting would be another. One of the practical problems with respect to human research is that epigenetic effects tend to be tissue and developmental phase–specific. Genes are expressed in the brain at a much higher rate than in other tissues, but there are substantial uncertainties about how far lymphocyte studies (for example) can be used as an index of what is happening in the brain. There is a need for animal models and for *postmortem* studies, and there are indications that the latter may be informative on biological factors involved in susceptibility to disease (McGowan et al., 2009).

There are strong reasons, too, for supposing that rGE are likely to be both common and influential (Jaffee & Price, 2007; Kendler & Baker, 2007). The point is that many of the key environmental risks/protective factors derive from human behavior, for example, marital conflict/breakup, social support, and loss of jobs. If human behavior influences environmental exposure, it follows that there will be genetic influences on environmental risk exposure simply because there are genetic influences on virtually all human behaviors. The first implication that follows is that risk factors that are defined in terms of measured environments may nevertheless operate, at least in part, by means of genetic mediation. As already indicated, that possibility gives rise to the need for the use of "natural experiments" that can take account of this possibility (Rutter, 2007). The second research implication is that investigations need to focus on *which* behaviors have *which* effects in *which* environments. This implication means that the focus in research has to be on the behaviors, with the extent to which there is a genetic influence on those behaviors as a secondary, rather than a primary, consideration. A somewhat different, but related, consideration is that research needs to take on board the demonstration that has been around for some half a century that experiences do not impinge on a passive organism. Rather, from infancy onward, children process their experiences and interpret them. This means that the environment that is effective for that individual may not be the same as the objective environment that applies similarly to everyone. What role active processing has in the shaping and selecting of environments should be a research priority, and it is surprising and regrettable that it has been the subject of so little systematic research. This research will need to distinguish objective environments from the interpretation of those environments and to identify the impact of each factor on behavioral outcomes.

BACKGROUND CONSIDERATIONS REGARDING INTERMEDIATE PHENOTYPES

For some time there has been an interest in the study of *endophenotypes*— meaning features thought to lie along the pathway from gene to psychiatric disorder but that are closer to the gene and therefore may have a simpler relation with a given gene (Cannon & Clarke, 2005; Gottesman & Gould, 2003). The idea is an interesting one and it may well have potential, but so far it has had a rather limited success in relation to mental disorders. In recent times, the focus has switched to "intermediate phenotypes." The concept is similar with respect to the assumption of a key role in the causal biological processes, but it differs in that there is no necessary expectation that they are more closely connected to gene action. With respect to G × E, they have been employed to study the environmental effect pathway by means of some kind of stress or challenge reaction. Their most important advantage is that the environment has an immediate effect without having to wait for some disease outcome to develop (Rutter, 2008). Why that is so important is that it enables the experimental study of G × E in humans. If there is a physiological response to the stress or challenge reaction that applies across species, it may also provide a most useful bridge between animal models and human experimental studies. That seems to be the case with respect to the use of response to inhalation of CO_2 as a way of inducing panic reactions (Battaglia, Marino, Maziade, Molteni, & D'Amato, 2008). Inhalation of CO_2 appears to have a comparable effect in mice. Similarly, Hariri and colleagues (2003, 2005; Hariri, Drabant, & Weinberger, 2006) used fear stimuli to examine amygdala reactivity, comparing short and long allelic variance of the serotonin transporter promoter gene. The Weinberger, Hariri, and Meyer-Lindenberg group have used other intermediate phenotypes to study G × E with respect to other genes and other outcomes (Meyer-Lindenberg & Weinberger, 2006). In addition, there is a range of examples of similar strategies in internal medicine (Rutter, 2008). The importance, therefore, of intermediate phenotypes is that it opens up major possibilities for studying G × E experimentally in humans—an essential need for the delineation of the biological pathways involved.

GENE–ENVIRONMENT INTERACTION

Expectations Regarding G × E

There are three strong reasons for expecting that G × E will be both relatively common and strongly influential (see Rutter, Thapar, & Pickles, 2009). First, genetically influenced differential response to the environment constitutes the mechanism thought to give rise to evolutionary change. This assertion is not just a historical perspective in relation to a great theory; it is contemporaneously operative as shown by the development in pathogenic organisms of resistance to antibiotics. Second, to suppose that there is no G × E would seem to require the assumption that environmental responsivity is the one biological feature that is uniquely outside of genetic influence. That would be a very strange assumption and certainly one that is highly implausible. Third, a wide range of human and animal naturalistic and experimental studies have shown huge heterogeneity in response to all manner of environmental features, both physical and psychosocial. Again, it is implausible that this variation involves no genetic influence. Accordingly, from a biological perspective, there has to be an expectation that G × E occurs and that it matters.

Empirical Evidence of G × E

The expectation that there is G × E is one thing, but the crucial question is whether there is sound empirical evidence of its occurrence. There is such evidence, and it is strong and compelling because it derives from several different strategies. Thus, G × E is implied in several different sorts of quantitative genetic studies (Rutter & Silberg, 2002). A recent example is provided by Hicks and colleagues' (2009) demonstration that variance accounted for by genetic factors increases as the level of environmental adversity goes up. Second, longitudinal/epidemiological studies show G × E with identified allelic variations of genes and measured environments. The Dunedin studies represent the best example of this research approach as shown by the findings in relation to depression (Caspi et al., 2003), antisocial behavior (Moffitt, Caspi, Harrington, & Milner, 2002), schizophrenia (Caspi et al., 2005), and cognitive functioning (Caspi et al., 2007). Third, evidence from animal models as represented by the findings from Suomi's group (see Barr et al., 2004) with rhesus macaque monkeys shows that an environmental feature, the contrast between peer-reared and mother-reared monkeys, altered the impact of genes. Fourth, human experimental studies as represented by the Weinberger, Hariri, and Meyer-Lindenberg group demonstrate G × E using the strategy of visually presented stimuli and measuring neural features by means of structural and functional brain imaging. In each case, the findings are assessed in relation to allelic variations of identified genes. The examples given are relevant in relation to G × E with respect to mental disorders, but it is important to note that similar evidence is available for a much wider range of biological and medical outcomes (Rutter, 2008).

Replications and Meta-Analyses

As in the whole of science, empirical findings require independent replication if there is to be acceptance of their validity. Meta-analyses constitute one way of putting together many different studies when the conclusions differ, or when the size of effects is in doubt. With respect to the epidemiological/longitudinal studies of G × E in the field of psychopathology, positive replications outnumber failures to replicate (see, e.g., Uher & McGuffin, 2008, 2010). Munafò, Durrant, Lewis, and Flint (2009) and Risch and colleagues (2009) have undertaken meta-analyses on a subgroup of studies with findings that claim to show that the effects of G × E could well be chance. There are numerous concerns about the assumptions in these meta-analyses (Rutter et al., 2009), but the main concern is that the focus ignores corresponding biological findings and experimental studies in humans and nonhuman animals.

Resistance of Some Behavioral Geneticists to the Reality of G × E

That some behavioral geneticists are, indeed, deeply resistant to accepting the reality of G × E is well demonstrated by the Eaves's (2006) paper showing that artifactual G × E could be produced by scaling variations (as has long been known but which raises the query not dealt with by Eaves as to whether the published studies have taken the necessary steps to check on this possibility). This is also shown by the tone of the Risch and colleagues (2009) article. Accordingly, it is necessary to consider the origins of this resistance. Two concrete facts are undeniable. First, behavioral geneticists have focused on G × E as a statistical rather than a biological concept. Second, some behavioral geneticists have focused exclusively on epidemiological studies and have refused to take account of either experimental studies with humans or animal models. The narrowness of the behavioral genetic approach could lead these scholars to fail to recognize the reality of G × E. Also, there has been a defensiveness over the long-standing, historical dismissal of G × E in the field of behavioral genetics.

Very importantly, adequate study of gene–environment co-action requires high-quality measures of the environment that have not received much attention in genetics research. If G × E holds true, large, ongoing longitudinal databases with rich measures of heritability may be rendered less valuable to the extent that they lack high-quality measures of the environment This reality is associated with an appreciation that any adequate study of gene–environment co-action requires new samples and new strategies. Brown and Harris (2008) have argued, for example, that G × E is more likely to apply to chronic than acute disorders and that the key environmental feature may be maltreatment rather than acute stressors.

Is All Well in G × E Research?

Unfortunately, the current, well-based enthusiasm for G × E does not mean that all is well. Much of the research, is of less-than-good quality and fails to deal adequately with crucial methodological hazards. Moreover, even with good G × E research, there are puzzling inconsistencies and nonreplications. It is essential that the inconsistencies are treated seriously and investigated properly. Inconsistencies in findings across studies might mean they are not robust, or they might indicate important moderation of G × E by other, not-yet-identified variables, as in G × E × G or G × E × E.

Turning to the parallel enthusiasm for genomewide association studies that require huge samples (half a million or so), if it is right that G × E is both common and important, does it make sense to focus on very large samples that almost inevitably lack sensitive discriminating measures of environment? Furthermore, it is necessary to ask whether, if the effects of individual genes are so tiny, what is the value of further gene hunting? Presumably, it is the hope that multiple genes will coalesce to operate on a common biological pathway. What justification is there that this will be the case? Is it likely?

Similarly, coming back to G × E, it has been argued that a key payoff of identifying G × E is that it will help the identification of both genetic and environmental mediating causal pathways (Caspi & Moffitt, 2006). What evidence is there that such breakthroughs are happening?

Advances in technology have made it possible to undertake research that was both scarcely conceivable and certainly completely impractical several decades ago. The challenge now is to use these exciting technological advances in a way that will truly increase biological understanding. The possibilities for success are very considerable, but so are the conceptual and methodological hazards. These possibilities and hazards will need careful consideration as we move into a reflection of implications for policy and practice.

REFERENCES

Academy of Medical Sciences. (2007). *Identifying the environmental causes of disease: How should we decide what to believe and when to take action?* London: Author.

Barr, C. S., Newman, T. K., Shannon, C., Parker, C., Dvoskin, R. L., Becker, M. L., et al. (2004). Rearing condition and *rh5–HTTLPR* interact to influence limbic–hypothalamic–pituitary–adrenal axis response to stress in infant macaques. *Biological Psychiatry, 55*, 733–738.

Bateson, P., Barker, D., Clutton-Brock, T., Deb, D., D'Udine, B., Foley, R. A., et al. (2004). Developmental plasticity and human health. *Nature, 430*, 419–421.

Battaglia, M., Marino, C., Maziade, M., Molteni, M., & D'Amato, F. (2008). Gene–environment interaction and behavioural disorders: A developmental perspective based on endophenotypes. In *Genetic effects on environmental vulnerability to disease* (pp. 103–119). Chichester, UK: Wiley.

Bishop, D. V. M. (2009). Genes, cognition, and communication: Insights from neurodevelopmental disorders. *Annals of the New York Academy of Sciences, 1156*, 1–18.

Bourgeois, J-P., Goldman-Rakic, P. S., & Rakic, P. (1999). Formation, elimination, and stabilization of synapses in the primate cerebral cortex. In M. S. Gazzaniga (Ed.), *The new cognitive neurosciences* (pp. 45–53). Cambridge, MA: MIT Press.

Brown, G. W., & Harris, T. O. (2008). Depression and the serotonin transporter 5-HTTLPR polymorphism: A review and a hypothesis concerning gene–environment interaction. *Journal of Affective Disorders, 111*, 1–12.

Cannon, M., & Clarke, M. C. (2005). Risk for schizophrenia—broadening the concepts, pushing back the boundaries. *Schizophrenia Research, 79*, 5–13

Caspi, A., Langley, K., Milne, B., Moffitt, T., O'Donovan, M., Owen, M., et al. (2008). A replicated molecular genetic basis for subtyping antisocial behavior in children with attention-deficit/hyperactivity disorder. *Archives of General Psychiatry, 65*, 203–210.

Caspi, A., & Moffitt, T. E. (2006). Gene–environment interactions in psychiatry: Joining forces with neuroscience. *Nature Reviews Neuroscience, 7*, 583–590.

Caspi, A., Moffitt, T. E., Cannon, M., McClay, J., Murray, R., Harrington H., et al. (2005). Moderation of the effect of adolescent-onset cannabis use on adult psychosis by a functional polymorphism in the catechol-O-methyltransferase gene: Longitudinal evidence of a gene–environment interaction. *Biological Psychiatry, 57*, 1117–1127.

Caspi, A., Sugden, K., Moffitt, T. E., Taylor, A., Craig, I. W., Harrington, H., et al. (2003). Influence of life stress on depression: Moderation by a polymorphism in the 5-HTT gene. *Science, 301*, 386–389.

Caspi, A., Williams, B., Kim-Cohen, J., Craig, I. W., Milne, B. J., Poulton, R., et al. (2007). Moderation of breastfeeding effects on the IQ by genetic variation in fatty acid metabolism. *Proceedings of the National Academy of Sciences of the USA, 107*, 18860–18865.

Eaves, L. J. (2006). Genotype × environment interaction in psychopathology: Fact or artefact? *Twin Research in Human Genetics, 9*, 1–8.

Gottesman, I. I., & Gould, T. D. (2003). The endophenotype concept in psychiatry: Etymology and strategic intentions. *American Journal of Psychiatry, 160*, 636–645.

Gunnar, M., & Vázquez, D. (2006). Stress neurobiology and developmental psychopathology. In D. Cicchetti & D. Cohen (Eds.), *Developmental psychopathology: Vol. 2. Developmental neuroscience* (pp. 533–577). Hoboken, NJ: Wiley.

Hariri, A. R., Drabant, E. M., Munoz, K. E., Kolachana, B. S., Mattay, V. S., Egan, M. F., et al. (2005). A susceptibility gene for affective disorders and the response of the human amygdala. *Archives of General Psychiatry, 62*, 146–152.

Hariri, A. R., Drabant, E. M., & Weinberger D. R. (2006). Imaging genetics: Perspectives from studies of genetically driven variation in serotonin function and corticolimibic affective processing. *Biological Psychiatry, 59*, 888–897.

Hariri, A. R., Mattay, V. S., Tessitore, A., Fera, F., & Weinberger, D. R. (2003). Neocortical modulation of the amygdala response to fearful stimuli. *Biological Psychiatry, 53*, 494–501.

Hicks, B. M., South, S. C., Dirago, A. D., Krueger, R. F., Iacono, W. G., & McGue, M. (2009). Environmental adversity and increasing genetic risk for externalizing disorders. *Archives of General Psychiatry, 66*, 640–648.

Hubel, D. H., & Wiesel, T. N. (2005). *Brain and visual perception*. Oxford, UK: Oxford University Press.

Jaffee, S. R., & Price, T. S. (2007). Gene–environment correlations: A review of the evidence and implications for prevention of mental illness. *Molecular Psychiatry, 12*, 432–442.

Jirtle, R. L., & Skinner, M. K. (2007). Environmental epigenomics and disease susceptibility. *Nature Reviews Genetics, 8*, 253–262.

Keller, M. C., & Miller, G. F. (2006). Resolving the paradox of common, harmful, heritable mental disorders: Which evolutionary genetic models work best? *Behavioral Brain Sciences, 29*, 385–452.

Kendler, K. S. (2005). "A gene for . . . "?: The nature of gene action in psychiatric disorders. *American Journal of Psychiatry, 162*, 1243–1252.

Kendler, K. S., & Baker, J. H. (2007). Genetic influences on measures of the environment: A systematic review. *Psychological Medicine, 37*, 615–626.

Kuhl, P. K., Andruski, J. E., Chistovich, I. A., Chistovich, L. A., Kozhevnikova, E. V., Ryskina, V. L., et al. (1997). Cross-language analysis of phonetic units in language addressed to infants. *Science, 277*, 684–686.

Maher, B. (2008). The case of the missing heritability. *Nature, 456*, 18–21.

Maye, J., Werker, J. F., & Gerken, L. (2002). Infant sensitivity to distributional information can affect phonetic discrimination. *Cognition, 82*, B101–B111.

McGowan, P. O., Sasaki, A., D'Alessio, A. C., Dymov, S., Labonté, B., Szyf, M., et al. (2009). Epigenetic regulation of the glucocorticoid receptor in human brain associates with childhood abuse. *Nature Neuroscience, 12*, 342–348.

Meaney, M. J. (2010). Epigenetics and the biological definition of gene × environment interactions. *Child Development, 81*, 41–79.

Meyer-Lindenberg, A., Buckholtz, J. W., Kolachana, B., Hariri, A. R., Pezawas, L., Blasi, G., et al. (2006). Neural mechanisms of genetic risk for impulsivity and violence in humans. *Proceedings of the National Academy of Sciences of the USA, 103*, 6269–6274.

Meyer-Lindenberg, A., & Weinberger, D. R. (2006). Intermediate phenotypes and genetic mechanisms of psychiatric disorders. *Nature Reviews Neuroscience, 7*, 818–827.

Mill, J., & Petronis, A. (2007). Molecular studies of major depressive disorder: The epigenetic perspective. *Molecular Psychiatry, 12*, 799–814.

Moffitt, T. E., Caspi, A., Harrington, H., & Milne, B. (2002). Males on the life-course persistent and adolescence-limited antisocial pathways: Follow-up at age 26. *Development and Psychopathology, 14*, 179–206.

Molenaar, P. C. M., Boomsma, D. I., & Dolan, C. V. (1993). A third source of developmental differences. *Behavioral Genetics, 23*, 519–524.

Munafò, M. R., Durrant, C., Lewis, G., & Flint, J. (2009). Environmental interactions at the serotonin transporter locus. *Biological Psychiatry, 25*, 211–219.

Plomin, R., De Fries, J. C., McClearn, G. E., & McGuffin, P. (Eds.). (2008). *Behavioral genetics* (5th ed.). New York: Worth.

Reichenberg, A., Gross, R., Weiser, M., Bresnahan, M., Silverman, J., Harlap, S., et al. (2006). Advancing paternal age and autism. *Archives of General Psychiatry, 63*, 1026–1032.

Risch, N., Herrell, R., Lehner, T., Liang, K. Y., Eaves, L., Hoh, J., et al. (2009). Interaction between the serotonin transporter gene (5-HTTLPR), stressful life events, and risk of depression: A meta-analysis. *Journal of the American Medical Association, 301*, 2462–2471.

Rutter, M. (2003). Categories, dimensions, and the mental health of children and adolescents. *Annals of the New York Academy of Sciences, 1008*, 11–21.

Rutter, M. (2006). *Genes and behavior: Nature–nurture interplay explained.* Oxford, UK: Blackwell.

Rutter, M. (2007). Proceeding from observed correlation to causal inference: The use of natural experiments. *Perspectives on Psychological Science, 2*, 377–395.

Rutter, M. (Ed.). (2008). *Genetic effects on environmental vulnerability to disease.* Chichester, UK: Wiley.

Rutter, M., Bishop, D. V., Pine, D., Scott, S., Stevenson, J., Taylor, E., et al. (Eds.). (2008). *Rutter's child and adolescent psychiatry* (5th ed.). Oxford, UK: Blackwell.

Rutter, M., Kim-Cohen, J., & Maughan, B. (2006). Continuities and discontinuities in psychopathology between childhood and adult life. *Journal of Child Psychology and Psychiatry, 163*, 1009–1018.

Rutter, M., & Pickles, A. (1991). Person-environment interactions: Concepts, mechanisms, and implications for data analysis. In T. D. Wachs & R. Plomin (Eds.), *Conceptualization and measurement of organism–environment interaction* (pp. 105–141). Washington, DC: American Psychological Association.

Rutter, M., & Silberg, J. (2002). Gene–environment interplay in relation to emotional and behavioral disturbance. *Annual Review of Psychology, 53*, 463–490.

Rutter, M., Thapar, A., & Pickles, A. (2009). Gene–environment interactions: Biologically valid pathway or artifact? *Archives of General Psychiatry, 66*, 1287–1289.

Skuse, D. H., & Seigal, A. (2008). Behavioral phenotypes and chromosomal disorders. In M. Rutter, D. Bishop, D. Pine, S. Scott, J. Stevenson, E. Taylor, et al. (Eds.), *Rutter's child and adolescent psychiatry* (5th ed., pp. 359–376). Oxford, UK: Blackwell.

Tabery, J. (2007). Biometric and developmental gene–environment interactions: Looking back, moving forward. *Development and Psychopathology, 19*, 961–976.

Tabery, J. (2008). R. A. Fisher, Lancelot Hogben, and the origin(s) of genotype-environment interaction. *Journal of Historical Biology, 41*, 717–761.

Thapar, A., & Rutter, M. (2008). Genetics. In M. Rutter, D. Bishop, D. Pine, S. Scott, J. Stevenson, E. Taylor, et al. (Eds.), *Rutter's child and adolescent psychiatry* (5th ed., pp. 339–358). Oxford, UK: Blackwell.

Tobias, E. S., & Black, D. M. (2002). The molecular biology of cancer. In D. L. Rimoin, J. M. Connor, R. E. Pyeritz, & B. R. Korf (Eds.), *Emery and Rimoin's principles and practice of medical genetics* (Vol. 1, 4th ed., pp. 514–570). London: Churchill Livingstone.

Uher, R., & McGuffin, P. (2008). The moderation by the serotonin transporter gene of environmental adversity in the aetiology of mental illness: Review and methodological analysis. *Molecular Psychiatry, 13*, 131–146.

Uher, R., & McGuffin, P. (2010). The moderation by the serotonin transporter gene of environmental adversity in the etiology of depression: 2009 update. *Molecular Psychiatry, 15*, 18–22

Werker, J. F. (2003). Baby steps to learning language. *Journal of Pediatrics, 143*, S62–S69.

CHAPTER 2

Genetic Sensitivity to the Environment

The Case of the Serotonin Transporter Gene and Its Implications for Studying Complex Diseases and Traits

Avshalom Caspi, Ahmad R. Hariri, Andrew Holmes, Rudolf Uher, *and* Terrie E. Moffitt

In 1996, it was reported that a repeat length polymorphism in the promoter region of the human serotonin transporter gene (*SLC6A4*; also known as *5-HTT*) regulates gene expression *in vitro*. Furthermore, individuals carrying one or two copies of the relatively low-expressing short (S) allele of the serotonin transporter–linked polymorphic region (*5-HTTLPR*) exhibit elevated neuroticism, a personality trait involved in the propensity to depression (Lesch et al., 1996). In 2002, it was reported that S-carriers exhibit elevated amygdala reactivity to threatening stimuli, as assessed by functional MRI (fMRI) (Hariri et al., 2002). In 2003, it was reported that S-carriers exhibit elevated depressive symptoms, diagnosable depression, and suicidality after experiencing stressful life events and childhood maltreatment (Caspi et al., 2003).

These three papers have influenced scientific and public discourse in three ways. First, the *5-HTTLPR* has become the most investigated genetic variant in psychiatry, psychology, and neuroscience. Second, these three papers and those following have generated evidence for validity of the construct of genetically driven individual differences in stress sensitivity.

Third, the *5-HTTLPR* gene–environment interaction (G × E) has captured the public imagination and framed contemporary discussions about how genes and environments shape who we are. In this chapter, we review the cumulative evidence base documenting the role of *5-HTT* in sensitivity to stress and vulnerability to psychopathology. Because the evidence base on *5-HTT* and stress sensitivity is currently advanced relative to other G × E investigations, this hypothesis constitutes a case study with lessons that extend to G × E research in general. The chapter begins with a review of studies and ends with lessons.

This chapter takes an inclusive approach to the literature on *5-HTT* and stress sensitivity, as opposed to an exclusive focus on papers attempting to approximate the methods of the initial report of a *5-HTTLPR* G × E (Caspi et al., 2003). An inclusive review is essential once it is understood that the hypothesis of interest is that variation in *5-HTT* influences reactivity to environmental stress exposure, and thereby brings about risk for depression. Accordingly, in many studies testing the *5-HTT* stress-sensitivity hypothesis, the outcome is not depression per se. Rather, inferential advantages are gained by studying intermediate phenotypes on the causal pathway from stress to depression that are considered to index stress sensitivity (e.g., stress hormones, amygdala reactivity). Likewise, stress is not narrowly construed as a count of stressful life events. Other stressors are examined in the field and in the laboratory, whenever doing so augments scientific inference (e.g., hurricane exposure rules out gene–environment correlation because victims' genes could not evoke this life event; officially recorded child abuse rules out recall bias; experimental stress induction allows titration of stress dosage). Because the outcome is not restricted to human depression, important information comes from studies of *5-HTT* and stress sensitivity in animals (e.g., genetically modified mice, rhesus macaques carrying an orthologous *5-HTTLPR* variant).

EVIDENCE FOR THE *5-HTT* STRESS-SENSITIVITY HYPOTHESIS

It is evident from research conducted with multiple species and from research using both observational and experimental methods that variation in *5-HTT* modifies organisms' stress responses to their environments (Figure 2.1). Complementary experimental and observational research designs are integral to testing not only the *5-HTT* stress-sensitivity hypothesis, but all G × E hypotheses (Caspi & Moffitt, 2006; van Os & Rutten, 2009). Experiments with humans, nonhuman primates, and rodents elucidate biological mechanisms behind the hypothesis and also validate findings from human observational studies by using designs with stronger internal valid-

Species	*5-HTT* Gene Variation	Biological Phenotype	Behavioral Phenotype
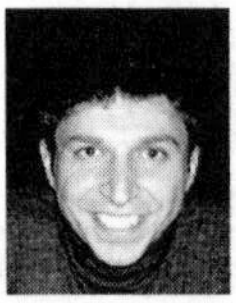 **Human** *Homo sapiens*	Repeat length polymorphism in the promoter region	Altered neural stress and threat circuitry. Increased HPA axis response to stress.	Intermediate phenotypes for depression and anxiety. Increased depression after stressful life events.
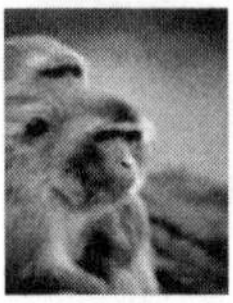 **Monkey** *Macaca mulatta*	Repeat length polymorphism in the promoter region	Altered neural stress and threat circuitry. Increased HPA axis response to stress.	Increased anxiety and stress reactivity after early life stress.
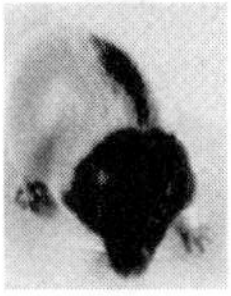 **Rat** *Rattus norvegicus*	Chemical mutagenesis "knockout"	Increased 5-HT signaling. Altered 5-HT receptor expression and function.	Increased anxiety-like behavior.
Mouse *Mus musculus*	Genetically engineered "knockout" or overexpression	Knockout: Increased 5-HT signaling. Altered 5-HT receptor expression and function. Increased amygdala dendritic spine density and PFC dendritic branching. Increased HPA axis response to stress.	Knockout: Increased anxiety-like behavior. Impaired fear extinction. Increased depression-related behavior after multiple stressors.
		Overexpression: Decreased 5-HT signaling. Altered 5-HT receptors.	Overexpression: Decreased anxiety-like behavior.

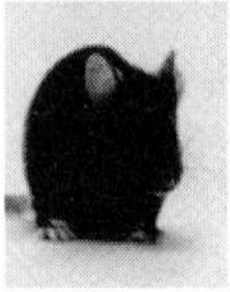

FIGURE 2.1. Role of *5-HTT* variation in stress sensitivity as underscored by the coherence of findings from hypothesis-driven studies in multiple species employing multiple methodologies.

ity (e.g., by random assignment to stress conditions). Observational studies use designs with stronger external validity (e.g., by studying real-world stressors), estimate the effect size of the *5-HTTLPR* G × E in the human population, and allow researchers to study clinical depression as the outcome.

Human Observational Studies

The initial G × E effect (Caspi et al., 2003) did not have an overwhelmingly impressive *P* value, but it was robust, having been (1) discovered in an epidemiologically sound longitudinal cohort study; (2) tested in a straightforward and transparent analysis; (3) reproduced across two stressors, child maltreatment and adult stressful life events; and (4) reproduced across four depression phenotypes. How has this hypothesis fared in observational studies since it was initially tested?

Table 2.1 and Table 2.2 list all human observational studies up to summer 2009 that tested the hypothesis that the *5-HTTLPR* moderates the effect of stress on depression phenotypes. Three observations emerge from the tables. First, multiple studies have reported that S-carriage moderates the influence of stress on depression. Whether or not the initial finding can be replicated has been answered in the affirmative. Second, positive findings have emerged from a variety of observational research designs used to test the hypothesis, including phenotype case-only designs, case–control designs, cross-sectional designs, longitudinal designs, and exposure designs. This suggests the finding is "sturdy," in the sense that its signal can be detected despite noise from varying research settings, sample characteristics, and study designs (Robins, 1978). Third, there have also been quite a few negative findings. The degree to which negative findings call the original result into question depends on whether differences in study designs are systematically related to differences in study findings. If failures to replicate are characterized by systematically different subject populations or systematically weaker methodologies, their challenge to the original result is greatly diminished.

We considered factors that might covary with positive versus negative findings, including subjects' sex, age, and nationality, and features of phenotype measurement, but these did not covary systematically with findings. However, positive and negative findings did closely track variation in methodological features related to the quality of environmental exposure measurement. Concerns have been expressed about standards of stress assessment in tests of this hypothesis (Brown & Harris, 2008; Monroe & Reid, 2008). We call attention to three issues.

(text resumes on page 30)

TABLE 2.1. Human Observational Studies Testing the Hypothesis That the *5-HTTLPR* Moderates the Effect of Stress on Depression Phenotypes in Studies of Specific Stressors

Specific stressor and study[a]	Design[b]	N	Female (%)	Mean age	Location	Stress assessment	Stressor	Outcome measure[c]	G × E interaction[d]
Childhood maltreatment									
Caspi (2003) [R, M]	Longitudinal	847	50	26	New Zealand	Objective/ interview	Child maltreatment	Diagnosis of depression	Yes: additive
Kaufman (2004/2006)[e]	Cross-sectional	196	51	9	U.S.	Objective	Child abuse	MFQ	Yes: recessive
Cicchetti (2007)	Cross-sectional	339	47	17	U.S.	Objective	Child abuse	Anxious/depressed symptoms (ASEBA)	Yes (sexual abuse): recessive
Wichers (2008)	Cross-sectional	394	100	18–64 years	Belgium	Questionnaire	Childhood Trauma Questionnaire (items concerning sexual and physical abuse were omitted)	SCL-90; SCID depressive symptoms	No (three-way interaction between *5-HTTLPR* S carriage, BDNF Met carriage, and childhood maltreatment)
Aguilera (2009)	Cross-sectional	534	55	23	Spain	Questionnaire	Childhood Trauma Questionnaire	SCL-90-R	Yes (sexual abuse): dominant
Aslund (2009)	Cross-sectional	1,482	48	17–18 years	Sweden	Questionnaire	Quarrels between parents: violence between parents; physical maltreatment; psychological maltreatment	Depression Self-Rating Scale	Yes (females): additive

Study	Design	N	%	Age	Country	Assessment	Population	Depression measure	G×E
Benjet (2010)	Cross-sectional	78	100	10–14 years	U.S.	Questionnaire	Victims of relational aggression	Children's Depression Inventory	Yes: recessive
Kumsta (in press)	Longitudinal	125	NA	Assessed at ages 11 and 15 years	England	Objective	Institution rearing between 6 and 42 months in Romanian orphanages	Depressive symptoms (CAPA, Rutter Child Scale; Strengths and Difficulties Questionnaire)	Yes: additive
Sugden (in press)	Longitudinal	2,017	51	12	England	Interview	Victims of bullying	Anxious/depressed symptoms (ASEBA)	Yes: additive
Medical conditions[f]									
Mossner (2001)	Exposed only	72	46	NA	Germany	Objective	Patients with idiopathic Parkinson's disease	Hamilton Rating Scale for Depression	Yes: additive
Grabe (2005) [R][g]	Cross-sectional	976	60	52	Germany	Questionnaire	Number of chronic diseases	von Zerssen's Complaints Scale (psychological and somatic symptoms)	Yes (females): dominant
Lenze (2005)	Exposed only	23	87	77	U.S.	Objective	Rehabilitation-hospital patients with hip fracture	Diagnosis of depression	Yes: dominant
Nakatani (2005)	Exposed only	2,509	25	64	Japan	Objective	Patients with acute myocardial infarction	Zung Self-Rating Depression Scale	Yes: dominant
Ramasubbu (2006)	Exposed only	51	NA	60	Canada	Objective	Stroke survivors	Diagnosis of depression	Yes: dominant
Otte (2007)	Exposed only	557	15	68	U.S.	Objective	Patients with documented coronary disease	Diagnosis of depression	Yes: dominant

(cont.)

23

TABLE 2.1. (cont.)

Specific stressor and study[a]	Design[b]	N	Female (%)	Mean age	Location	Stress assessment	Stressor	Outcome measure[c]	G × E interaction[d]
Medical conditions (cont.)									
Kohen (2008)	Exposed only	150	37	60	U.S.	Objective	Stroke survivors	Geriatric Depression Scale	Yes: recessive
McCaffery (2008)	Exposed only	977	21	59	Canada	Objective	Patients with established cardiovascular disease	BDI	No
Kim (2009)	Longitudinal	521	55	72	Korea	Questionnaire	Number of chronic health problems	Diagnosis of depression	Yes: recessive
Other stressors									
Kilpatrick (2007)	Cross-sectional	589	64–77	> 60	U.S.	Objective/questionnaire	Hurricane exposure + low social support 6 months before the hurricane	Diagnosis of depression	Yes: additive
Brummet (2008)	Cross-sectional	288	75	58	U.S.	Objective	Caregivers of patients with Alzheimer's disease/dementia	CES-D	Yes (females): additive

24

[a]Full references are available in a data supplement that accompanies the online version of the original article. Studies included in the Risch et al. meta-analysis are marked with an [R]; studies included in the Munafò et al. meta-analysis are marked with an [M].

[b]Case-only designs studied depressed patients, and the parameter of interest was whether genotype distinguished cases who had environmental exposure. Case-control designs compared depressed patients and healthy subjects on genetic and environmental risk factors. Cross-sectional designs studied the association between genetic and environmental factors and depression phenotypes at a point time. All three designs are prone to bias because information about exposure is assessed retrospectively. Information bias can be minimized by careful instrument construction, by seeking an objective record of the exposure, or by obtaining information about the exposure and the outcome from independent sources. Longitudinal designs usually assess the environmental exposure before the outcome, thereby minimizing some biases. However, many G × E studies that have been carried out in the context of prospective longitudinal studies have collected exposure information retrospectively at the same time as collecting outcome information, thereby undermining the strength of the design. Exposed-only designs studied individuals selected on the basis of their environmental exposure, and the parameter of interest was whether genotype was associated with depression outcome.

[c]BDI, Beck Depression Inventory; CES-D, Center for Epidemiologic Studies Depression Scale; MFQ, Mood and Feelings Questionnaire; ASEBA, Achenbach System of Empirically Based Assessment; SCL-90, Symptom Checklist; CAPA, Child and Adolescent Psychiatric Assessment.

[d]Information in parentheses indicates whether the interaction was conditional (e.g., for one sex only, for a specific measure, etc.). Genetic models are generally not systematically compared in the reports and our rating is based on having read the Method and Results sections of each paper.

[e]The initial report contained 101 children. The second report contained 196 children, including those in the original report.

[f]A consideration in studies of depression-inducing medical illnesses is whether these illnesses index "psychological stress" or an independent biological mechanism that is part and parcel of the medical illness. The latter possibility is suggested by evidence that depression is linked to abnormalities in endogenous cytokines and that stimulating proinflammatory cytokines induces depression, especially among 5-HTTLPR S-carriers (in some [Bull, 2008; Lotrich, 2009] but not all [Kraus, 2007] studies). Because the etiology of depression following medical illness is multifactorial, involving both psychological and biological mechanisms, it is not yet possible to tell what part of the "stress of being ill" is moderated by the 5-HTTLPR in these studies.

[g]This report also analyzed unemployment as a stressor and found that unemployed S carriers reported more psychological and somatic symptoms. This interaction was observed among females, but not among males.

TABLE 2.2. Human Observational Studies Testing the Hypothesis That the *5-HTTLPR* Moderates the Effect of Stress on Depression Phenotypes in Studies of Stressful/Adverse Life Events

Study[a]	Design[b]	N	Female (%)	Mean age	Location	Stress assessment	Stressor	Outcome measure[c]	G×E interaction[d]
Caspi (2003) [R, M]	Longitudinal	845	50	26	New Zealand	Interview	Past 5 years	Diagnosis of depression	Yes: additive
Eley (2004) [R, M]	Case–control	377	58	12–19 years	England	Questionnaire	Family environmental risk assessed with three variables: the Social Problems Questionnaire, parental education, and adverse life events	MFQ	Yes (females): additive
Kendler (2005)	Longitudinal	572	NA	35	U.S.	Interview	Nearest month of stressful life events	Diagnosis of depression	Yes: recessive
Jacobs (2006)	Longitudinal	374	100	27	Holland	Questionnaire	Past 3 months	SCL-90	Yes: additive
Mandelli (2006)	Case only	670	68	48	Italy	Interview	12 months preceding onset of first depression	Diagnosis of depression	Yes: dominant
Taylor (2006)	Cross-sectional	118	57	21	U.S.	Questionnaire	Adverse childhood experiences/past 6 months	BDI	Yes: recessive
Sjoberg (2006)	Cross-sectional	180	63	16–19 years	Sweden	Interview	Lifetime: 6 questions about psychosocial circumstances in the family	Depression Self-Rating Scale	Yes (females): additive

Study	Design	N	%	Age	Country	Method	Life events	Depression measure	Result
Wilhelm (2006) [R]	Longitudinal	127	67	48	Australia	Interview	1 year and 5 years prior to depression	Diagnosis of depression	Yes (for events in past 5 years): additive
Zalsman (2006)	Case–control	316	68	38	U.S.	Interview	Past 6 months	Hamilton Depression Rating Scale	Yes: dominant
Cervilla (2007)	Case–control	737	72	49	Spain	Questionnaire	Past 6 months	Diagnosis of depression	Yes: recessive
Dick (2007)	Family-based association study	1,913	NA	NA	U.S.	Questionnaire	Unemployment in past 12 months; divorced, widowed or separated; and reporting fair or poor health	Diagnosis of depression	Yes, family-based analyses, overtransmission of the short allel concentrated among individuals who experienced stressful life events
Kim (2007) [R, M]	Cross-sectional	732	NA	65+	Korea	Interview	Past 12 months	Diagnosis of depression	Yes: dominant
Scheid (2007) [M]	Cross-sectional	495 pregnant women	100	20–34 (81%)	U.S.	Questionnaire	Lifetime events, grouped by type	CES-D	Yes (abuse, but not other stressful life events): recessive
Lazary (2008)	Cross-sectional	567	79	31	Hungary	Questionnaire	Past 2 years	Zung Self-Rating Depression Scale	Yes: additive

(cont.)

TABLE 2.2. (cont.)

Study[a]	Design[b]	N	Female (%)	Mean age	Location	Stress assessment	Stressor	Outcome measure[c]	G × E interaction[d]
Bukh (2009)	Case only	290	66	39	Denmark	Interview	6 months preceding onset of the patients' first episode of depression	Diagnosis of depression	Yes: recessive
Goldman (in press)	Longitudinal	984	45	66	Taiwan	Interview	Lifetime	CES-D	Yes: additive (extended to include the XL genotype)
Gillespie (2005) [R]	Cross-sectional	1,091	NA	39	Australia	Questionnaire	Past 12 months	Diagnosis of depression	No
Surtees (2006) [R, M]	Cross-sectional; selected for high and low extreme Neuroticism scores	4,175	47	60	England	Questionnaire	Childhood adverse experiences/up to 6 stressful life events in past 5 years	Diagnosis of depression	Opposite (childhood adverse experiences); Negative (adult life events)
Chipman (2007) [R]	Cross-sectional	2,095	52	20–24	Australia	Questionnaire	Past 6 months	Goldman Depression Scale	No
Chorbov (2007) [R]	Longitudinal	236	100	22	U.S.	Questionnaire	History of traumatic events	Diagnosis of depression	Opposite

Study	Design	N		Age	Country	Method	Exposure	Outcome	Result
Araya (2009)	Longitudinal	4,334	NA	7	England	Questionnaire	Past 2 years (list of events that children found upsetting, according to maternal checklist)	SDQ emotional symptom five-item subscale	No
Laucht (2009) [R]	Cross-sectional	309	54	19	Germany	Questionnaire	Past 5 years	Diagnosis of depression; BDI	No
Power (2009) [R]	Cross-sectional	1,421	NA	65+	France	Questionnaire	Past 12 months	Case-level depression, according to MINI and CES-D	No
Zhang (2009)	Case–control	792	54	33	China	Questionnaire	Negative life events (in family life, working problems, and social life)	Diagnosis of depression	Opposite

[a] Full references are available in a data supplement that accompanies the online version of the original article. Studies included in the Risch et al. meta-analysis are marked with an [R]; studies included in the Munafò et al. meta-analysis are marked with an [M]. A study by Middeldorp et al. was included in the meta-analysis by Risch et al. although no test of G × E was reported in available publications.

[b] Case-only designs studied depressed patients, and the parameter of interest was whether genotype distinguished cases who had environmental exposure. Case-control designs compared depressed patients and healthy subjects on genetic and environmental risk factors. Cross-sectional designs studied the association between genetic and environmental factors and depression phenotypes at a point in time. All three designs are prone to bias because information about the exposure is assessed retrospectively. Information bias can be minimized by careful instrument construction, by seeking an objective record of the exposure, or by obtaining information about the exposure and the outcome from independent sources. Longitudinal designs usually assess the environmental exposure before the outcome, thereby minimizing some biases. However, many G × E studies that have been carried out in the context of prospective longitudinal studies have collected exposure information retrospectively at the same time as collecting outcome information, thereby undermining the strength of the design.

[c] BDI, Beck Depression Inventory; CES-D, Center for Epidemiologic Studies Depression Scale; MFQ, Mood and Feelings Questionnaire; SCL-90, Symptom Checklist; MINI, Mini International Neuropsychiatric Interview; SDQ, Strengths and Difficulties Questionnaire.

[d] Information in parentheses indicates whether the interaction was conditional (e.g., for one sex only, for a specific measure, etc.). Genetic models are generally not systematically compared in the reports and our rating is based on having read the Method and Results sections of each paper.

First, almost all nonreplications rely on brief self-report measures of stress, whereas studies using objective indicators or face-to-face interviews to assess stress exposure yield positive replications ("Stress Assessment" column in Tables 2.1 and 2.2). Face-to-face interviewers can clarify the meaning of a reported life event and enhance memory for life events by probing and by using techniques such as life event calendars, as did the initial study (Caspi et al., 2003). In contrast, it is known that self-report event checklists gather idiosyncratic and inaccurate information (Dohrenwend, 2006; Monroe, 2008).

Second, studies of specific stressors consistently yield positive findings. Why are these studies so consistent? One possibility is that their focus on a specific, homogeneous, developmentally relevant, and clearly operationalized depression-inducing event decreased between-subject heterogeneity in the exposure and enhanced internal validity of the study design. Table 2.1 groups studies of two specific stressors that are established causes of depression: childhood maltreatment and medical illness. Nine studies report about depression that follows childhood experiences associated with maltreatment and victimization. Although exposure measurement is not uniform, the studies are united by focusing on threatening events in which physical, sexual, or relational harm were carried out or intended. Virtually all of these studies focus on children, adolescents, and young adults. All of them show that S-carriage moderates the association between child maltreatment and depression. Another nine studies report about depression following medical illness. Virtually all focus on middle-age and elderly participants. Studies of patients suffering hip fractures, strokes, Parkinson's disease, heart disease, and chronic disease load show that S-carriage moderates the association between medical illness and depression.

Third, whereas studies of specific stressors consistently generate positive findings, studies of stressful/adverse life events yield mixed results (Table 2.2). This inconsistency could result from the highly variable measurement of stressful life events (Monroe & Reid, 2008; Shanahan & Bauldry, in press). The pool of studies exemplifies five difficulties in stress measurement: (1) Stress measures are sometimes noncomparable and fall prey to the fallacy that because measures have the same name they measure the same construct (Block, 1995). For example, some studies count death of a spouse as a stressor, whereas others count being the child of a father in an unskilled job as a stressor. Some studies count stress events, others model event severity. Some stressors are chronic, others acute. Some studies define a "stressor" by its level of distress, others do not. Some studies examine events that happened to the proband, others examine events among the proband's friends and relatives. (2) Some studies assess stress through currently depressed individuals' self-reports, which are biased by mood-congruent memory revision and thus overcount events (Joormann,

Hertel, LeMoult, & Gotlib, 2009). Moreover, humans seek explanations, a phenomenon termed "effort after meaning," which leads respondents who have been depressed to misattribute their illness to a life event. Some studies assess events through long-term retrospective reports (sometimes over decades), which are flawed by forgetting and undercount life events, particularly among respondents who lack depression. In addition, respondents often overcount trivial and undercount severe events (Monroe, 2009). These cognitive processes (mood-congruent memory revision, effort after meaning, and retrospective forgetting) working together can artifactually influence a study's association between life events and depression. Thus, a correlation between life events and depression does not indicate validity, contrary to claims (Merikangas & Risch, 2009). (3) Some studies test the connection between stress and depression contemporaneously, others across years or decades. (4) Some studies are unable to rule out reverse causation, in which depression precipitates stressful events; for example, one study measured depression over the respondents' lifetime, but ascertained life stress during only the past year (Gillespie, Whitfield, Williams, Heath, & Martin, 2005). (5) Most studies do not consider variation in participants' depression history, despite evidence that stress is more relevant for initial than recurrent depression episodes.

In the first decade of research about the *5-HTTLPR* G × E, scientists have frequently taken advantage of existing data sets, quickly adding genotype data to studies that had previously measured depression and life events for other purposes. Not all of these studies' designs and measures are well suited to testing the G × E hypothesis. Covariation between poor measurement quality and negative findings was observed early on (Uher & McGuffin, 2008) and has been confirmed with the increasing number of published G × E studies (Uher & McGuffin, 2010). Notably, many of the largest studies in Table 2.1 and Table 2.2 were obliged to collect brief retrospective self-reports of stress through telephone interviews or postal questionnaires in order to contain data collection costs. Thus, unfortunately, large sample size tends to coincide with poor measurement quality, and meta-analyses that give larger samples greater weight in estimating an effect across studies further compound this problem. There is hope that a new generation of cohort studies purpose-built for testing G × E will improve replicability, but these must correct the problems of exposure measurement discussed in the previous paragraph, lest they merely repeat the problems on a far larger scale.

Most observational G × E research on *5-HTT* in humans has focused on depression. However, additional evidence links the *5-HTTLPR* to a broader range of stress-reactive phenotypes, including PTSD (Xie et al., 2009), posttrauma suicide attempt (Roy, Hu, Janal, & Goldman, 2007), aggressive reactions to a cold-pressor test (Verona, Joiner, Johnson, &

Bender, 2006), stress-linked alcohol consumption (Barr, Newman, Lindell, et al., 2004; Covault et al., 2007) and substance use (Brady et al., 2009a, 2009b), stress-related sleep disturbance (Brummett et al., 2007), and even premature ejaculation (Safarinejad, 2009). Research on quantitative endophenotypes shows that S-carriers with high levels of childhood maltreatment and adversity exhibit enhanced anxiety sensitivity (Stein, Schork, & Gelernter, 2008) and a bias toward perceiving and expecting negative outcomes (Williams et al., 2009). Moreover, S-carrying children who are raised by unresponsive or nonsupportive mothers exhibit poor self-regulation of negative affect (Barry, Kochanska, & Philibert, 2009; Fox et al., 2005; Kochanska, Philibert, & Barry, 2009; Pauli-Pott, Friedl, Hinney, & Hebebrand, 2009), which predicts a variety of adult psychiatric disorders (Caspi, Moffitt, Newman, & Silva, 1996). Finally, research that monitors affective experiences on a daily basis shows that S-carriers experience anxious mood on days with more intense stressors (Gunthert et al., 2007) and larger increases in negative affect while trying to quit smoking (Gilbert et al., 2009). To claim that these diverse outcomes are heterotypic manifestations of a unifying genetic vulnerability to stress reflected in the 5-HTTLPR S allele requires a theory that specifies the unifying mechanism. The leading theory (Jacobs et al., 2006; Lesch et al., 1996) is that the 5-HTTLPR is a genetic substrate for a latent personality trait, termed "negative affectivity" or "neuroticism." Negative affectivity prospectively predicts risk for all stress-related psychiatric disorders (Krueger, Caspi, Moffitt, Silva, & McGee, 1996). In theory, 5-HTTLPR S-carriers are characterized by the stable trait of negative affectivity that is converted to psychopathology only under conditions of stress, just as glass is always characterized by the trait of brittleness but shatters only when a stone is thrown. Negative affectivity represents the potential for excitability of anxiety and fear neural circuits, and is characterized by an attentional bias toward negatively valenced information and a cognitive sensitivity to perceive threat (Watson & Clark, 1984). This trait is operationalized in all experimental tests of the 5-HTTLPR G × E hypothesis, reviewed next.

Experimental Neuroscience Studies

In 2002, a synergy emerged between research in human affective neuroscience and genetic research into the 5-HTTLPR. Specifically, noninvasive fMRI, which assays information processing within distinct neuronal circuits, revealed relatively exaggerated threat-related amygdala reactivity in carriers of the 5-HTTLPR S allele (Hariri et al., 2002). This initial finding has since been replicated in independent samples of both healthy volunteers and psychiatric patients, using a multitude of threatening stimuli and neuroimaging modalities (Bertolino et al., 2005; Brown & Hariri, 2006; Canii et al., 2005; Dannlowski, Ohrmann, Bauer, Deckert, et al., 2007; Dannlowski, Ohrmann, Bauer, Kugel, et al., 2007; Domschke et al., 2006; Furmark et al., 2004; Hariri et al., 2005; Heinz et al., 2005, 2007; Smolka et al., 2007). This effect on the magnitude of amygdala reactivity has recently been extended, with S-carriers also exhibiting a relatively faster response than L-allele homozygotes (Furman, Hamilton, Joormann, & Gotlib, in press). Consistent with the heightened sensitivity to environmental threat documented in S-carriers, recent work suggests that the effects of the S allele on amygdala function may be unique to stimulus-provoked amygdala reactivity and not elevated baseline levels of activation (Canli et al., 2006; Rao et al., 2007; Viviani et al., 2010).

The bias in threat-related amygdala reactivity associated with the 5-HTTLPR S allele is positioned to drive the polymorphism's associations with altered mood and affective disorders, especially in interaction with exposure to environmental stressors and trauma. Evidence from animal and human studies demonstrates that the amygdala mediates both physiological (e.g., autonomic reactivity) and behavioral (e.g., reallocation of attentional resources) effects that allow an individual to respond to environmental and social challenges (Whalen & Phelps, 2009). Neuroimaging studies have reported positive correlations between indices of anxiety and amygdala reactivity to affective stimuli (especially threatening stimuli) (Hariri, 2009). Such findings demonstrate that variability in the magnitude of threat-related amygdala reactivity predicts individual differences in sensitivity to environmental threat and stress.

Human neuroimaging research suggests that relatively increased amygdala reactivity associated with the 5-HTTLPR S allele is likely to reflect both the functional and the structural architecture of a distributed network of brain regions. Research suggests that this network communicates information about the environment to the amygdala and relays signals between the amygdala and regulatory circuits in the medial prefrontal cortex. This putative mechanism is further underscored by the significant role serotonin signaling plays in the general development and function of this extended neural network (Hariri & Holmes, 2006). The S allele has been associated with altered functional coupling (as indexed by correlated fMRI signal strength) between the amygdala and regions of the medial prefrontal cortex (Heinz et al., 2005; Pezawas et al., 2005). These medial prefrontal regions integrate amygdala-mediated arousal and downregulate amygdala reactivity. Medial prefrontal regions are also involved in the extinction of conditioned fear responses, which are dependent on amygdala circuitry.

The pattern of 5-HTTLPR-associated differences in the functional dynamics of the amygdala and medial prefrontal cortex is echoed in structural measures within this same network. Specifically, the S allele has been associated with relatively decreased gray matter volume in the amygdala and medial prefrontal cortex (Canii et al., 2005; Pezawas et al., 2005). The

S allele has also been associated with alterations in the microstructure of the uncinate fasciculus, the white matter fiber bundle providing the majority of connections between the amygdala and the medial prefrontal cortex (Pacheco et al., 2009). Individual differences in uncinate fasciculus microstructure correlate with trait anxiety (Kim & Whalen, 2009). In addition, postmortem tissue analyses have associated the 5-HTTLPR S allele with relative enlargement of the pulvinar, which relays visual information to subcortical and higher cortical brain regions (Young et al., 2007). Consistent with this, as well as with amygdala-mediated behavioral arousal, numerous studies have reported increased cortical activity in response to experimental provocation in S-carriers (Battaglia et al., 2005; Fallgatter, Jatzke, Bartsch, Hamelbeck, & Lesch, 1999; Fallgatter et al., 2004; Gallinai et al., 2003; Hensch et al., 2006; Strobel et al., 2003).

In addition, a growing group of studies has begun to document effects of the 5-HTTLPR on intermediate behavioral and physiological processes that map onto these alterations in brain structure and function. The S allele is associated with increased acquisition of conditioned fear responses (Lonsdorf et al., 2009), increased auditory startle response (Armbruster et al., 2009; Brocke et al., 2006), and greater sympathetic reactivity when simply observing another person receiving shock (Crisan et al., 2009). Moreover, the 5-HTTLPR S allele has been associated with increased HPA axis reactivity to aversive or threatening stimuli in a number of studies (Alexander et al., 2009; Gotlib, Joormann, Minor, & Hallmayer, 2008; Mueller, Brocke, Fries, Lesch, & Kirschbaum, 2010; Way & Taylor, 2010). The S allele typically has no impact on baseline levels of HPA function in these studies, underscoring its documented effect on threat-related amygdala reactivity. In addition, the S allele has been linked with difficulty disengaging from, or preferential attention toward, threat-related stimuli (Beevers, Gibb, McGeary, & Miller, 2007; Beevers, Wells, Ellis, & McGeary, 2009; Fox, Ridgewell, & Ashwin, 2009; Gibb, Benas, Grassia, & McGeary, 2009; Osinsky et al., 2008), a more negative information-processing bias (Hayden et al., 2008), emotion-induced retrograde amnesia (Strange, Kroes, Roiser, Tan, & Dolan, 2008), sensitivity to financial loss (Crisan et al., 2009; Roiser et al., 2009), and even social blushing (Domschke et al., 2009). Although this literature is not without inconsistencies (e.g., some reported associations are sex-specific and others have not replicated), it does suggest that the effects of the 5-HTTLPR S allele on the brain's neural circuitry for responding to environmental threat and stress translate to biases in both behavioral and physiological processes which may, in turn, shape individual risk for depression upon exposure to acute trauma or chronic stressors (Figure 2.2). Multiple components of this ongoing research were highlighted in one report of increases in threat-related amygdala and medial prefrontal cortical activation as well as heart rate and startle amplitude in 5-HTTLPR

S-carriers who also exhibited a self-reported sensitivity to perceived danger in the environment (Williams et al., 2009).

Nonhuman Primate Studies

Rhesus monkeys have an orthologue of the human *5-HTTLPR*, making them an excellent model species for G × E studies. Like the human variant, the rhesus S allele is associated with decreased transcriptional efficiency *in vitro* (Barr et al., 2003). The modulating influence of the polymorphism on early life stress has been tested by separating infant rhesus monkeys from their mothers and rearing them with other infants (a long-established model of early life adversity in this species). During initial episodes of separation, monkeys carrying the *rh5-HTTLPR* S allele exhibit less "protest" and self-directed behaviors that are considered active coping responses to this stressor (Spinelli et al., 2007). Instead, separated S-allele monkeys display greater anxiety, agitation, stereotypies, and an exaggerated HPA axis response (Barr, Newman, Shannon, et al., 2004; Spinelli et al., 2007).

The modulating influence of the *rh5-HTTLPR* on separation in infancy persists into later life, manifesting, for example, as higher ACTH responses to stress in S-carrier monkeys than LL homozygotes (Barr, Newman, Schwandt, et al., 2004). It is important to underscore that these long-lasting phenotypic effects of the S allele only occur in monkeys exposed to maternal separation early life stress, echoing the G × E observed in relation to human depression.

Another major parallel between the human and monkey data has been the finding that, as in humans, the stress-related S allele phenotype in monkeys is related to an intermediate neural phenotype characterized by abnormal corticolimbic structure and function. For example, the S allele in monkeys also has been mapped onto reduced gray matter volumes in the amygdala, medial prefrontal and orbitofrontal cortex, and pulvinar (Jedema et al., 2010). Moreover, monkeys with the S allele exhibit greater metabolic activity than LL homozygotes in the amygdala and its networked cortical regions, including orbitofrontal cortex, in response to the stress of relocation (Kalin et al., 2008). Given the importance of the orbitofrontal cortex in social behavior, abnormalities in this region might also account for the finding that S-carriers engage in less eye gaze with high-status conspecifics and are more risk-averse in their presence (Watson, Ghodrasa, & Piatt, 2009). An intriguing development is recent data from S-carrier monkeys (Jedema et al., 2010) and *5-HTT* mutant mice (Brigman et al., 2010) demonstrating that reversal learning, a measure of cognitive flexibility subserved by the orbitofrontal cortex (Schoenbaum & Shaham, 2008), is enhanced as a function of relative *5-HTT* gene deficiency. This may reflect increased sensitivity to negative environmental stimuli, although further work will be needed to substantiate this. Notwithstanding, these data indicate that altered *5-HTT* gene function may influence multiple higher behaviors, as would be predicted if it affects a core corticolimbic neural circuitry.

Studies Involving Genetically Engineered *5-HTT* Mutations in Rodents

Research using rodents allows for experimental control over genetic background and the environment to a degree that is neither practically nor ethically feasible in human or even nonhuman primate studies (Cryan & Holmes, 2005). Although there is functional gene variation in the murine *5-HTT* (*slc6a4*) (Carneiro et al., 2009), there is no rodent orthologue of the *5-HTTLPR*. As an alternative approach, mice and rats have been genetically engineered with loss-of-function mutations in the *5-HTT* gene. Studying the consequences of these mutations for behavior and brain function has greatly complemented the work on the *5-HTTLPR* in primates and provided some key insights into the mechanisms that mediate the influence of *5-HTT* on negative affect and stress reactivity (Hariri & Holmes, 2006; Murphy & Lesch, 2008).

Mice in which the *5-HTT* has been functionally excised either by targeted mutation or chemical mutagenesis exhibit heightened anxiety-like behavior, impaired fear extinction, and exaggerated HPA-axis responses to acute stress. While it is far less common to engineer mutant rats than mice, a *5-HTT*-null mutant rat has been generated and also shows increased anxiety-like behavior (Homberg et al., 2007). Furthermore, providing an interesting counterpoint to these "knockout" mutants, mice with transgenic overexpression of the *5-HTT* actually produce decreased anxiety-like behavior (Jennings et al., 2006). The consistency of these findings across models, laboratories, and species is rarely seen in the field of rodent behavioral genetics and illustrates the strong penetrance of the mutation's effects.

The "depression-related" consequences of rodent *5-HTT* knockout mice are, at first blush, less consistent than the anxiety-related consequences, in that they are seen in some of the standard rodent assays for this behavior but not others. This variability may, however, be a legitimate reflection of differences in the level of stress evoked under varying test conditions. In support of this hypothesis, following repeated exposure to stress (e.g., forced swimming, tail suspension), *5-HTT* knockout mice develop a depression-related "despair-like" phenotype that is not seen with single exposure (Jennings et al., 2006). The parallels with the primate data showing that the S-allele influence on depression is contingent upon repeated stress exposure are clear.

Much of our understanding of the functional role of the *5-HTT* as a master modulator of the 5-HT system has been built upon work in rodents (Torres & Amara, 2007). As such, researchers have a ready platform and toolset from which to perform certain neural and molecular analyses in *5-HTT* mutant rodents (e.g., *in vivo* measurement of brain 5-HT availability) that cannot be employed in humans. One of the key themes to emerge from this work is that the neural consequences of *5-HTT* gene mutation extend well beyond the *5-HTT* and its role as a regulator of 5-HT availability. *5-HTT* null mutation leads to alterations throughout the 5-HT system that include changes in 5-HT receptor binding and 5-HT synthesis (Hariri & Holmes, 2006; Murphy & Lesch, 2008). At the systems level, *5-HTT* knockout mice exhibit an abnormally high density of excitatory dendritic spines on amygdala neurons and an increase in dendritic arborization of prefrontal cortex neurons (Hariri & Holmes, 2006). The implication here is that influence of *5-HTT* variation may not be limited to effects on 5-HT availability or even on the 5-HT system. Recently, this implication was confirmed in a rhesus macaque model (Jedema et al., 2010), in which the *rh5-HTTLPR* S allele affected behavior and brain morphology but not *5-HTT* (Christian et al., 2009) or 5-HT_{1A} concentrations *in vivo*. Similar complexities in the likely molecular consequences of the *5-HTTLPR* have been documented in humans (David et al., 2005; Heinz et al., 2000; Lee et al., 2005; Parsey et al., 2006; Reimold et al., 2007; Shioe et al., 2003). Collectively, mouse, monkey, and human findings suggest that *5-HTTLPR*'s behavioral effects on stress reactivity may be most consistently rooted in neural development.

An intriguing line of enquiry in this context has centered on the hypothesis that *5-HTT* variation may in part modulate the capacity to cope with stress by shaping the early life development of corticolimbic circuitry (Hariri & Holmes, 2006). In fact, the importance of the 5-HT system in neurodevelopment has long been recognized, and the *5-HTT* is known to be critical for the formation of cortical systems in particular (Esaki et al., 2005; Gaspar, Cases, & Maroteaux, 2003). Pharmacological inhibition of the *5-HTT* during early life mimics the anxiety-like phenotype of *5-HTT* knockout (Ansorge, Zhou, Lira, Hen, & Gingrich, 2004). Moreover, poor maternal care produces heightened anxiety-like behavior in mice with a partial (heterozygous) *5-HTT* null mutation, which are phenotypically normal under conditions of good maternal care (Carola et al., 2008).

These findings raise the question of whether the effects of *5-HTT* knockout are developmentally driven. It has been hypothesized that the *5-HTTLPR* G × E observed in relation to adult stressful life events should selectively affect people already "primed" by childhood adversity (Brown & Harris, 2008). This opens up some very interesting avenues for future animal studies. For example, would *5-HTT* loss restricted to early life devel-

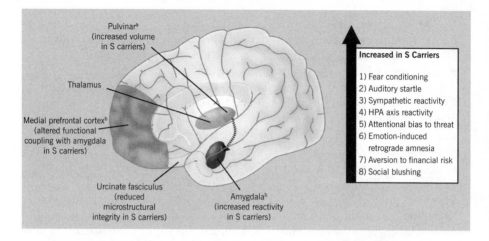

FIGURE 2.2. How the *5-HTTLPR* affects neural circuitry for responding to environmental threat and stress. [a]Implicated in humans and nonhuman primates. [b]Implicated in humans, nonhuman primates, and rodents.

opment be sufficient to increase anxiety and impair stress coping? If so, is there a critical window and what is the corresponding ontogenic period in humans? Researchers could then elucidate the key neural and molecular changes underlying these effects. This could, in turn, "square the circle" by nominating mechanisms to target with novel therapeutic approaches in humans.

LESSONS FOR G × E RESEARCH

In the previous section, we reviewed evidence about the *5-HTT* stress-sensitivity hypothesis. Lessons learned in this research apply broadly to all G × E research. In this section, we draw on these lessons to dispel some misconceptions and offer some constructive recommendations.

G × E Hypotheses Can Be Tested with Large and Small Samples

Statistical power is critical for theory-free, exploratory scans for G × E (Burton et al., 2009). This realization has prompted the creation of large case–control consortia and massive biobanks. A question that puzzles many readers is how to reconcile the obvious benefits of huge samples with evidence that G × E have been reported in many small-sample studies of

5-HTT and stress sensitivity, particularly in studies comparing stress-exposed versus matched nonexposed groups (e.g., abused children) and in experimental studies of humans and animals. There are statistical reasons for this.

The problem has to do with the approach to testing interactions (McClelland & Judd, 1993): If the product term (i.e., the interaction term in multiple regression) is calculated from two normally distributed symmetrical variables, it has restricted variance but is uncorrelated with the first-order predictors (Figure 2.3, top row). However, a product term of two categorical variables (e.g., minor allele frequency [MAF] of 25% and rate of exposure [P_{exp} of 25%) is significantly correlated with the first-order predictors (Figure 2.3, middle row). Such is the case in practically all observational G × E studies of psychiatric phenotypes. As a result, the residual variance of the product term after factoring out first-order predictors—and the corresponding power to detect interactions—declines rapidly with minor allele frequencies and rates of exposure departing from 50%. The full power for testing interactions between categorical variables is only preserved in the optimal case where minor allele frequency and exposure rate equal 50% (bottom of Figure 2.3). An implication of this insight is that hypothesis-driven G × E studies that recruit participants on the basis of their genotype and their environmental exposure (e.g., experimental G × E studies with balanced cell sizes) are better powered to test for genetically moderated exposure effects than are observational field studies, which must make do with unequal-sized groups since these occur in nature.

G × E Research Can Be Carried Out Before as Well as After Replicated Gene Discovery

Some researchers claim that G × E studies should only be carried out if there exists a genotype-to-phenotype main effect, but this claim is statistically unwarranted (Rutter, Thapar, & Pickles, 2009). Such a strategy also precludes identification of environmentally dependent genetic effects that are small in absolute size or are contingent on relatively uncommon environmental factors (Figure 2.4). Moreover, genotype–phenotype association studies may not replicate if G × E are operating and research samples differ on environmental risk exposure. Waiting for genomewide association studies (GWAS) to throw up candidate genes may be ill-advised because G × E may conceal good candidates from GWAS. Inconsistent genotype–phenotype associations have inspired successful searches for G × E in different fields of medicine, from asthma (Martinez, 2007) to cardiovascular disease (Ordovas & Tai, 2008). Inconsistent associations between the *5-HTTLPR* S allele and depression (Hoefgen et al., 2005; Lasky-Su, Faraone, Glatt, & Tsuang, 2005; Sen, Burmeister, & Ghosh, 2004) prompted

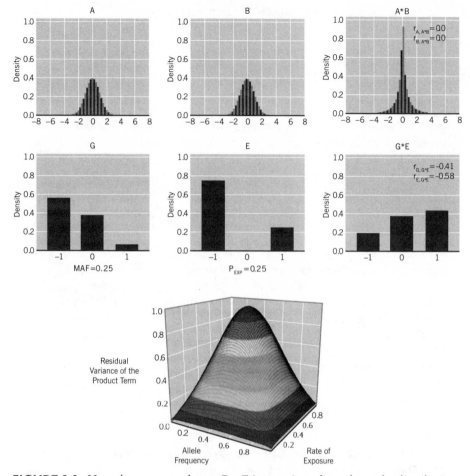

FIGURE 2.3. How the power to detect G × E interactions depends on the distributions of the genotypes and exposures in the sample. The two rows of graphs demonstrate a key difference between interactions involving normally distributed continuous variables (top row) and those involving asymmetrically distributed categorical ones (middle row). If the product term A*B (i.e., the term that represents interaction in a multiple regression) is calculated from two normally distributed symmetrical variables A and B, it has a restricted variance (leptokurtic distribution) but is uncorrelated with the first-order predictors (i.e., the correlations between A and A*B [$r_{A,A*B}$] and between B and A*B [$r_{B,A*B}$] are zero). However, the product term G*E that represents two categorical variables (G: genotype with a minor allele frequency [MAF] of 25%; and E: categorical exposure in the population [P_{EXP}] of 25%) is strongly correlated with the first-order predictors (i.e., the correlations between G and G*E [$r_{G,G*E}$] and between E and G*E [$r_{E,G*E}$] are substantial). As a result, the residual variance of the product term (bottom of figure) after factoring out first-order predictors, and the power to detect interactions, declines rapidly as the rates of exposure and minor allele frequency depart from 50%. The full power for testing interactions between categorical variables is only preserved in the special case of minor allele frequency equal to 50% and exposure rate of 50% (the top segment). "Density" reflects the proportion of individuals falling within each narrow band of values of the variable on the x axis.

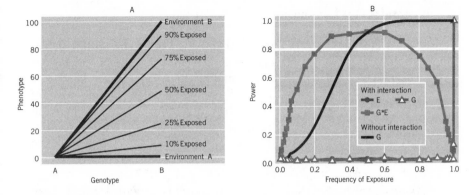

FIGURE 2.4. How the frequency of an environmental exposure in a sample influences the ability to detect genetic effects and G × E interactions. Panel A shows the influence of environmental exposure frequency on the ability to identify genetic effects, in two genotypes of equal prevalence. Genotype A shows no phenotypic response to the environmental exposure. Genotype B shows a response to the environmental exposure. What would happen if the association between genotype and phenotype were studied without knowledge of the environmental exposure and its frequency (shown from 10% to 90%)? A sample having many exposed subjects will report a genetic effect on the phenotype, whereas a sample having few exposed subjects will not, and if exposure is not ascertained, the source of nonreplication will remain a mystery. Panel B shows the influence of the rate of environmental exposure on statistical power to detect G × E interactions and main effects of genes. Each point is based on 10,000 simulations of samples of 1000 drawn from a population with equal distributions of two genotypes, with a continuous outcome generated as a moderately strong G × E (i.e., the difference in the environment–phenotype correlation between genetic strata = 0.3), and no main effect. In samples with exposure frequency close to 0, there is no detectable interaction or main effect. For exposure frequency below 50%, there is greater power to detect a G × E interaction (-■-) than to detect a main effect of genes (—). With rates of exposure exceeding 50%, the power of detecting a direct effect of genes (—) increases above that of detecting an interaction, even though interaction is the data-generating mechanism. The probability of detecting a spurious main effect of genes (or environments) remains at the 2.5% chance level across the range of exposure frequency if the interaction term is retained in the equation.

us to consider G × E in our initial studies of the *5-HTTLPR* and depression.

The Psychiatric GWAS Consortium Steering Committee (2008) recommends conducting G × E studies only after convincing genotype–phenotype associations have been identified by (1) finding the disease susceptibility gene by conducting a GWAS, then (2) identifying the functional consequences of the putative causal variant, and only then (3) testing interactions between the variant and environmental factors. This strategy is presumed to offer a foolproof approach to detecting replicable G × E. However, research in obesity illustrates that this strategy may not work. *FTO* was found to be a susceptibility gene through GWAS (Frayling et al., 2007), and *FTO*'s functional consequences were identified (Cecil, Tavendale, Watt, Hetherington, & Palmer, 2008; Fredriksson et al., 2008; Gerken et al., 2007; Wardle et al., 2008). G × E research then documented that an active lifestyle mitigates obesity risk from *FTO* (Andreasen et al., 2008; Rampersaud et al., 2008; Ruiz et al., in press; Vimaleswaran et al., 2009). However, this G × E interaction has not been universally replicated (Hakanen et al., 2009; Jonsson et al., 2009), in part because of cross-study differences in the quality of physical activity measurement. The moral is that a robust genotype–phenotype association cannot guarantee a robust G × E finding, because the study of G × E requires more appropriate and high-quality exposure measurement.

G × E Research Is a Helpful Tool for Gene Discovery

Although most G × E research uses candidate genes, environmental exposures can also be used to discover novel loci. Indeed, one possible reason for the paucity of susceptibility genes in psychiatry is that gene discovery studies have been searching for genetic effects on disease rather than for genetic effects on vulnerability to environmental causes of disease (Rutter, 2008). Whereas in genetic association studies, a candidate gene is a gene suspected of being involved in a trait or disease—either because its protein product is relevant or because it has been uncovered in the course of association or linkage analysis of the phenotype—in G × E research a candidate gene is one plausibly related to the organisms' reactivity to the environmental risk or pathogen (Moffitt, Caspi, & Rutter, 2005). The idea that genes may moderate the effect of environmental risk has direct implications for hypothesis-driven selection of novel candidate genes. For example, genes associated with the physiological response to psychological stress, particularly in the HPA axis, are natural candidates for G × E research on stress and depression (Bradley et al., 2008). Genes regulated by hypoxia are candidates for G × E research on obstetric complications and schizophrenia (Nicodemus et al., 2008). Genes involved in biosynthesis of fatty acids are candidates for G × E research on nutrition and brain development (Caspi et al., 2007). Genes involved in lead absorption are relevant for research on attention deficits and hyperactivity (Hopkins et al., 2008). Genes involved in ototoxicity are relevant for research on learning difficulties (Ross et al., 2009).

Research on "candidate environmental risks" can be combined with theory-free genetics to discover novel loci in two ways. One way is to turn GWAS into gene–environment-wide interaction studies (Khoury & Wacholder, 2009). Theoretically, the ability to measure G × E interactions should sharpen measurement of gene–disease associations in subsets of the population and even potentially increase statistical power to detect such associations (Khoury & Wacholder, 2009). This will become increasingly possible as researchers seek to integrate genomewide information with information about environmental exposures gathered in the context of epidemiological studies. But sample sizes will become prohibitive when testing gene–environment-wide interactions because (1) more tests are involved, (2) tests for interactions have less power compared to tests for main effects, and (3) environmental exposures introduce additional measurement error. If genetic epidemiologists embrace purely agnostic, theory-free approaches and data-mining tools in studying G × E, the "fishing expedition" may net little. The new generation of purpose-built gene–environment-wide interaction studies may be an improvement over opportunistic studies published in these early years of G × E research, but even these will fall short unless they attend to the measurement of environmental exposures. An alternative is to pursue study designs that use confirmed environmental effects on disease. Such "exposed-only designs" will test genomewide associations comparing equally exposed individuals who do versus do not develop a disease in order to discover novel susceptibility loci. Examples of this design can be seen in research on infectious disease, whose starting point is pathogen exposure (Kotb et al., 2002). The environmental risks (i.e., pathogens) for many psychiatric conditions are well established, if not always well measured. As such, the strong prior probabilities for environmental risks can be harnessed in psychiatry to design genomewide studies focused on identifying genetic differences in responses to well-defined environmental risks. This approach to gene discovery will involve entirely different designs and sampling frames than currently used in case–control studies and biobanks.

A second way in which environmental exposures can be used to discover novel loci is to study gene expression (mRNA levels) as a quantitative phenotype, although attention needs to be paid to tissue informativeness (Dimas et al., 2009). Gene expression profiling offers a powerful tool to identify genomic responses to the environment by investigating responses to specific, well-operationalized, and reliably measured pathogens and stressors, including exposures to social adversities (Miller et al., 2009). By assessing genotype effects on gene expression levels (Cheung &

Spielman, 2009), polymorphisms in environmentally responsive genes may be identified and then used to study why some people become ill when challenged by the environment and others do not. Incorporating environmental genomics into psychiatry may facilitate identifying susceptibility factors in environmentally induced psychiatric conditions.

Construct Validation Is a Useful Way to Evaluate G × E Research

There are two distinct cultures vying to evaluate the worth of the 5-HTTLPR G × E findings: a purely statistical (theory-free) approach that relies wholly on meta-analysis (Munafò, Durrant, Lewis, & Flint, 2009; Risch et al., 2009) versus a construct-validity (theory-guided) approach that looks for a nomological network of convergent evidence (this chapter). The statistical approach is essential for confirming direct genotype–phenotype association discoveries. This approach is driven by the imperative to avoid false positives when evaluating associations sifted from huge amounts of data in theory-free, genomewide testing with nil prior probability of gene–disease association (Moonesinghe, Khoury, Liu, & Ioannidis, 2008). Naturally, the statistical approach prizes exact replication. In the statistical approach, replication attempts' elements should match the original report's elements, including sample, phenotype, polymorphism, genetic model, and direction of effect. Larger samples are given greater weight in statistical evaluation, because with all other study elements held equal, power is decisive (Chanock et al., 2007).

It is our contention that the purely statistical approach is not sufficient, or necessary, for evaluating research into G × E hypotheses involving candidate genes. In such G × E research, the prior probability of association is far from nil, thus mitigating the risk of false positives. For example, the 5-HTTLPR stress-sensitivity hypothesis was informed by knowledge about the serotonin system's role in depression and the transporter gene's function (Lesch et al., 1996), by inconsistent associations between the 5-HTTLPR and depression suggesting environmental moderation might be operating (Lesch, 2003), by evidence that stress causes depression (Monroe & Simons, 1991), and by initial reports that 5-HTT variation influenced stress reactivity (Bennett et al., 2002; Hariri et al., 2002; Murphy et al., 2001). In G × E research, replication attempts' elements need not match those of the original report. G × E research involves not only polymorphism and phenotype, but another element: the environment. Whereas genetic measurements are standard and unchanging across time and across studies and phenotypic measurements can also be standardized to a high degree, environmental exposure measurements vary markedly across studies (Ioannides, Loy, Poulton, & Chia, 2009). Two kinds of heterogeneity should be distinguished: heterogeneity in the types of stress exposure versus heterogeneity in the quality of exposure measurements. Regarding exposure types, stressful experiences come in many forms (Table 2.1 and Table 2.2) and studies of the 5-HTTLPR G × E have rightly gone beyond the original report to incorporate them. This environmental measurement heterogeneity has implications for matching the genetic model across studies, because the "correct" genetic model could vary depending on severity of the environmental exposure or other factors such as developmental stage and course of illness (e.g., first-onset vs. recurrent depression). By insisting that all results must conform to one genetic model, the meta-analysis approach conceals potentially informative patterns, if they exist. Regarding measurement quality, in G × E research it is folly to give greater weight to larger samples, because many large samples are afflicted by poor exposure measurement. Overall, heterogeneity in both the type of stress exposures and in the quality of exposure measurements renders the studies in Table 2.1 and Table 2.2 inappropriate for drawing one simple conclusion about statistical replication (Chanock et al., 2007).

Meta-analysis can be a useful tool for interpreting multiple tests of a G × E hypothesis, when best practice is followed. Meta-analyses should table the universe of publications testing the G × E, explaining in a transparent way why each was analyzed or omitted. The subsample analyzed should represent the distribution of positive and negative results in the literature. Metaregression should be undertaken to evaluate methodological sources of variation among findings. Methodological evaluation should be guided by long-established cautions. For example, large samples often suffer poor measurement quality, and large exposure-to-outcome correlations often signal measurement bias, not validity. It should be appreciated that when the sample of studies is small, a statistical test for heterogeneity is underpowered and its nonsignificance does not contraindicate metaregression. If methodological heterogeneity is ruled out, metaregression should investigate substantive sources of variation among findings (e.g., sex, age, exposure severity), and if these are uncovered, variation in genetic model should be considered in relation to the substantive findings. Meta-analyses of the 5-HTTLPR G × E hypothesis have been reported (Munafò et al., 2009; Risch et al., 2009), but did not follow best practice (Kaufman, Gelernter, Kaffman, Caspi, & Moffitt, 2010; Koenen & Galea, 2009; Lotrich & Lenze, 2009; Rutter, 2010; Schwahn & Grabe, 2009; Uher & McGuffin, 2010).

In any case, whether G × E studies can meet prerequisite standards for statistical meta-analysis is immaterial, since replicating a theory-free association is not the goal. The goal is to evaluate the construct validity of a theory-guided hypothesis (Strauss & Smith, 2009). In contrast to the statistical approach, the construct validation approach prizes design heterogeneity (although it requires high-quality samples and measures) (Vandenbroucke, 2008). Construct validation seeks "sturdy" findings (Robins, 1978), defined as results that emerge repeatedly despite variation in sample characteristics, phenotype measurement, and environmental exposure, and that are validated across human epidemiology, experimental neuroscience, and animal models. We have attempted to show that this is the case with evidence for the *5-HTT* stress-sensitivity hypothesis.

Public Understanding of Genetic Science

One of G × E research's important contributions is often overlooked by scientists: teaching the falsehood of genetic (and environmental) determinism (Moffitt, Caspi, & Rutter, 2006). For over a century the public has been fed a diet of determinism, beginning with early 20th-century eugenics policies to correct all human flaws by culling the breeding stock. Midcentury opinions swung back toward naive environmental determinism, exemplified by B. F. Skinner's 1948 *Walden Two*. In the late 20th century, public opinion was compelled toward genetic determinism again when high heritability estimates were taken to imply that nongenetic factors have little importance for mental health and behavior. Discoveries of single mutations causing rare disorders strengthened the public's belief that knowing one's genetic makeup is tantamount to knowing one's future. Deterministic beliefs, environmental or genetic, are dangerous. Determinism encourages policies that violate human rights (at worst) and waste resources on ill-conceived mental health improvement programs (at best). Media coverage of this century's new findings of G × E interaction (and environmental effects on gene expression) is persuading the public to embrace a more realistic, nuanced understanding of the causes of behavior, in which some genes' effects depend on lifestyle choices that are often under human control. That understanding will be the best defense against misuse of genetic information. Interdependence between life stress and the *5-HTTLPR* leads this shift in understanding, because stress and depression touch almost everyone.

ACKNOWLEDGMENTS

This chapter is reprinted from the *American Journal of Psychiatry*, May 2010, Vol. 167, No. 5, pp. 509–527. Copyright 2010 by the American Psychiatric Association. Reprinted by permission. Work on this chapter was supported by grants from the U.K. Medical Research Council (Nos. G0100527 and G0601483), the National Institute on Aging (No. AG032282), the National Institute of Mental Health (Nos. MH077874 and MH072837), the National Institute of Child Health and Human Development (No. HD061298), and the Intramural Research Program of the National Institute on Alcohol Abuse and Alcoholism. Avshalom Caspi is a Royal Society–Wolfson Merit Award holder. We thank Eric Lenze, Richie Poulton, and David Reiss for helpful discussions of the research literature.

REFERENCES

Alexander, N., Kuepper, Y., Schmitz, A., Osinsky, R., Kozyra, E., & Hennig, J. (2009). Gene–environment interactions predict Cortisol responses after acute stress: Implications for the etiology of depression. *Psychoneuroendocrinology, 34*, 1294–1303.

Andreasen, C. H., Stender-Petersen, K. L., Mogensen, M. S., Torekov, S. S., Wegner, L., Andersen, G., et al. (2008). Low physical activity accentuates the effect of the FTO rs9939609 polymorphism on body fat accumulation. *Diabetes, 57*, 95–101.

Ansorge, M., Zhou, M., Lira, A., Hen, R., & Gingrich, J. (2004). Early-life blockade of 5-HT transporter alters emotional behavior in adult mice. *Science, 306*, 879–881.

Armbruster, D., Moser, D. A., Strobel, A., Hensch, T., Kirschbaum, C., Lesch, K. P., et al. (2009). Serotonin transporter gene variation and stressful life events impact processing of fear and anxiety. *International Journal of Neuropsychopharmacology, 12*, 393–401.

Barr, C. S., Newman, T. K., Becker, M. L., Parker, C. C., Champoux, M., Lesch, K. P., et al. (2003). The utility of the non-human primate model for studying gene by environment interactions in behavioral research. *Genes, Brain and Behavior, 2*, 336–340.

Barr, C. S., Newman, T. K., Lindell, S., Shannon, C., Champoux, M., Lesch, K. P., et al. (2004). Interaction between serotonin transporter gene variation and rearing condition in alcohol preference and consumption in female primates. *Archives of General Psychiatry, 61*, 1146–1152.

Barr, C. S., Newman, T. K., Schwandt, M., Shannon, C., Dvoskin, R. L., Lindell, S., et al. (2004). Sexual dichotomy of an interaction between early adversity and the serotonin transporter gene promoter variant in rhesus macaques. *Proceedings of the National Academy of Sciences USA, 101*, 12358–12363.

Barr, C. S., Newman, T. K., Shannon, C., Parker, C., Dvoskin, R. L., Becker, M. L., et al. (2004). Rearing condition and rh5-HTTLPR interact to influence limbic–hypothalamic–pituitary–adrenal axis response to stress in infant macaques. *Biological Psychiatry, 55*, 733–738.

Barry, R. A., Kochanska, G., & Philibert, R. A. (2008). G–E interaction in the organization of attachment: Mothers' responsiveness as a moderator of children's genotypes. *Journal of Child Psychology and Psychiatry and Allied Disciplines, 49*, 1313–1320.

Battaglia, M., Ogliari, A., Zanoni, A., Citterio, A., Pozzoli, U., Giorda, R., et al. (2005). Influence of the serotonin transporter promoter gene and shyness on children's cerebral responses to facial expressions. *Archives of General Psychiatry, 62*, 85–94.

Beevers, C. G., Gibb, B. E., McGeary, J. E., & Miller, I. W. (2007). Serotonin transporter genetic variation and biased attention for emotional word stimuli among psychiatric inpatients. *Journal of Abnormal Psychology, 116,* 208–212.

Beevers, C. G., Wells, T. T., Ellis, A. J., & McGeary, J. E. (2009). Association of the serotonin transporter gene promoter region (5-HTTLPR) polymorphism with biased attention for emotional stimuli. *Journal of Abnormal Psychology, 118,* 670–681.

Bennett, A. J., Lesch, K. P., Heils, A., Long, J. C., Lorenz, J. G., Shoaf, S. E., et al. (2002). Early experience and serotonin transporter gene variation interact to influence primates CNS function. *Molecular Psychiatry, 7,* 118–122.

Bertolino, A., Arciera, G., Rubino, V., Latorre, V., De Candia, M., Mazzola, V., et al. (2005). Variation of human amygdala response during threatening stimuli as a function of 5-HTTLPR genotype and personality style. *Biological Psychiatry, 57,* 1517–1525.

Block, J. (1995). A contrarian view of the five-factor approach to personality description. *Psychological Bulletin, 117,* 187.

Bradley, R. G., Binder, E. B., Epstein, M. P., Tang, Y., Nair, H. P., Liu, W., et al. (2008). Influence of child abuse on adult depression: Moderation by the corticotropin-releasing hormone receptor gene. *Archives of General Psychiatry, 65,* 190–200.

Brady, G. H., Beach, S. R., Philibert, R. A., Chen, Y. F., Lei, M. K., Murry, V. M., et al. (2009a). Parenting moderates a genetic vulnerability factor in longitudinal increases in youths' substance use. *Journal of Consulting Clinical Psychology, 77,* 1–11.

Brady, G. H., Beach, S. R., Philibert, R. A., Chen, Y. F., & Murry, V. M. (2009b). Prevention effects moderate the association of 5-HTTLPR and youth risk behavior initiation: Gene & environment hypotheses tested via a randomized prevention design. *Child Development, 80,* 645–661.

Brigman, J., Mathur, P., Harvey-White, J., Izquierdo, A., Saksida, L., Bussey, T. J., et al. (2010). Pharmacological or genetic inactivation of the serotonin transporter improves reversal learning in mice. *Cerebral Cortex, 20,* 1955–1963.

Brocke, B., Armbruster, D., Muller, J., Hensch, T., Jacob, C. P., Lesch, K. P., et al. (2006). Serotonin transporter gene variation impacts innate fear processing: Acoustic startle response and emotional startle. *Molecular Psychiatry, 11,* 1106–1112.

Brown, G. W., & Harris, T. O. (2008). Depression and the serotonin transporter 5-HTTLPR polymorphism: A review and a hypothesis concerning gene–environment interaction. *Journal of Affective Disorders, 111,* 1–12.

Brown, S. M., & Hariri, A. R. (2006). Neuroimaging studies of serotonin gene polymorphisms: Exploring the interplay of genes, brain, and behavior. *Cognitive, Affective, and Behavioral Neuroscience, 6,* 44–52.

Brummett, B. H., Krystal, A. D., Ashley-Koch, A., Kuhn, C. M., Zuchner, S., Siegler, I. C., et al. (2007). Sleep quality varies as a function of 5-HTTLPR genotype and stress. *Psychosomatic Medicine, 69,* 621–624.

Burton, P. R., Hansell, A. L., Fortier, I., Manolio, T. A., Khoury, M. J., Little, J., et al. (2009). Size matters: Just how big is BIG?: Quantifying realistic sample size requirements for human genome epidemiology. *International Journal of Epidemiology, 38*, 263–273.

Canii, T., Omura, K., Haas, B. W., Fallgatter, A., Constable, R. T., & Lesch, K. P. (2005). Beyond affect: A role for genetic variation of the serotonin transporter in neural activation during a cognitive attention task. *Proceedings of the National Academy of Sciences USA, 102*, 12224–12229.

Canli, T., Qiu, M., Omura, K., Congdon, E., Haas, B. W., Amin, Z., et al. (2006). Neural correlates of epigenesis. *Proceedings of the National Academy of Sciences USA, 103*, 16033–16038.

Carneiro, A., Airey, D., Thompson, B., Zhu, C., Lu, L., Chester, E., et al. (2009). Functional coding variation in recombinant inbred mouse lines reveals multiple serotonin transporter-associated phenotypes. *Proceedings of the National Academy of Sciences USA, 106*, 2047–2052.

Carola, V., Frazzetto, G., Pascucci, T., Audero, E., Puglisi-Allegra, S., Cabib, S., et al. (2008). Identifying molecular substrates in a mouse model of the serotonin transporter × environment risk factor for anxiety and depression. *Biological Psychiatry, 63*, 840–846.

Caspi, A., & Moffitt, T. E. (2006). Gene–environment interactions in psychiatry: Joining forces with neuroscience. *Nature Reviews Neuroscience, 7*, 583–590.

Caspi, A., Moffitt, T. E., Newman, D. L., & Silva, P. A. (1996). Behavioral observations at age 3 years predict adult psychiatric disorders: Longitudinal evidence from a birth cohort. *Archives of General Psychiatry, 53*, 1033–1039.

Caspi, A., Sugden, K., Moffitt, T. E., Taylor, A., Craig, I. W., Harrington, H., et al. (2003). Influence of life stress on depression: Moderation by a polymorphism in the 5-HTT gene. *Science, 301*, 386–389.

Caspi, A., Williams, B., Kim-Cohen, J., Craig, I. W., Milne, B. J., Poulton, R., et al. (2007). Moderation of breastfeeding effects on the IQ by genetic variation in fatty acid metabolism. *Proceedings of the National Academy Sciences USA, 104*, 18860–18865.

Cecil, J. E., Tavendale, R., Watt, P., Hetherington, M. M., & Palmer, C. N. (2008). An obesity-associated FTO gene variant and increased energy intake in children. *New England Journal of Medicine, 359*, 2558–2566.

Chanock, S., Manolio, T., Boehnke, M., Boerwinkle, E., Hunter, D., Thomas, G., et al. (2007). Replicating genotype–phenotype associations. *Nature, 447*, 655–660.

Cheung, V. G., & Spielman, R. S. (2009). Genetics of human gene expression: Mapping DNA variants that influence gene expression. *Nature Reviews Genetics, 10*, 595–604.

Christian, B. T., Fox, A. S., Oler, J. A., Vandehey, N. T., Murali, D., Rogers, J., et al. (2009). Serotonin transporter binding and genotype in the nonhuman primate brain using [C-11]DASB PET. *NeuroImage, 47*, 1230–1236.

Covault, J., Tennen, H., Armeli, S., Conner, T. S., Herman, A. L., Cillessen, A. H., et al. (2007). Interactive effects of the serotonin transporter 5-HTTLPR polymorphism and stressful life events on college student drinking and drug use. *Biological Psychiatry, 61*, 609–616.

Crisan, L. G., Pana, S., Vulturar, R., Heilman, R. M., Szekely, R., Druga, B., et al.

(2009). Genetic contributions of the serotonin transporter to social learning of fear and economic decision making. *Socical Cognitive and Affective Neurosciences, 4*, 399–408.

Cryan, J., & Holmes, A. (2005). The ascent of mouse: Advances in modelling human depression and anxiety. *Nature Reviews Drug Discovery, 4*, 775–790.

Dannlowski, U., Ohrmann, P., Bauer, J., Deckert, J., Hohoff, C., Kugel, H., et al. (2007). 5-HTTLPR biases amygdala activity in response to masked facial expressions in major depression. *Neuropsychopharmacology, 33*, 418–424.

Dannlowski, U., Ohrmann, P., Bauer, J., Kugel, H., Baune, B. T., Hohoff, C., et al. (2007). Serotonergic genes modulate amygdala activity in major depression. *Genes, Brain and Behavior, 6*, 672–676.

David, S. P., Murthy, N. V., Rabiner, E. A., Munafò, M. R., Johnstone, E. C., Jacob, R., et al. (2005). A functional genetic variation of the serotonin (5-HT) transporter affects 5-HT1A receptor binding in humans. *Journal of Neuroscience, 25*, 2586–2590.

Dimas, A. S., Deutsch, S., Stranger, B. E., Montgomery, S. B., Borei, C., Attar-Cohen, H., et al. (2009). Common regulatory variation impacts gene expression in a cell type-dependent manner. *Science, 325*, 1246–1250.

Dohrenwend, B. P. (2006). Inventorying stressful life events as risk factors for psychopathology: Toward resolution of the problem of intracategory variability. *Psychological Bulletin, 132*, 477–495.

Domschke, K., Braun, M., Ohrmann, P., Suslow, T., Kugel, H., Bauer, J., et al. (2006). Association of the functional -1019C/G 5-HT1A polymorphism with prefrontal cortex and amygdala activation measured with 3 T fMRI in panic disorder. *International Journal of Neuropsychopharmacology, 9*, 349–355.

Domschke, K., Stevens, S., Beck, B., Baffa, A., Hohoff, C., Deckert, J., et al. (2009). Blushing propensity in social anxiety disorder: Influence of serotonin transporter gene variation. *Journal of Neural Transmission, 116*, 663–666.

Esaki, T., Cook, M., Shimoji, K., Murphy, D. L., Sokoloff, L., & Holmes, A. (2005). Developmental disruption of serotonin transporter function impairs cerebral responses to whisker stimulation in mice. *Proceedings of the National Academy of Sciences USA, 102*, 5582–5587.

Fallgatter, A. J., Herrmann, M. J., Roemmler, J., Ehlis, A. C., Wagener, A., Heidrich, A., et al. (2004). Allelic variation of serotonin transporter function modulates the brain electrical response for error processing. *Neuropsychopharmacology, 29*, 1506–1511.

Fallgatter, A. J., Jatzke, S., Bartsch, A. J., Hamelbeck, B., & Lesch, K. P. (1999). Serotonin transporter promoter polymorphism influences topography of inhibitory motor control. *International Journal of Neuropsychopharmacology, 2*, 115–120.

Fox, E., Ridgewell, A., & Ashwin, C. (2009). Looking on the bright side: Biased attention and the human serotonin transporter gene. *Proceedings of the Royal Society of London: Series B. Biological Sciences, 276*, 1747–1751.

Fox, N. A., Nichols, K. E., Henderson, H. A., Rubin, K., Schmidt, L., Hamer, D., et al. (2005). Evidence for a gene–environment interaction in predicting behavioral inhibition in middle childhood. *Psychological Sciences and Social Sciences, 16*, 921–926.

Frayling, T. M., Timpson, N. J., Weedon, M. N., Zeggini, E., Freathy, R. M., Lindgren, C. M., et al. (2007). A common variant in the FTO gene is associated with body mass index and predisposes to childhood and adult obesity. *Science, 316*, 889–894.

Fredriksson, R., Hagglund, M., Olszewski, P. K., Stephansson, O., Jacobsson, J. A., Ojszewska, A. M., et al. (2008). The obesity gene, FTO, is of ancient origin, up-regulated during food deprivation and expressed in neurons of feeding-related nuclei of the brain. *Endocrinology, 149*, 2062–2071.

Furman, D., Hamilton, P., Joormann, J., & Gotlib, I. (in press). Altered timing of amygdala activation during sad mood elaboration as a function of 5-HTTLPR. *Social Cognitive and Affective Neuroscience.*

Furmark, T., Tillfors, M., Garpenstrand, H., Marteinsdottir, I., Langström, B., Oreland, L., et al. (2004). Serotonin transporter polymorphism related to amygdala excitability and symptom severity in patients with social phobia. *Neuroscience Letters, 362*, 189–192.

Gallinai, J., Senkowski, D., Wernicke, C., Juckel, G., Becker, I., Sander, T., et al. (2003). Allelic variants of the functional promoter polymorphism of the human serotonin transporter gene is associated with auditory cortical stimulus processing. *Neuropsychopharmacology, 28*, 530–532.

Gaspar, P., Cases, O., & Maroteaux, L. (2003). The developmental role of serotonin: News from mouse molecular genetics. *Nature Reviews Neuroscience, 4*, 1002–1012.

Gerken, T., Girard, C. A., Tung, Y. C., Webby, C. J., Saudek, V., Hewitson, K. S., et al. (2007). The obesity-associated FTO gene encodes a 2-oxoglutarate-dependent nucleic acid demethylase. *Science, 318*, 1469–1472.

Gibb, B. E., Benas, J. S., Grassia, M., & McGeary, J. (2009). Children's attentional biases and 5-HTTLPR genotype: Potential mechanisms linking mother and child depression. *Journal of Clinical Child and Adolescent Psychology, 38*, 415–426.

Gilbert, D. G., Zuo, Y., Rabinovich, N. E., Riise, H., Needham, R., & Huggenvik, J. I. (2009). Neurotransmission-related genetic polymorphisms, negative affectivity traits, and gender predict tobacco abstinence symptoms across 44 days with and without nicotine patch. *Journal of Abnormal Psychology, 118*, 322–334.

Gillespie, N. A., Whitfield, J. B., Williams, B., Heath, A. C., & Martin, N. G. (2005). The relationship between stressful life events, the serotonin transporter (5-HTTLPR) genotype and major depression. *Psychological Medicine, 35*, 101–111.

Gotlib, I. H., Joormann, J., Minor, K. L., & Hallmayer, J. (2008). HPA axis reactivity: A mechanism underlying the associations among 5-HTTLPR, stress, and depression. *Biological Psychiatry, 63*, 847–851.

Gunthert, K. C., Conner, T. S., Armeli, S., Tennen, H., Covault, J., & Kranzler, H. R. (2007). Serotonin transporter gene polymorphism (5-HTTLPR) and anxiety reactivity in daily life: A daily process approach to gene–environment interaction. *Psychosomatic Medicine, 69*, 762–768.

Hakanen, M., Raitakari, O. T., Lehtimaki, T., Peltonen, N., Pahkala, K., Sillanmaki, L., et al. (2009). FTO genotype is associated with body mass index after the age of seven years but not with energy intake or leisure-time physical activity. *Journal of Clinical Endocrinology and Metabolism, 94,* 1281–1287.

Hariri, A. R. (2009). The neurobiology of individual differences in complex behavioral traits. *Annual Review of Neuroscience, 32,* 225–247.

Hariri, A. R., Drabant, E. M., Munoz, K. E., Kolachana, B. S., Mattay, V. S., Egan, M. F., et al. (2005). A susceptibility gene for affective disorders and the response of the human amygdala. *Archives of General Psychiatry, 62,* 146–152.

Hariri, A. R., & Holmes, A. (2006). Genetics of emotional regulation: The role of the serotonin transporter in neural function. *Trends in Cognitive Science, 10,* 182–191.

Hariri, A. R., Mattay, V. S., Tessitore, A., Kolachana, B., Fera, F., Goldman, D., et al. (2002). Serotonin transporter genetic variation and the response of the human amygdala. *Science, 297,* 400–404.

Hayden, E. P., Dougherty, L. R., Maloney, B., Olino, T. M., Sheikh, H., Durbin, C. E., et al. (2008). Early-emerging cognitive vulnerability to depression and the serotonin transporter promoter region polymorphism. *Journal of Affective Disorders, 107,* 227–230.

Heinz, A., Braus, D. F., Smolka, M. N., Wrase, J., Puis, I., Hermann, D., et al. (2005). Amygdala–prefrontal coupling depends on a genetic variation of the serotonin transporter. *Nature Neuroscience, 8,* 20–21.

Heinz, A., Jones, D. W., Mazzanti, C., Goldman, D., Ragan, P., Hommer, D., et al. (2000). A relationship between serotonin transporter genotype and in vivo protein expression and alcohol neurotoxicity. *Biological Psychiatry, 47,* 643–649.

Heinz, A., Smolka, M. N., Braus, D. F., Wrase, J., Beck, A., Flor, H., et al. (2007). Serotonin transporter genotype (5-HTTLPR): Effects of neutral and undefined conditions on amygdala activation. *Biological Psychiatry, 61,* 1011–1014.

Hensch, T., Wargelius, H. L., Herold, U., Lesch, K. P., Oreland, L., & Brocke, B. (2006). Further evidence for an association of 5-HTTLPR with intensity dependence of auditory-evoked potentials. *Neuropsychopharmacology, 31,* 2047–2054.

Hoefgen, B., Schulze, T. G., Ohlraun, S., von Widdern, O., Höfeis, S., Gross, M., et al. (2005). The power of sample size and homogenous sampling: Association between the 5-HTTLPR serotonin transporter polymorphism and major depressive disorder. *Biological Psychiatry, 57,* 247–251.

Homberg, J., Olivier, J., Smits, B., Mul, J., Mudde, J., Verheul, M., et al. (2007). Characterization of the serotonin transporter knockout rat: A selective change in the functioning of the serotonergic system. *Neuroscience, 146,* 1662–1672.

Hopkins, M. R., Ettinger, A. S., Hernández-Avila, M., Schwartz, J., Téllez-Rojo, M. M., Lamadrid-Figueroa, H., et al. (2008). Variants in iron metabolism genes predict higher blood lead levels in young children. *Environmental Health Perspectives, 116,* 1261–1266.

Ioannidis, J. P., Loy, E. Y., Poulton, R., & Chia, K. S. (2009). Researching genetic versus nongenetic determinants of disease: A comparison and proposed unification. *Science Translational Medicine, 1*, 1–6.

Jacobs, N., Kenis, G., Peeters, F., Derom, C., Vlietinck, R., & van Os, J. (2006). Stress-related negative affectivity and genetically altered serotonin transporter function: Evidence of synergism in shaping risk of depression. *Archives of General Psychiatry, 63*, 989–996.

Jedema, H. P., Gianaros, P. J., Greer, P. J., Kerr, D. D., Liu, S., Higley, J. D., et al. (2010). Cognitive impact of genetic variation of the serotonin transporter in primates is associated with differences in brain morphology rather than serotonin neurotransmission. *Molecular Psychiatry, 15*, 512–522.

Jennings, K., Loder, M., Sheward, W., Pei, Q., Deacon, R., Benson, M., et al. (2006). Increased expression of the 5-HT transporter confers a low-anxiety phenotype linked to decreased 5-HT transmission. *Journal of Neuroscience, 26*, 8955–8964.

Jonsson, A., Renström, F., Lyssenko, V., Brito, E., Isomaa, B., Berglund, G., et al. (2009). Assessing the effect of interaction between an FTO variant (rs9939609) and physical activity on obesity in 15,925 Swedish and 2,511 Finnish adults. *Diabetologie, 52*, 1334–1338.

Joormann, J., Hertel, P. T., LeMoult, J., & Gotlib, I. H. (2009). Training forgetting of negative material in depression. *Journal of Abnormal Psychology, 118*, 34–43.

Kalin, N. H., Shelton, S. E., Fox, A. S., Rogers, J., Oakes, T. R., & Davidson, R. J. (2008). The serotonin transporter genotype is associated with intermediate brain phenotypes that depend on the context of eliciting stressor. *Molecular Psychiatry, 13*, 1021–1027.

Kaufman, J., Gelernter, J., Kaffman, A., Caspi, A., & Moffitt, T. E. (2010). Arguable assumptions, debatable conclusions (Letter). *Biological Psychiatry, 67*, e19–e20.

Khoury, M. J., & Wacholder, S. (2009). Invited commentary: From genomewide association studies to gene–environment-wide interaction studies: Challenges and opportunities. *American Journal of Epidemiology, 169*, 227–230.

Kim, M. J., & Whalen, P. J. (2009). The structural integrity of an amygdalaprefrontal pathway predicts trait anxiety. *Journal of Neuroscience, 29*, 11614–11618.

Kochanska, G., Philibert, R. A., & Barry, R. A. (2009). Interplay of genes and early mother and child relationship in the development of self-regulation from toddler to preschool age. *Journal of Child Psychology and Psychiatry and Allied Disciplines, 50*, 1331–1338.

Koenen, K. C., & Galea, S. (2009). Gene–environment interactions and depression (Letter). *Journal of the American Medical Association, 302*, 1859.

Kotb, M., Norrby-Teglund, A., McGeer, A., El-Sherbini, H., Dorak, S. T., Khurshid, A., et al. (2002). An immunogenetic and molecular basis for differences in outcomes of invasive group A streptococcal infections. *Nature Medicine, 8*, 1398–1404.

Krueger, R. F., Caspi, A., Moffitt, T. E., Silva, P. A., & McGee, R. (1996). Personality traits are differentially linked to mental disorders: A multitraitmultidiagnosis study of an adolescent birth cohort. *Journal of Abnormal Psychology, 105,* 299–312.

Lasky-Su, J. A., Faraone, S. V., Glatt, S. J., & Tsuang, M. T. (2005). Meta-analysis of the association between two polymorphisms in the serotonin transporter gene and affective disorders. *American Journal of Medical Genetics, 133B,* 110–115.

Lee, M., Bailer, U. F., Frank, G. K., Henry, S. E., Meltzer, C. C., Price, J. C., et al. (2005). Relationship of a 5-HT transporter functional polymorphism to 5-HT1A receptor binding in healthy women. *Molecular Psychiatry, 10,* 715–716.

Lesch, K. P. (2003). Neuroticism and serotonin: A developmental genetic perspective. In R. Plomin, J. DeFries, I. Craig, & P. McGuffin (Eds.), *Behavioral genetics in the postgenomic era.* Washington, DC: American Psychological Association.

Lesch, K. P., Bengel, D., Heils, A., Sabol, S. Z., Greenberg, B. D., Petri, S., et al. (1996). Association of anxiety-related traits with a polymorphism in the serotonin transporter gene regulatory region. *Science, 274,* 1527–1531.

Lonsdorf, T. B., Weike, A. L., Nikamo, P., Schalling, M., Hamm, A. O., & Ohman, A. (2009). Genetic gating of human fear learning and extinction: Possible implications for gene–environment interaction in anxiety disorder. *Psychological Science, 20,* 198–206.

Lotrich, F. E., & Lenze, E. (2009). Gene–environment interactions and depression (Letter). *Journal of the American Medical Association, 302,* 1860.

Martinez, F. D. (2007). Gene–environment interactions in asthma. *Proceedings of the American Thoracic Society, 4,* 26–31.

McClelland, G. H., & Judd, C. M. (1993). Statistical difficulties of detecting interactions and moderator effects. *Psychological Bulletin, 114,* 376.

Merikangas, K. R., & Risch, N. (2009). Gene–environment interactions and depression (Letter). *Journal of the American Medical Association, 302,* 1861–1862.

Miller, G. E., Chen, E., Fok, A. K., Walker, H., Um, A., Nicholls, E. F., et al. (2009). Low early-life social class leaves a biological residue manifested by decreased glucocorticoid and increased proinflammatory signaling. *Proceedings of the National Academy Sciences USA, 106,* 14716–12721.

Moffitt, T. E., Caspi, A., & Rutter, M. (2005). Strategy for investigating interactions between measured genes and measured environments. *Archives of General Psychiatry, 62,* 473–481.

Moffitt, T. E., Caspi, A., & Rutter, M. (2006). Measured gene–environment interactions in psychopathology. *Perspectives on Psychological Science, 1,* 5–27.

Monroe, S. M. (2008). Modern approaches to conceptualizing and measuring human life stress. *Annual Review of Clinical Psychology, 4,* 33–52.

Monroe, S. M., & Reid, M. W. (2008). Gene–environment interactions in depression research: Genetic polymorphisms and life-stress polyprocedures. *Psychological Science, 19,* 947–956.

Monroe, S. M., & Simons, A. D. (1991). Diathesis–stress theories in the context of life stress research: Implications for the depressive disorders. *Psychological Bulletin, 110,* 406–425.

Moonesinghe, R., Khoury, M. J., Liu, T., & Ioannidis, J. P. (2008). Required sample size and nonreplicability thresholds for heterogeneous genetic associations. *Proceedings of the National Academy of Sciences USA, 105,* 617–622.

Mueller, A., Brocke, B., Fries, E., Lesch, K. P., & Kirschbaum, C. (2010). The role of the serotonin transporter polymorphism for the endocrine stress response in newborns. *Psychoneuroendocrinology, 35,* 289–296.

Munafò, M. R., Durrant, C., Lewis, G., & Flint, J. (2009). Gene × environment interactions at the serotonin transporter locus. *Biological Psychiatry, 65,* 211–219.

Murphy, D. L., & Lesch, K. P. (2008). Targeting the murine serotonin transporter: Insights into human neurobiology. *National Review of Neuroscience, 9,* 85–96.

Murphy, D. L., Li, Q., Engel, S., Wichems, C., Andrews, A., Lesch, K. P., et al. (2001). Genetic perspectives on the serotonin transporter. *Brain Research Bulletin, 56,* 487–494.

Nicodemus, K. K., Marenco, S., Batten, A. J., Vakkalanka, R., Egan, M. F., Straub, R. E., et al. (2008). Serious obstetric complications interact with hypoxia-regulated/vascular-expression genes to influence schizophrenia risk. *Molecular Psychiatry, 13,* 873–877.

Ordovas, J., & Tai, E. S. (2008). Why study gene–enviroment interactions? *Current Opinion in Lipidology, 19,* 1 58–167.

Osinsky, R., Reuter, M., Kapper, Y., Schmitz, A., Kozyra, E., Alexander, N., et al. (2008). Variation in the serotonin transporter gene modulates selective attention to threat. *Emotion, 8,* 584–588.

Pacheco, J., Beevers, C. G., Benavides, C., McGeary, J., Stice, E., & Schnyer, D. M. (2009). Frontal–limbic white matter pathway associations with the serotonin transporter gene promoter region (5-HTTLPR) polymorphism. *Journal of Neuroscience, 29,* 6229–6233.

Parsey, R. V., Hastings, R. S., Oquendo, M. A., Hu, X., Goldman, D., Huang, Y.-y., et al. (2006). Effect of a triallelic functional polymorphism of the serotonin-transporter-linked promoter region on expression of serotonin transporter in the human brain. *American Journal of Psychiatry, 163,* 48–51.

Pauli-Pott, U., Friedl, S., Hinney, A., & Hebebrand, J. (2009). Serotonin transporter gene polymorphism (5-HTTLPR), environmental conditions, and developing negative emotionality and fear in early childhood. *Journal of Neural Transmission, 116,* 503–512.

Pezawas, L., Meyer-Lindenberg, A., Drabant, E. M., Verchinski, B. A., Munoz, K. E., Kolachana, B. S., et al. (2005). 5-HTTLPR polymorphism impacts human cingulate-amygdala interactions: A genetic susceptibility mechanism for depression. *Nature Neuroscience, 8,* 828–834.

Psychiatric GWAS Consortium Steering Committee. (2008). A framework for interpreting genome-wide association studies of psychiatric disorders. *Molecular Psychiatry, 14,* 10–17.

Rampersaud, E., Mitchell, B. D., Pollin, T. I., Fu, M., Shen, H., O'Connell, J. R., et al. (2008). Physical activity and the association of common FTO gene variants with body mass index and obesity. *Archives of Internal Medicine, 168,* 1791–1797.

Rao, H., Gillihan, S. J., Wang, J., Korczykowski, M., Sankoorikal, G. M., Kaercher, K. A., et al. (2007). Genetic variation in serotonin transporter alters resting brain function in healthy individuals. *Biological Psychiatry, 62,* 600–606.

Reimold, M., Smolka, M. N., Schumann, G., Zimmer, A., Wrase, J., Mann, K., et al. (2007). Midbrain serotonin transporter binding potential measured with [11C]DASB is affected by serotonin transporter genotype. *Journal of Neural Transmission, 114,* 635–639.

Risch, N., Herrell, R., Lehner, T., Liang, K. Y., Eaves, L., Hoh, J., et al. (2009). Interaction between the serotonin transporter gene (5-HTTLPR), stressful life events, and risk of depression: A meta-analysis. *Journal of the American Medical Association, 301,* 2462–2471.

Robins, L. N. (1978). Sturdy childhood predictors of adult antisocial behavior: Replications from longitudinal studies. *Psychological Medicine, 8,* 611–622.

Roiser, J. P., de Martino, B., Tan, G. C. Y., Kumaran, D., Seymour, B., Wood, N. W., et al. (2009). A genetically mediated bias in decision making driven by failure of amygdala control. *Journal of Neuroscience, 29,* 5985–5991.

Ross, C. J., Katzov-Eckert, H., Dube, M. P., Brooks, B., Rassekh, S. R., Barhdadi, A., et al. (2009). Genetic variants in TPMT and COMT are associated with hearing loss in children receiving cispiatin chemotherapy. *Nature Genetics, 41,* 1345–1349.

Roy, A., Hu, X. Z., Janal, M. N., & Goldman, D. (2007). Interaction between childhood trauma and serotonin transporter gene variation in suicide. *Neuropsychopharmacology, 32,* 2046–2052.

Ruiz, J. R., Labayen, I., Ortega, F. B., Legry, V., Moreno, L. A., Dallongeville, J., et al. (in press). Physical activity attenuates the effect of the FTO rs9939609 polymorphism on total and central body fat in adolescents: The HELENA Study. *Archives of Pediatrics and Adolescent Medicine.*

Rutter, M. (Ed.). (2008). *Genetic effects on environmental vulnerability to disease.* Chichester, UK: Wiley

Rutter, M. (2010). Commentary in "Cutting Edge" series of "Depression and Anxiety" gene–environment interplay. *Depression and Anxiety, 27,* 1–4.

Rutter, M., Thapar, A., & Pickles, A. (2009). Gene–environment interactions: Biologically valid pathway or artifact? *Archives of General Psychiatry, 66,* 1287–1289.

Safarinejad, M. R. (2009). Polymorphisms of the serotonin transporter gene and their relation to premature ejaculation in individuals from Iran. *Journal of Urology, 181,* 2656–2661.

Schoenbaum, G., & Shaham, Y. (2008). The role of orbitofrontal cortex in drug addiction: A review of preclinical studies. *Biological Psychiatry, 63,* 256–262.

Schwahn, C., & Grabe, H. J. (2009). Gene–environment interactions and depression [Letter]. *Journal of the American Medical Association, 302,* 1860.

Sen, S., Burmeister, M., & Ghosh, D. (2004). Meta-analysis of the association between a serotonin transporter promoter polymorphism (5-HTTLPR) and anxiety-related personality traits. *American Journal of Medical Genetics, 127B,* 85–89.

Shanahan, M. J., & Bauldry, S. (in press). Improving environmental markers in gene–environment research: Insights from life course sociology. In K. S. Kendler, S. Jaffee, & D. Romer (Eds.), *The dynamic genome and mental health: The role of genes and environments in development.* New York: Oxford University Press.

Shioe, K., Ichimiya, T., Suhara, T., Takano, A., Sudo, Y., Yasuno, F., et al. (2003). No association between genotype of the promoter region of serotonin transporter gene and serotonin transporter binding in human brain measured by PET. *Synapse, 48,* 184–188.

Smolka, M. N., Buhler, M., Schumann, G., Klein, S., Hu, X. Z., Moayer, M., et al. (2007). Gene–gene effects on central processing of aversive stimuli. *Molecular Psychiatry, 12,* 307–317.

Spinelli, S., Schwandt, M., Lindell, S., Newman, T. K., Heilig, M., Suomi, S. J., et al. (2007). Association between the recombinant human serotonin transporter linked promoter region polymorphism and behavior in rhesus macaques during a separation paradigm. *Developmental Psychopathology, 19,* 977–987.

Stein, M. B., Schork, N. J., & Gelernter, J. (2008). Gene-by-environment (serotonin transporter and childhood maltreatment) interaction for anxiety sensitivity, an intermediate phenotype for anxiety disorders. *Neuropsychopharmacology, 33,* 312–319.

Strange, B. A., Kroes, M. C., Roiser, J. P., Tan, G. C., & Dolan, R. J. (2008). Emotion-induced retrograde amnesia is determined by a 5-HTT genetic polymorphism. *Journal of Neuroscience, 28,* 7036–7039.

Strauss, M. E., & Smith, G. T. (2009). Construct validity: Advances in theory and methodology. *Annual Review of Clinical Psychology, 5,* 1–25.

Strobel, A., Debener, S., Schmidt, D., Hünnerkopf, R., Lesch, K. P., & Brocke, B. (2003). Allelic variation in serotonin transporter function associated with the intensity dependence of the auditory evoked potential. *American Journal of Medical Genetics, 118B,* 41–47.

Torres, G., & Amara, S. (2007). Glutamate and monoamine transporter: New visions of form and function. *Current Opinion in Neurobiology, 17,* 8955–8964.

Uher, R., & McGuffin, P. (2008). The moderation by the serotonin transporter gene of environmental adversity in the aetiology of mental illness: Review and methodological analysis. *Molecular Psychiatry, 13,* 131–146.

Uher, R., & McGuffin, P. (2010). The moderation by the serotonin transporter gene of environmental adversity in the aetiology of mental illness: 2009 update. *Molecular Psychiatry, 15,* 18–22.

van Os, J., & Rutten, B. P. (2009). Gene–environment-wide interaction studies in psychiatry. *American Journal of Psychiatry, 166,* 964–966.

Vandenbroucke, J. P. (2008). Observational research, randomised trials, and two views of medical science. *PLoS Med, 5,* e67.

Verona, E., Joiner, T. E., Johnson, F., & Bender, T. W. (2006). Gender specific gene–environment interactions on laboratory-assessed aggression. *Biological Psychology, 71,* 33–41.

Vimaleswaran, K. S., Li, S., Zhao, J. H., Luan, J., Bingham, S. A., Khaw, K. T., et al. (2009). Physical activity attenuates the body mass index-increasing influence of genetic variation in the FTO gene. *American Journal of Clinical Nutrition, 90*, 425–428.

Viviani, R., Sim, E. J., Lo, H., Beschoner, P., Osterfeld, N., Maier, C., et al. (2010). Baseline brain perfusion and the serotonin transporter promoter polymorphism. *Biological Psychiatry, 67*, 317–322.

Wardle, J., Carnell, S., Haworth, C. M., Farooqi, I. S., O'Rahilly, S., & Piomin, R. (2008). Obesity associated genetic variation in RO is associated with diminished satiety. *Journal of Clinical Endocrinology and Metabolism, 93*, 3640–3643.

Watson, D., & Clark, L. A. (1984). Negative affectivity: The disposition to experience aversive emotional states. *Psychological Bulletin, 96*, 465–490.

Watson, K., Ghodasra, J., & Piatt, M. (2009). Serotonin transporter genotype modulates social reward and punishment in rhesus macaques. *PLoS One, 4*, e4156.

Way, B., & Taylor, S. (2010). The serotonin transporter promoter polymorphism (5-HTTLPR) is associated with cortisol response to psychosocial stress. *Biological Psychiatry, 67*, 487–492.

Whalen, P. J., & Phelps, E. A. (Eds.). (2009). *The human amygdala*. New York: Guilford Press.

Williams, L. M., Gatt, J. M., Schofield, P. R., Olivieri, G., Peduto, A., & Gordon, E. (2009). "Negativity bias" in risk for depression and anxiety: Brain–body fear circuitry correlates 5-HTT-LPR and early life stress. *NeuroImage, 47*, 804–814.

Xie, P., Kranzler, H., Poling, J., Stein, M., Anton, R., Brady, K., et al. (2009). The interactive effect of stressful life events and serotonin transporter 5-HTTLPR genotype on PTSD diagnosis in two independent populations. *Archives of General Psychiatry, 66*, 1201–1209.

Young, K. A., Holcomb, L. A., Bonkale, W. L., Hicks, P. B., Yazdani, U., & German, D. C. (2007). 6HTTLPR polymorphism and enlargement of the pulvinar: Unlocking the backdoor to the limbic system. *Biological Psychiatry, 61*, 813–818.

CHAPTER 3

Neurobiological Mechanisms Supporting Gene–Environment Interaction Effects

Ahmad R. Hariri

Individual differences in trait affect, personality, and temperament are critical in shaping complex human behaviors, successfully navigating social interactions, and overcoming challenges from our ever-changing environments. Such individual differences may also serve as important predictors of vulnerability to developmental psychopathology, including depression, anxiety, and addiction, especially upon exposure to environmental adversity. Accordingly, identifying the neural mechanisms that give rise to trait individual differences affords a unique opportunity to develop a deeper understanding of complex human behaviors as well as related disease liability and treatment. Having established multiple modal neural processes supporting specific aspects of complex behavioral processes, human neuroimaging studies, especially those employing blood oxygen level–dependent (BOLD) functional magnetic resonance imaging (fMRI), have now begun to reveal the neural substrates of interindividual variability in these and related constructs. Recent studies have established that BOLD fMRI measures represent temporally stable and reliable indices of brain function. Thus, much like their behavioral counterparts, patterns of brain activation represent enduring, trait-like phenomenon, which in and of themselves may serve as important markers of individual differences.

As neuroimaging studies continue to illustrate the predictive relation between regional brain activation and trait-like behaviors (e.g., increased amygdala reactivity predicts trait anxiety), an important next step is to identify the underlying mechanisms driving variability in brain circuit function. Using common functional genetic variation to model variability in brain chemistry is one emerging approach to mapping individual differences in behaviorally relevant brain function. Identifying links between genes and brain function is important not only for establishing a mechanistic foundation for individual differences in behavior but also for explicating the pathways through which gene–environment interactions (G × E) shape risk for psychopathology.

This chapter describes the mapping of behaviorally relevant neural processes and how genetically driven differences in these processes may support interactions between genes and environments that shape variability in behavior and risk for psychopathology. The potential of integrating measures of genes, brain, and behavior is highlighted by a series of studies whose collective results demonstrate that a common functional polymorphism in the human serotonin transporter gene (*SLC6A4*) biases the processing of environmental threat within a distributed corticolimbic neural circuitry supporting trait anxiety and stress reactivity. The mapping of these links highlights a specific neural mechanism through which this polymorphism may increase risk for psychopathology upon exposure to environmental stressors—that is, G × E.

ANXIETY, AMYGDALA REACTIVITY, AND SEROTONIN

The experience of anxiety is commonplace among both human and nonhuman primates as well as other highly social animals. In the context of social interactions, especially within delimited social hierarchies consisting of dominant and subordinate individuals, anxiety serves to shape appropriate and often opposing responses to precipitating events such as competition for limited resources (e.g., food, water, reproductive partners). Anxiety is a direct response to threat, and chronic anxiety may be a response to chronic or severe threat. However, sensitivity to potentially threatening social cues (e.g., affective facial expressions) varies considerably between individuals and represents a core component of commonly employed constructs representing trait anxiety. Individuals with high trait anxiety exhibit a propensity to more frequently appraise situations as more threatening than do others and are generally more sensitive to social cues, including those representing both explicit and implicit threat (e.g., angry and fearful facial expressions). In turn, these individuals are at increased risk for developing psychopathology characterized by abnormal social and emotional behaviors such as depression and often precipitated by exposure to chronic or severe stressors (Kendler, Kuhn, & Prescott, 2004). Examining the neural correlates of individual variability in dispositional temperament such as trait anxiety represents an important step in understanding key socioemotional behaviors and an effective means of elucidating processes mediating $G \times E$.

Converging evidence from animal and human studies clearly demonstrates that the amygdala is centrally involved in mediating both physiological (e.g., autonomic reactivity) and behavioral (e.g., reallocation of attentional resources) effects that allow an individual to respond adaptively to varied environmental and social challenges (LeDoux, 2000). A large corpus of human neuroimaging research reveals that the amygdala is robustly engaged by varied biologically salient environmental stimuli, most notably emotional facial expressions, especially those representing threat. However, individuals differ appreciably in the magnitude of amygdala activation on exposure to emotionally expressive facial expressions, and these individual differences appear to be stable over time (Johnstone et al., 2005; Manuck, Brown, Forbes, & Hariri, 2007).

Recent neuroimaging studies have reported positive relations between the magnitude of amygdala reactivity to affective, especially threatening, stimuli and interindividual variability in indices of trait (Dickie & Armony, 2008; Etkin et al., 2004; Haas, Omura, Constable, & Canli, 2007; Killgore & Yurgelun-Todd, 2005; Most, Chun, Johnson, & Kiehl, 2006; Ray et al., 2005) and also state (Bishop, Duncan, & Lawrence, 2004; Somerville, Kim, Johnstone, Alexander, & Whalen, 2004) anxiety. In one study, Stein et al. report that high trait anxiety is associated with greater amygdala reactivity not only to angry and fearful but also to happy facial expressions (Stein, Simmons, Feinstein, & Paulus, 2007). Consistent with this pattern of normal variability, various mood and anxiety disorders (e.g., unipolar and bipolar depression, generalized anxiety disorder, social phobia) have been linked with greater amygdala responses to facial expressions depicting fear and anger, as well as sadness and disgust, and, more variably, to emotionally neutral facial expressions (Cooney, Atlas, Joormann, Eugene, & Gotlib, 2006; Evans et al., 2008; Phan, Fitzgerald, Nathan, & Tancer, 2006; Phillips, Drevets, Rauch, & Lane, 2003; Stein, Goldin, Sareen, Zorrilla, & Brown, 2002; Whalen, Shin, Somerville, McLean, & Kim, 2002). Such findings demonstrate that anxiety-related psychopathology is associated with a heightened amygdala response to diverse affective stimuli. Furthermore, in the absence of such disorders, variability in the magnitude of threat-related amygdala reactivity is an important predictor of individual differences in trait anxiety.

Having first established a predictive link between amygdala reactivity and trait anxiety, factors that drive such behaviorally relevant variability in brain function can now be identified in the broader context of detailing the biological mechanisms mediating individual differences in temperamental anxiety. Converging preclinical and clinical evidence indicates that amygdala functioning is sensitive to the effects of central serotonin (Sadikot & Parent, 1990), whose principle forebrain innervation is provided by the midbrain dorsal raphe nuclei (DRN). Available data from animal studies indicate that relative increases in local serotonin (5-HT) result in potentiation of amygdala activation and associated behavioral phenomenon, such as fear conditioning (Amat, Matus-Amat, Watkins, & Maier, 1998; Amat et al., 2004; Burghardt, Bush, McEwen, & LeDoux, in press; Burghardt, Sullivan, McEwen, Gorman, & LeDoux, 2004; Forster et al., 2006; Maier & Watkins, 2005). Recent neuroimaging studies using multimodal positron emission tomography (PET)/fMRI or pharmacological challenge BOLD fMRI have provided direct evidence for parallel effects of 5-HT in humans. Specifically, *in vivo* PET has revealed that decreased endogenous capacity for local 5-HT reuptake (Rhodes et al., 2007) or negative feedback autoregulation of 5-HT neurons (Fisher et al., 2009) is associated with relatively increased amygdala reactivity. Acute IV administration of a selective serotonin reuptake inhibitor, which reduces capacity for 5-HT reuptake, during BOLD fMRI is likewise associated not only with increased amygdala reactivity but also with decreased habituation of amygdala reactivity over time (Bigos et al., 2008). These data clearly indicate that variability in the regulation of 5-HT signaling is an important source of individual differences in amygdala reactivity.

A NEURAL MECHANISM FOR GENE–ENVIRONMENT EFFECTS ON DEPRESSION

Since its identification in the mid-1990s the serotonin transporter (*5-HTT*) gene–linked polymorphic region (*5-HTTLPR*) has been the focus of extensive and often contentious research. Although the exact molecular mechanism remains unclear and there are relatively few replicated associations between the *5-HTTLPR* and myriad behavioral and clinical measures, the *5-HTTLPR* short allele, which presumably results in relatively increased 5-HT signaling, has been consistently linked to risk for psychopathology, especially depression, in interaction with environmental stress (for a review, see Caspi, Hariri, Holmes, Uher, & Moffitt, Chapter 2, this volume). In 2002, a synergy emerged between ongoing research in human affective neuroscience and that focused on explicating the biological and behavioral impact of the *5-HTTLPR* gene. Specifically, fMRI was used to establish a clear neural systems-level signature of the *5-HTTLPR* gene: relatively exaggerated threat-related amygdala reactivity in carriers of the short allele (Hariri et al., 2002). This initial finding has since been replicated in numerous independent samples of both healthy volunteers and psychiatric patients using a multitude of threatening stimuli and neuroimaging modalities. Meta-analysis of all available findings in 2008 confirmed a significant association between the *5-HTTLPR* short allele and increased amygdala activation (Munafò, Brown, & Hariri, 2008). More remarkable than the robustness and consistency of this association, which is already one of the strongest in the literature, is the mapping of the *5-HTTLPR* gene onto a clear bias in the brain's canonical circuitry for marshalling resources in response to environmental threat and stress. The bias in threat-related amygdala reactivity associated with the *5-HTTLPR* short allele is positioned to drive the polymorphisms associations with altered mood and risk for affective disorders, especially in interaction with exposure to environmental stressors and trauma.

The mapping of amygdala reactivity onto individual differences in anxiety is a direct reflection of a network of afferent and efferent connections that uniquely position this subcortical structure to transduce a convergence of multimodal sensory inputs into an orchestrated and often reflexive behavioral and physiological response to environmental threat and stress. Recent human neuroimaging research has revealed that the *5-HTTLPR* gene impacts the structure and function of multiple brain regions within this network in a manner consistent with the increased threat-related amygdala reactivity associated with the short allele. The *5-HTTLPR* short allele has been associated with altered functional coupling (as indexed by correlated fMRI signal strength) between the amygdala and regions of the medial prefrontal cortex (Heinz et al., 2005; Pezawas et al., 2005). These medial prefrontal regions are critical for the proper integration of amygdala-mediated arousal and subsequent down-regulation of amygdala, reactivity as well as the extinction of conditioned fear responses that are dependent on amygdala circuitry. The pattern of *5-HTTLPR*-associated differences in the functional dynamics of the amygdala and medial prefrontal cortex are echoed in structural measures within this same network. Specifically, the *5-HTTLPR* short allele has been associated with relatively decreased gray matter volume in the amygdala and medial prefrontal cortex (Canli et al., 2005; Pezawas et al., 2005). Most recently, the *5-HTTLPR* short allele was associated with alterations in the microstructure of the uncinate fasciculus, the white matter fiber system providing the majority of afferent and efferent connections between the amygdala and the medial prefrontal cortex (Pacheco et al., 2009). In addition, post-mortem tissue analyses have associated the *5-HTTLPR* short allele with relative enlargement of the pulvinar, the principal thalamic nucleus for relaying visual information to higher cortical and subcortical brain regions (Young et al., 2007).

The collection of findings reviewed above suggest that the consistent pattern of relatively increased amygdala reactivity associated with the *5-HTTLPR* short allele is likely grounded in pronounced and discrete alterations in both the structural and functional architecture of a distributed network of brain regions involved not only in communicating information about the environment to the amygdala but also in relaying signals between the amygdala and higher order regulatory cortical circuits in the medial prefrontal cortex. This putative mechanism is further underscored by the significant role *5-HTTLPR* signaling play in the general development and function of this extended neural network (for a review, see Hariri & Holmes, 2006). A growing group of studies have begun to document effects of the *5-HTTLPR* gene on intermediate behavioral and physiological processes that map in an impressively consistent fashion onto these alterations in brain structure and function. For example, the *5-HTTLPR* short allele has been associated with increased hypothalamus–pituitary–adrenal (HPA) axis reactivity (Alexander et al., 2009; Chen, Joormann, Hallmayer, & Gotlib, 2009; Goodyer, Bacon, Ban, Croudace, & Herbert, 2009; Gotlib, Joormann, Minor, & Hallmayer, 2008; Mueller, Brocke, Fries, Lesch, & Kirschbaum, 2010; Wust et al., 2009), greater difficulty disengaging from or preferential attention toward threat-related stimuli (Beevers, Ellis, Wells, & McGeary, 2010; Beevers, Gibb, McGeary, & Miller, 2007; Beevers, Wells, Ellis, & McGeary, 2009; Fox et al., 2005; Gibb, Benas, Grassia, & McGeary, 2009; Osinsky et al., 2008; Perez-Edgar et al., 2010), emotion-induced retrograde amnesia (Strange, Kroes, Roiser, Tan, & Dolan, 2008), and even greater levels of social blushing (Domschke et al., 2009; Fox et al., 2005). Although this literature is not without inconsistencies (e.g., some reported associations have been sex-specific and others have not been replicated), it does suggest that the clear effects of the *5-HTTLPR* short allele on the brain's neural circuitry for responding to environmental threat and stress likely translate to a myriad of biases in both behavioral and physiological processes which may, in turn, shape individual risk trajectories for psychosocial dysfunction such as depression upon exposure to acute trauma or chronic stressors. Multiple components of this ongoing research were highlighted in a recent study reporting overlapping increases in threat-related amygdala and medial prefrontal cortical activation as well as heart rate and startle amplitude in *5-HTTLPR* short allele carriers also exhibiting a self-reported sensitivity to perceived danger in the environment (Williams et al., 2009).

LOOKING FORWARD

An important consideration for the future of this research is the need to conduct large-scale prospective studies beginning in childhood to determine any developmental shifts in neurogenetic pathways mediating individual differences in behavior as well as their predictive utility in identifying neuropsychiatric disease risk as a function of environmental or other stressors. All of the studies described above and most of the studies available in the literature as a whole have been conducted in adults carefully screened for the absence of psychopathology. Because of this, these findings identify mechanisms contributing to variability in the normative range of behavior only. Predictive utility is ideally tested through prospective studies beginning with premorbid populations that account for the moderating effects of environmental stress in the emergence of clinical disorder over time (Caspi & Moffitt, 2006; Viding, Williamson, & Hariri, 2006).

There also is tremendous potential in developing large databases (again preferably thousands of subjects) with detailed measures of behavioral traits, neuroimaging-based measures of multiple brain circuitries, and extensive genotyping. One of the most exciting applications of molecular genetics is in identifying novel biological pathways contributing to the emergence of complex traits (Gibson & Goldstein, 2007; McCarthy et al., 2008). The continued refinement of a detailed map of sequence variation across the entire human genome (i.e., single-nucleotide polymorphisms that "tag" every gene) and production of technologies supporting efficient high-throughput identification of such variation in individuals have dramatically accelerated the discovery of genes involved in the emergence of complex disease processes (Fellay et al., 2007; Link et al., 2008), as well as normal variability in continuous traits (Lettre et al., 2008). Many of the genes identified in such studies have illuminated novel pathways not previously implicated in these processes or traits, spurring intensive efforts to understand the potential biological effects of the proteins produced by these genes. As such, these "genomewide" screens represent an opportunity to leap forward beyond the available pool of candidate molecules and pathways in parsing the mechanisms of complex biological processes. In addition, these efforts may lead to improving our understanding of neurobiological pathways mediating G × E effects on risk for psychopathology.

REFERENCES

Alexander, N., Kuepper, Y., Schmitz, A., Osinsky, R., Kozyra, E., & Hennig, J. (2009). Gene–environment interactions predict cortisol responses after acute stress: Implications for the etiology of depression. *Psychoneuroendocrinology, 34*(9), 1294–1303.

Amat, J., Matus-Amat, P., Watkins, L. R., & Maier, S. F. (1998). Escapable and inescapable stress differentially alter extracellular levels of 5-HT in the basolateral amygdala of the rat. *Brain Research, 812*(1–2), 113–120.

Amat, J., Tamblyn, J. P., Paul, E. D., Bland, S. T., Amat, P., Foster, A. C., et al. (2004). Microinjection of urocortin 2 into the dorsal raphe nucleus activates serotonergic neurons and increases extracellular serotonin in the basolateral amygdala. *Neuroscience, 129*(3), 509–519.

Beevers, C. G., Ellis, A. J., Wells, T. T., & McGeary, J. E. (2010). Serotonin transporter gene promoter region polymorphism and selective processing of emotional images. *Biological Psychology, 83*, 260–265.

Beevers, C. G., Gibb, B. E., McGeary, J. E., & Miller, I. W. (2007). Serotonin transporter genetic variation and biased attention for emotional word stimuli among psychiatric inpatients. *Journal of Abnormal Psychology, 116*(1), 208–212.

Beevers, C. G., Wells, T. T., Ellis, A. J., & McGeary, J. E. (2009). Association of the serotonin transporter gene promoter region (5-HTTLPR) polymorphism with biased attention for emotional stimuli. *Journal of Abnormal Psychology, 118*(3), 670–681.

Bigos, K. L., Pollock, B. G., Aizenstein, H., Fisher, P. M., Bies, R. R., & Hariri, A. R. (2008). Acute 5-HT reuptake blockade potentiates human amygdala reactivity. *Neuropsychopharmacology, 33*(13), 3221–3225.

Bishop, S. J., Duncan, J., & Lawrence, A. D. (2004). State anxiety modulation of the amygdala response to unattended threat-related stimuli. *Journal of Neuroscience, 24*(46), 10364–10368.

Burghardt, N. S., Bush, D. E. A., McEwen, B. S., & LeDoux, J. E. (2007). Acute selective serotonin reuptake inhibitors increase conditioned fear expression: Blockade with a 5-HT2C receptor antagonist. *Biological Psychiatry, 62*(10), 1111–1118.

Burghardt, N. S., Sullivan, G. M., McEwen, B. S., Gorman, J. M., & LeDoux, J. E. (2004). The selective serotonin reuptake inhibitor citalopram increases fear after acute treatment but reduces fear with chronic treatment: A comparison with tianeptine. *Biological Psychiatry, 55*(12), 1171–1178.

Canli, T., Omura, K., Haas, B. W., Fallgatter, A., Constable, R. T., & Lesch, K. P. (2005). Beyond affect: A role for genetic variation of the serotonin transporter in neural activation during a cognitive attention task. *Proceedings of the National Academy of Sciences of the USA, 102*(34), 12224–12229.

Caspi, A., & Moffitt, T. E. (2006). Gene–environment interactions in psychiatry: Joining forces with neuroscience. *Nature Reviews: Neuroscience, 7*(7), 583–590.

Chen, M. C., Joormann, J., Hallmayer, J., & Gotlib, I. H. (2009). Serotonin transporter polymorphism predicts waking cortisol in young girls. *Psychoneuroendocrinology, 34*(5), 681–686.

Cooney, R. E., Atlas, L. Y., Joormann, J., Eugene, F., & Gotlib, I. H. (2006).

Amygdala activation in the processing of neutral faces in social anxiety disorder: Is neutral really neutral? *Psychiatry Research, 148*(1), 55–59.

Dickie, E. W., & Armony, J. L. (2008). Amygdala responses to unattended fearful faces: Interaction between sex and trait anxiety. *Psychiatry Research, 162*(1), 51–57.

Domschke, K., Stevens, S., Beck, B., Baffa, A., Hohoff, C., Deckert, J., et al. (2009). Blushing propensity in social anxiety disorder: Influence of serotonin transporter gene variation. *Journal of Neural Transmission, 116*(6), 663–666.

Etkin, A., Klemenhagen, K. C., Dudman, J. T., Rogan, M. T., Hen, R., Kandel, E. R., et al. (2004). Individual differences in trait anxiety predict the response of the basolateral amygdala to unconsciously processed fearful faces. *Neuron, 44*(6), 1043–1055.

Evans, K. C., Wright, C. I., Wedig, M. M., Gold, A. L., Pollack, M. H., & Rauch, S. L. (2008). A functional MRI study of amygdala responses to angry schematic faces in social anxiety disorder. *Depression and Anxiety, 25*(6), 496–505.

Fellay, J., Shianna, K. V., Ge, D., Colombo, S., Ledergerber, B., Weale, M., et al. (2007). A whole-genome association study of major determinants for host control of HIV-1. *Science, 317*, 944–947.

Fisher, P. M., Meltzer, C. C., Price, J. C., Coleman, R. L., Ziolko, S. K., Becker, C., et al. (2009). Medial prefrontal cortex 5-HT(2A) density is correlated with amygdala reactivity, response habituation, and functional coupling. *Cerebral Cortex, 19*(11), 2499–2507.

Forster, G. L., Feng, N., Watt, M. J., Korzan, W. J., Mouw, N. J., Summers, C. H., et al. (2006). Corticotropin-releasing factor in the dorsal raphe elicits temporally distinct serotonergic responses in the limbic system in relation to fear behavior. *Neuroscience, 141*(2), 1047–1055.

Fox, N. A., Nichols, K. E., Henderson, H. A., Rubin, K., Schmidt, L., Hamer, D., et al. (2005). Evidence for a gene–environment interaction in predicting behavioral inhibition in middle childhood. *Psychological Science, 16*(12), 921–926.

Gibb, B. E., Benas, J. S., Grassia, M., & McGeary, J. (2009). Children's attentional biases and 5-HTTLPR genotype: Potential mechanisms linking mother and child depression. *Journal of Clinical Child and Adolescent Psychology, 38*(3), 415–426.

Gibson, G., & Goldstein, D. B. (2007). Human genetics: The hidden text of genome-wide associations. *Current Biology, 17*(21), R929–R932.

Goodyer, I. M., Bacon, A., Ban, M., Croudace, T., & Herbert, J. (2009). Serotonin transporter genotype, morning cortisol and subsequent depression in adolescents. *British Journal of Psychiatry, 195*(1), 39–45.

Gotlib, I. H., Joormann, J., Minor, K. L., & Hallmayer, J. (2008). HPA axis reactivity: A mechanism underlying the associations among 5-HTTLPR, stress, and depression. *Biological Psychiatry, 63*(9), 847–851.

Haas, B. W., Omura, K., Constable, R. T., & Canli, T. (2007). Emotional conflict and neuroticism: Personality-dependent activation in the amygdala and subgenual anterior cingulate. *Behavioral Neuroscience, 121*(2), 249–256.

Hariri, A. R., & Holmes, A. (2006). Genetics of emotional regulation: The role of the serotonin transporter in neural function. *Trends in Cognitive Science,* *10*(4), 182–191.

Hariri, A. R., Mattay, V. S., Tessitore, A., Kolachana, B., Fera, F., Goldman, D., et al. (2002). Serotonin transporter genetic variation and the response of the human amygdala. *Science, 297,* 400–403.

Heinz, A., Braus, D. F., Smolka, M. N., Wrase, J., Puls, I., Hermann, D., et al. (2005). Amygdala–prefrontal coupling depends on a genetic variation of the serotonin transporter. *Nature Neuroscience, 8*(1), 20–21.

Johnstone, T., Somerville, L. H., Alexander, A. L., Oakes, T. R., Davidson, R. J., Kalin, N. H., et al. (2005). Stability of amygdala BOLD response to fearful faces over multiple scan sessions. *NeuroImage, 25*(4), 1112–1123.

Kendler, K. S., Kuhn, J., & Prescott, C. A. (2004). The interrelationship of neuroticism, sex, and stressful life events in the prediction of episodes of major depression. *American Journal of Psychiatry, 161*(4), 631–636.

Killgore, W. D., & Yurgelun-Todd, D. A. (2005). Social anxiety predicts amygdala activation in adolescents viewing fearful faces. *NeuroReport, 16*(15), 1671–1675.

LeDoux, J. E. (2000). Emotion circuits in the brain. *Annual Review of Neuroscience, 23,* 155–184.

Lettre, G., Jackson, A. U., Gieger, C., Schumacher, F. R., Berndt, S. I., Sanna, S., et al. (2008). Identification of ten loci associated with height highlights new biological pathways in human growth. *Nature Genetics, 40*(5), 584–591.

Link, E., Parish, S., Armitage, J., Bowman, L., Heath, S., Matsuda, F., et al. (2008). SLCO1B1 variants and statin-induced myopathy—a genomewide study. *New England Journal of Medicine, 359*(8), 789–799.

Maier, S. F., & Watkins, L. R. (2005). Stressor controllability and learned helplessness: The roles of the dorsal raphe nucleus, serotonin, and corticotropin-releasing factor. *Neuroscience and Biobehavioral Reviews, 29*(4–5), 829–841.

Manuck, S. B., Brown, S. M., Forbes, E. E., & Hariri, A. R. (2007). Temporal stability of individual differences in amygdala reactivity. *American Journal of Psychiatry, 164*(10), 1613–1614.

McCarthy, M. I., Abecasis, G. R., Cardon, L. R., Goldstein, D. B., Little, J., Ioannidis, J. P., et al. (2008). Genome-wide association studies for complex traits: Consensus, uncertainty and challenges. *Nature Reviews: Genetics, 9*(5), 356–369.

Most, S. B., Chun, M. M., Johnson, M. R., & Kiehl, K. A. (2006). Attentional modulation of the amygdala varies with personality. *NeuroImage, 31*(2), 934–944.

Mueller, A., Brocke, B., Fries, E., Lesch, K. P., & Kirschbaum, C. (2010). The role of the serotonin transporter polymorphism for the endocrine stress response in newborns. *Psychoneuroendocrinology, 35*(2), 289–296.

Munafò, M. R., Brown, S. M., & Hariri, A. R. (2008). Serotonin transporter (5-HTTLPR) genotype and amygdala activation: A meta-analysis. *Biological Psychiatry, 63*(9), 852–857.

Osinsky, R., Reuter, M., Kupper, Y., Schmitz, A., Kozyra, E., Alexander, N., et al. (2008). Variation in the serotonin transporter gene modulates selective attention to threat. *Emotion, 8*(4), 584–588.

Pacheco, J., Beevers, C. G., Benavides, C., McGeary, J., Stice, E., & Schnyer, D. M. (2009). Frontal–limbic white matter pathway associations with the serotonin transporter gene promoter region (5-HTTLPR) polymorphism. *Journal of Neuroscience, 29*(19), 6229–6233.

Perez-Edgar, K., Bar-Haim, Y., McDermott, J. M., Gorodetsky, E., Hodgkinson, C. A., Goldman, D., et al. (2010). Variations in the serotonin-transporter gene are associated with attention bias patterns to positive and negative emotion faces. *Biological Psychology, 83*(3), 269–271.

Pezawas, L., Meyer-Lindenberg, A., Drabant, E. M., Verchinski, B. A., Munoz, K. E., Kolachana, B. S., et al. (2005). 5-HTTLPR polymorphism impacts human cingulate–amygdala interactions: A genetic susceptibility mechanism for depression. *Nature Neuroscience, 8*(6), 828–834.

Phan, K. L., Fitzgerald, D. A., Nathan, P. J., & Tancer, M. E. (2006). Association between amygdala hyperactivity to harsh faces and severity of social anxiety in generalized social phobia. *Biological Psychiatry, 59*(5), 424–429.

Phillips, M. L., Drevets, W. C., Rauch, S. L., & Lane, R. (2003). Neurobiology of emotion perception, II: Implications for major psychiatric disorders. *Biological Psychiatry, 54*(5), 515–528.

Ray, R. D., Ochsner, K. N., Cooper, J. C., Robertson, E. R., Gabrieli, J. D., & Gross, J. J. (2005). Individual differences in trait rumination and the neural systems supporting cognitive reappraisal. *Cognitive, Affective, and Behavioral Neuroscience, 5*(2), 156–168.

Rhodes, R. A., Murthy, N. V., Dresner, M. A., Selvaraj, S., Stavrakakis, N., Babar, S., et al. (2007). Human 5-HT transporter availability predicts amygdala reactivity in vivo. *Journal of Neuroscience, 27*(34), 9233–9237.

Sadikot, A. F., & Parent, A. (1990). The monoaminergic innervation of the amygdala in the squirrel monkey: An immunohistochemical study. *Neuroscience, 36*(2), 431–447.

Somerville, L. H., Kim, H., Johnstone, T., Alexander, A. L., & Whalen, P. J. (2004). Human amygdala responses during presentation of happy and neutral faces: Correlations with state anxiety. *Biological Psychiatry, 55*(9), 897–903.

Stein, M. B., Goldin, P. R., Sareen, J., Zorrilla, L. T., & Brown, G. G. (2002). Increased amygdala activation to angry and contemptuous faces in generalized social phobia. *Archives of General Psychiatry, 59*(11), 1027–1034.

Stein, M. B., Simmons, A. N., Feinstein, J. S., & Paulus, M. P. (2007). Increased amygdala and insula activation during emotion processing in anxiety-prone subjects. *American Journal of Psychiatry, 164*(2), 318–327.

Strange, B. A., Kroes, M. C., Roiser, J. P., Tan, G. C., & Dolan, R. J. (2008). Emotion-induced retrograde amnesia is determined by a 5-HTT genetic polymorphism. *Journal of Neuroscience, 28*(28), 7036–7039.

Viding, E., Williamson, D. E., & Hariri, A. R. (2006). Developmental imaging genetics: Challenges and promises for translational research. *Development and Psychopathology, 18*(3), 877–892.

Whalen, P. J., Shin, L. M., Somerville, L. H., McLean, A. A., & Kim, H. (2002). Functional neuroimaging studies of the amygdala in depression. *Seminars on Clinical Neuropsychiatry, 7*(4), 234–242.

Williams, L. M., Gatt, J. M., Schofield, P. R., Olivieri, G., Peduto, A., & Gordon, E. (2009). "Negativity bias" in risk for depression and anxiety: Brain–body fear circuitry correlates, 5-HTT-LPR and early life stress. *NeuroImage, 47*(3), 804–814.

Wust, S., Kumsta, R., Treutlein, J., Frank, J., Entringer, S., Schulze, T. G., et al. (2009). Sex-specific association between the 5-HTT gene-linked polymorphic region and basal cortisol secretion. *Psychoneuroendocrinology, 34*(7), 972–982.

Young, K. A., Holcomb, L. A., Bonkale, W. L., Hicks, P. B., Yazdani, U., & German, D. C. (2007). 5HTTLPR polymorphism and enlargement of the pulvinar: Unlocking the backdoor to the limbic system. *Biological Psychiatry, 61*(6), 813–818.

CHAPTER 4

Neurogenetic Mechanisms of Gene–Environment Interactions

Andreas Meyer-Lindenberg

Severe neuropsychiatric disorders such as schizophrenia and autism seem, on first view, to be largely the domain of genetic risk factors. The *heritability*, that is, that proportion of disease liability that is ascribed to genetic factors, is estimated from twin studies to be in the range of around 80%. However, heritability estimates, derived from genetic epidemiological studies such as these, may not model the contribution of the gene–environment interaction (G × E) effect correctly, largely because it is often not feasible to include measures of environmental risk in the study, which precludes their quantification. Simulation work (van Os & Poulton, 2008) shows that under a range of assumptions, interactions of genes with the environment may in fact make up a considerable proportion of the risk proportion ascribed to genetics—in other words, genetic risk factors that interact with the environment, although largely uncharacterized, certainly form an important research frontier.

In this chapter, we pursue a translational genetic approach toward characterizing mechanisms of G × E, studying genetic risk factors that have been shown to interact with environmental risk on the level of categorical disease categories. These genetic risk variants and environmental risk factors will be studied in human brain. In other words, we will not ask whether a given genetic variant or environmental risk factor impacts, by itself, on disease risk—this information will be taken from genetic epidemiology; rather, we will ask how a given genetic risk factor or environmental stressor acts on human brain, in an attempt to elucidate neuromechanisms mediating genetic risk in interaction with the environment. We will largely focus on risk for schizophrenia, a paradigmatic disease with high heritability.

A convenient starting point into an inquiry into genetic mechanisms in schizophrenia is afforded by asking which brain abnormalities in schizophrenia are known to be pronounced and have evidence for heritability. In brain structure, reductions in volume have been consistently observed in lateral and medial temporal lobe as well as in dorsolateral prefrontal cortex (DLPFC) (Honea et al., 2007). However, that by itself does not imply that this abnormality is heritable. In a recent study, we examined cortical thickness in patients with schizophrenia, their first-degree relatives, who share 50% of genetic risk, and in a large sample of controls (Goldman et al., 2009). While we found unambiguous evidence for a reduction of thickness with maximum in both lateral and medial prefrontal cortex, the evidence for heritability was less clear; while it was apparent that patients with thin prefrontal cortex also tended to have relatives with thin prefrontal cortex (a measure quantified as Risch's lambda for siblings), thin cortices were not, at a statistically stringent threshold, more prevalent in siblings compared to normal controls. Based on these findings, we argued that brain volume, at least as measured by cortical thickness, may not be an ideal intermediate phenotype in schizophrenia. Similar findings were derived from a voxel-based morphometry study of the same subjects (Honea et al., 2007); studies of subcortical structures using an automated segmentation procedure, however, provided evidence for heritability for some of these phenotypes— for example, hippocampal volume, a measure that is not captured by cortical thickness (Goldman et al., 2007).

While structural intermediate phenotypes provide only an ambiguous evidence base for studying genetic risk, a much clearer picture emerges when the function of the DLPFC is being considered. A large body of work has consistently shown that if prefrontal cortex is activated, for example, by a working memory task, such as the so-called n-back paradigm (a working memory task), reliable abnormalities in DLPFC are observed in schizophrenia that often extend into other parts of the so-called working memory network, which also includes the parietal lobule and cerebellum (Callicott et al., 2000). Recent evidence from the study of genetically high-risk individuals (in this case, again in siblings) did provide clear evidence that this abnormality in DLPFC is found in siblings, at a degree intermediate between that seen in patients and controls, providing, for function, evidence for heritability and an incentive to pursue this intermediate phenotype in genetic studies (Callicott et al., 2003; Rasetti et al., 2009). While the exact extent and directionality of the abnormality in DLPFC has been somewhat debated and depends on the exact paradigm used, using the n-back task, in our hand, we observed an "inefficient" response, meaning that patients with schizophrenia show a much stronger activation compared to controls, and siblings, as a representative population at high genetic risk, show an intermediate increase in activation. We interpret this inefficiency as indicative of worse signal-to-noise ratio in prefrontal cortex during working memory in schizophrenia. Recent work has made significant contributions to understanding the neurochemical mechanisms underlying these functional abnormalities. According to an influential model first proposed by Durstewitz, Seamans, and Sejnowski (2000), a primary role is ascribed to dopamine, which interacts with other neurotransmitter systems, especially the excitatory neurotransmitter glutamate and the inhibitory neurotransmitter GABA, in modulating signal-to-noise ratio in prefrontal cortex. This is assumed to act primarily through D_1 receptors. When D_1 receptors in prefrontal cortex are optimally stimulated, during working memory, the signal, which in modeling corresponds to an activation peak representing the token of information "held in mind," is maximal, while noise level in the rest of cortex is minimal; conversely, suboptimal D_1 stimulation corresponds to a state in which signal is slow and multiple unrelated peaks, corresponding to the noise level, rise, reflecting an increase in task-irrelevant noise. This line of work is directly linked to current models of the pathophysiology of schizophrenia, because abnormalities in dopamine synthesis and turnover have been consistently found to be abnormal in the disorder (Laruelle & Abi-Dargham, 1999). A large body of evidence shows that dopamine synthesis and release is increased (disinhibited) subcortically, especially in striatum and to some degree also in midbrain, and shown to be related to genetic risk (Huttunen et al., 2008). In cortex, where measurement of dopamine is much more difficult, the evidence is less clear; on balance, however, researchers assume that dopaminergic stimulation in cortex is abnormally decreased (Laruelle & Abi-Dargham, 1999), corresponding to the signal-to-noise ratio observed in neuroimaging.

What underlies this complex dysregulation? A large body of work indicates that a feedback loop exists that links DLPFC to the dopamine-synthesizing neurons in midbrain, regulating both their synthesizing activity and the amount of dopamine that they release back into DLPFC and into striatum. This circuit, for which evidence accrues mainly from preclinical studies (Sesack, Carr, Omelchenko, & Pinto, 2003), is potentially very important for understanding neurogenetic risk and G × E in schizophrenia because it links two very well-established pathophysiological phenomena in this disorder, namely, DLPFC dysfunction and disinhibited dopamine release. This prompts the question whether these two phenomena might be related in schizophrenia. Early work from our lab showed that this is indeed likely (Meyer-Lindenberg et al., 2002). In this study, we measured presynaptic dopamine synthesis using positron emission tomography (PET) and a tracer, [18F]-DOPA, which allows quantification of an aspect of dopamine synthesis. In the same subjects, we measured DLPFC activity during working memory, this time again using PET, with an O^{15} water tracer, and a different activation paradigm, the Wisconsin Card Sorting Test. We replicated previous work showing abnormal activation in DLPFC and disinhibited striatal dopamine synthesis; as a novel contribution, we then went on to provide evidence that in patients with schizophrenia, these two measures were strongly correlated: the more abnormal DLPFC activity was, the more disinhibited the striatal dopamine synthesis. Conversely, we found no such relation in healthy controls, indicating that these two pathophysiological phenomena are indeed linked via feedback circuit, specifically leading to the hypothesis that pathological prefrontal cortex function might lead to disinhibited dopamine release, although, of course, the directionality of the finding cannot be proven from a correlational observation.

How do these neural systems-level findings relate to the psychopathology of schizophrenia and the mechanisms of psychosis in interaction with environmental adversity? This can be elucidated taking a point of departure from the seminal paper by Schultz (1998) and coworkers, which identified a neural mechanism for the attribution of salience, or important events in the environment. In the context of reward processing, Schultz observed that a dopaminergic peak in midbrain was linked to the timing of an expected reward (reward being paradigmatic here because rewarding events are salient in the environment). This so-called error prediction signal is essential for adaptive learning because learning can only occur if the need to readjust to the environment is signaled when a discrepancy between the expectation of the individual and the environmental occurrence is noted. Clearly, the occurrence of a midbrain dopaminergic signal depends on the adequate processing of environmental information in cortex; evidence suggests that this is related to midbrain through glutamatergic efference from DLPFC. In other words, the same circuit just discussed from the point of view of homeostasis of the dopaminergic system in psychosis is the system processing salience information in human brain in general, suggesting that abnormal attribution of salience through the system could occur in schizophrenia and be related to the processing of environmental stimuli. So, the system would be a prime candidate for mediation of environmental risk factors. Indeed, a convergent body of evidence produced by the laboratory of Paul Fletcher in Cambridge has shown that midbrain dopaminergic salience signals, using reward paradigms, can be reliably measured with fMRI and are profoundly abnormal in patients with schizophrenia, in subjects at risk for schizophrenia, and in healthy controls under ketamine-induced psychosis (Murray et al., 2008). Intriguingly, patients with schizophrenia did not show the expected activation of the salience signal to a rewarding stimulus, as is observed in healthy controls (Murray et al., 2008). This phenomenon might be related to some aspects of the schizophrenic negative syndrome, such as anhedonia and apathy. Most strikingly, however, schizophrenic patients showed abnormal activation to explicitly nonrewarding, controlled stimuli, a condition in which healthy controls showed no such effect. This suggests that the salience attribution system in schizophrenia is chaotically up-regulated, attributing salience to events of no behavioral relevance—a circumstance that provides a plausible neurophysiological–psychopathological explanation for the emergence of delusions in schizophrenia. It has been proposed that this mesolimbic dopaminergic salience system may be "sensitized" (Featherstone, Kapur, & Fletcher, 2007) in schizophrenia. Indeed, it has been shown that dopamine-agonistic drugs and stress sensitize mesolimbic dopamine release (Arnsten & Goldman Rakic, 1998) and that dopaminergic reactivity to stress is increased in the disorder (Brunelin et al., 2008). Interestingly, in our own work, we have recently applied a multimodal neuroimaging approach to a reward paradigm, measuring dopamine synthesis in midbrain and striatal structures using [^{18}F]-DOPA PET and cortical activation during a word paradigm using fMRI (Dreher, Meyer-Lindenberg, Kohn, & Berman, 2008). We found that during reward expectation, dopamine synthesis was in fact related to DLPFC activation. Intriguingly, the directionality of this interaction was positive in young but negative in older males. This suggests that the tuning of this regulatory circuit linking DLPFC and midbrain is affected by age, potentially contributing to an explanation of why symptoms of schizophrenia emerge after puberty, typically in the second and third decade in men, and in the third and fourth decade in women.

If dopaminergic mechanisms in the circuit are critical for genetic risk and G × E, a useful approach would be to investigate candidate genetic variation in the dopaminergic system for an impact on functioning and connectivity in the outlying structures. Turning to this research approach now, we will discuss COMT, the gene encoding the enzyme catecholamine-O-methyltransferase, the major enzyme degrading dopamine in prefrontal cortex. Throughout the brain, dopaminergic function at the synapse is terminated either by reuptake into the presynapse through the dopamine transporter or by diffusion out of the synapse and catabolism by COMT. Since in prefrontal cortex dopamine transporters are scarce, COMT emerges as the critical determinant of how much extra-neuronal dopamine prefrontal cortex neurons are exposed to (Lewis et al., 2001). The COMT gene has been linked to schizophrenia by genetic evidence: it is located at 22q on 11.2, a region that exhibits a positive linkage signal for schizophrenia (Owen, Williams, & O'Donovan, 2004; Stefansson et al., 2009). Even more compellingly, a microdeletion syndrome, 22q 11.2 syndrome or velocardio facial syndrome (Mendelian inheritance in man: MIM 192430), is well known to be associated with a very strongly increased risk of psychosis, indicating that this region harbors risk genes for the disease (Murphy, 2002). In

COMT, a variety of genetic variants have been described that have been linked to schizophrenia through functional and association studies. Most work has focused on a common substitution at amino acid 158 of the membrane form of the protein found in brain, corresponding to a single nucleotide polymorphism (rs4680) that results in a substitution of valine (VAL), the amino acid found in the wild type form, by methionine (MET). This common polymorphism affects the stability of the protein at body temperature, which in the wild type form is stable at 37 degrees Celsius, in the *MET* form partially denatured. This leads to a considerable and significant decrease in enzyme activity in brain and lymphocytes in the *MET* form and a corresponding strong increase of dopamine in brain areas in which *COMT* is the primary means of degrading dopamine, that is, in DLPFC, but not in striatum (Chen et al., 2004). Using working memory probes such as the n-back task, a convergent body of evidence shows that carriers of the *VAL* allele have impaired signal-to-noise ratio in cortex, compared to carriers of the *MET* allele (Mier, Kirsch, & Meyer-Lindenberg, 2010). In agreement with this, variation in *COMT* has also been shown to modulate cognitive performance depending on the prefrontal cortex, and the cortical response to dopaminergic stimulation, for example, by amphetamine (Mattay et al., 2003) or by the *COMT* inhibitor tolcapone (Apud et al., 2007). The latter line of work showed that *COMT* genotype places individuals at a predictable point on the curve linking prefrontal function to extraneuronal dopaminergic stimulation, a curve that is well known from the work by Goldman-Rakic and others (Goldman-Rakic, Muly, & Williams, 2000) to follow an "inverted-u" shape. This corresponds to the fact that an optimum range of dopaminergic stimulation for these neurons exists, both under- and overstimulation leading to reduced activation efficiency. Homozygotes for the *VAL* allele are positioned on the left ascending limb of this inverted-u-shape curve, heterozygotes, carrying a *VAL* and a *MET* allele, further to the right, but not yet at the optimum, whereas homozygotes for the *MET* allele are nearer even to the right of the optimum of that curve (Meyer-Lindenberg & Weinberger, 2006). This could be directly confirmed by a multimodal PET study that showed that *COMT* genotype impacted on the prefrontal regulation of midbrain dopamine synthesis in the genotype-dependent directionality consistent with the inverted-u-shape model, and that subjects with more *MET* alleles were positioned to the right of their genetic controls (Meyer-Lindenberg et al., 2005). This consistent evidence on the level of brain functional intermediate phenotypes nominates the *CMT-VAL* allele as a biological factor shifting prefrontal signal to noise and processing in cortical striatal circuits in the direction observed in overt schizophrenia, suggesting an association of the *VAL* allele with schizophrenia. While this was indeed found in many studies, current meta-analytic evidence only shows a marginal, nonsignificant increase in schizophrenia risk associated with the *VAL* allele (Fan et al., 2005). This is a consistent issue in the study of candidate genes in schizophrenia. While the origins of this wide discrepancy between consistent intermediate phenotype results and inconsistent, variable, and often statistically nonsignificant association findings when disease phenotypes are used are being debated (Flint & Munafò, 2007; Meyer-Lindenberg & Weinberger, 2006), one clear reason, in our estimation, lies in the nature of psychiatric phenotypes as such. These phenotypes are based on behavioral observation in clinical history and therefore are far removed from the underlying biology, which, if the experience from other disease phenotypes such as this is a guide, will be biologically heterogeneous. Using intermediate phenotypes closer to the level of genetic biology, it is therefore plausible that genetic penetrance will be higher and the picture more consistent on the level of brain; this has recently been confirmed for the *COMT-VAL-MET* variant by a meta-analysis from our group (Mier et al., 2010) and resonates with the finding of the other existing meta-analysis on imaging genetic findings (Munafò, Brown, & Hariri, 2008), both of which show that the degree of penetrance is considerably higher than that observed for behavioral phenotypes for the same variant.

Returning to G × E, is there evidence that the *CMT-VAL* variant increases risk for schizophrenia through interaction with environmental adversity? This is indeed so. Starting with a seminal paper by Caspi, Moffitt, and coworkers (Caspi et al., 2005), a consistent literature has emerged showing that the effect of adolescent-onset cannabis use on the risk for psychosis, a well-established environmental risk factor for schizophrenia, is strongly moderated by the *COMT-VAL-MET* genotype. In the original Caspi study and to some degree in subsequent studies, only carriers of the *VAL* allele showed a significantly increased risk for psychosis under cannabis use. This suggests that cannabis use had an impact on the dopaminergic-salience system and that the effect of cannabis on that system should be modulated by the *COMT* polymorphism, two research topics meriting further study.

At this point an important note of caution is in order. The genetics of schizophrenia is complex; while heritability is high, recent results from genomewide association studies strongly suggest that no frequent variant exists that by itself increases disease risk by more than 30% (Purcell et al., 2009; Shi et al., 2009; Stefansson et al., 2009). In fact, simulation studies indicate that thousands of risk alleles may be related to heritability in this genetically complex disorder (Purcell et al., 2009). This implies that interactions between genes, *epistasis*, may play an important role in the disorder, and may also contribute to the interactions with the environment. Is there evidence that interacting dopaminergic variance increases the risk for schizophrenia? This is indeed suggested by a recent large study focusing on functional effects delineating epistasis in candidate dopaminergic risk polymorphisms (Talkowski et al., 2008). This evidence on the level of disease association is again strongly complimented by evidence on the level of imaging genetics.

A convenient example is afforded by considering the postsynaptic transduction of dopamine signals, mediated through D_2 receptors. Neuropharmacology has described a signal transduction pathway in which these receptors couple through G-alpha I/O proteins to reduce cAMP production and regulate PKA activity. A critical regulatory molecule in this pathway is dopamine and CMT-regulated phosphoprotein of molecular weight 32 (DARPP-32). The seminal work of Paul Greenguard and associates has shown that DARPP-32 is a key signaling molecule in dopamine receptive neurons, regulating an array of subsequent neurophysiological processes in the response to psychotomimetic drugs, drugs of abuse, and neuroleptics, affecting striatal and cortical function and plasticity (Svenningsson et al., 2004). However this "canonical" CIMP–DARPP-32 pathway is not the only way in which dopamine signals are transduced in neurons, since the two receptors may also use an AKT1–GSK-3 signaling cascade via beta-arestin-2, which is independent of cAMP. Since genetic variation in both AKT1 and the gene-encoding DARPP-32 called PPP1R1B have been linked to schizophrenia risk, an imaging genetics approach is available to examine the neurosystems responsive to this variant in an attempt to delineate the neural systems relevant for schizophrenia genetic and G × E risk that are related to dopaminergic postsynaptic signal transduction. In fact, convergent evidence showed that these signal transduction pathways impact on the activation of striatum and functional connectivity of striatum with prefrontal cortex (Meyer-Lindenberg et al., 2007; Tan et al., 2008). This again highlighted prefrontal, striatal interactions, nominating not only a system for salience attribution but also basic neuropsychological functions such as gating, ascribed to the striatum, which in this view acts as a "filter" for environmental information. Deficiencies of this "filter" have been associated with liability for psychosis and cognitive impairment in the disorder (Swerdlow, Geyer, & Braff, 2001).

As expected and predicted, interactions of these genes with other dopaminergic risk genes, such as *COMT*, are observed (Bertolino et al., 2006), as are interactions with risk genes not from the dopaminergic pathway such as the glutamatergic risk gene *GRM3* (Tan et al., 2007). Even in *COMT* itself, evidence supports the existence of multiple variants within the genes which show epistatic interactions. In a large sample of Israelis of Ashkenazi descent, combining the *VAL-MET* polymorphism with two single-nucleotide polymorphisms at other loci, one in a promoter region (*rs165599*), the other downstream in intron 1 (*rs737865*) delineated a haplotype highly associated with schizophrenia risk (Shifman et al., 2002).

We found that interactions between these risk alleles, summarized as haplotypes across the gene, have increased explanatory power in prefrontal function in a pattern that was again reminiscent of the inverted-u-shaped curve (Meyer-Lindenberg, Nichols, et al., 2006). Furthermore, interactions between pre- and postsynaptic signal regulatory proteins, such as RGS4, have been observed in human imaging (Buckholtz et al., 2007), as have been interactions between COMT and the dopamine transporter, the alternative way of clearing dopamine from the synapse (Bertolino et al., 2006). Taken together, clear evidence suggests both the existence of epistatic interactions in the dopaminergic system, their relevance for functional circuits relevant for psychosis and environmental risk factors, especially through a processing of salience and psychosocial stress, and genetic and neural interactions of this system going beyond the dopaminergic system, notably glutamatergic risk variance.

Translating the treasure trove of epidemiologically secure environmental risk factors will require an experimental approach to try and isolate the neurobiology indexed by these risk factors (if any) to identify features that can be manipulated, can be quantified, and which lends itself to eliciting an immediate response that allows brain imaging to be used as the tool. In other words, pushing the area of neuromechanisms of G × E further will require an understanding of the neuromechanisms mediating the environmental risk factors themselves.

This is certainly easier if the risk factors themselves have a clear biological mode of action. As we have seen, a model can be presented for cannabis abuse being linked to the neural processing of environmental salience in general, potentially through a sensitization process and subject to dopaminergic modulation. However, other well-established environmental risk factors exist that do not easily fit into this explanatory scheme. Among those, notable examples are migration, urbanicity, and social status, all of which are associated with strong impact on schizophrenia disease risk with meta-analytic support (van Os & Poulton, 2008). In all these cases, the epidemiological variable itself, in our view, is likely to be a proxy for an underlying factor, or factors, that interact with genetic risk through neurosystems that remain to be characterized. Taking migration as an example, the fact that migration is associated with schizophrenia risk could be associated with a wide range of (not mutually exclusive!) underlying factors such as infectious and immunological differences between the country of origin and the host country, genetic and personality variation making a subset of the population more or less likely to migrate, and differences in social interaction styles and cues that differentially impose stress on migrants. If these factors are identified, again, their impact on the brain is likely to be pleiotropic and depend on when in the lifespan these environmental risk factors impact, to what degree, and in what context. While it is easy to feel intimidated by this complexity, it is nevertheless possible to sift epi-demiological data to arrive at falsifiable mechanistic hypotheses amenable to experimental testing with systems neuroscience methods. For example, epidemiological data on migration, urbanicity, and social status are all con-sistent with the assumption that an underlying problem is attributable to specific social stressors that are inappropriately processed by neural circuits biased through a schizophrenia-risk genetic background.

As a first step to elucidate such circuits, we have studied the neural cor-relates of social status (Zink et al., 2008). Given the stated a priori hypoth-esis, it makes sense to start with status since it already occupies a social dimension. Human social hierarchies are prominent in multiple domestic, work, and recreational settings, where they define implicit expectations and action dispositions that drive appropriate social behavior. Further-more, while the relevance of social status for schizophrenia risk has been debated, there is no doubt that social status by itself increases and modu-lates a large variety of both somatic and psychiatric disorders (Sapolsky, 2004), and social status strongly predicts well-being, morbidity, and even survival. Social hierarchies spontaneously and stably emerge in children as young as 2 years. Status within a particular social hierarchy is often made explicit (e.g., via uniforms, honorifics, verbal assignment, or in some lan-guages even through status-specific grammar, but can also be inferred from cues such as facial features, height, gender, age, and dress).

Social status is an attractive phenotype for a translational genetics approach because status is a feature of social hierarchies that are found throughout the animal kingdom, suggesting the existence of neuromech-anisms to efficiently extract and process status information. In humans, dominance has been linked to heritable personality traits that interact with multiple neurotransmitter and neuroendocrine systems, and can be automatically and efficiently inferred, indicating the existence of biological systems that process social rank information. Finally, status is an attrac-tive environmental risk factor to study because prior data link the specif-ics of status to disease risk in primates. In primate hierarchies, the alpha (top) position is associated with lower disease risk in stable hierarchies, but higher disease risk in unstable hierarchies (Sapolsky, 2004), suggesting that by manipulating the hierarchy experimentally, neural systems can be iso-lated that are selectively responsive in an unstable hierarchy, delineating a system that would be an attractive start target for studying $G \times E$. In other words, the epidemiological data showing a differential impact of stable and unstable hierarchy can be translated into a neuroscience experiment. If we can find neural systems exclusively active during unstable hierarchy, we can link those systems back, via the epidemiological data that formed our point of departure, to health risk.

In a first study of this phenomenon, we simulated a social hierarchy by inviting subjects to play a rewarding game in the scanner (Zink et al., 2008). Subjects were informed that two other participants were playing the game at the same time and were shown the responses of the other "participants" while being informed that these responses did not matter for their own reward, that is, we created an explicitly nonconfrontational, yet strongly hierarchical, context by assigning subjects three stars for the best, one star for the worst, and two stars for the intermediate player—the proband. Using functional resonance imaging, we showed that the presence of a social superior in the simulated context strongly differentially engaged perceptual attentional systems, as well as DLPFC and key nodes of the salience attribution system. Conversely, viewing a social inferior led to no activation at all, suggesting that social hierarchies in humans are processed linearly by allocating attention and salience resources to social superiors in good agreement with behavioral evidence. In a second step, we then made the hierarchy unstable by informing subjects that their positional rank would change based on their performance during the game. While we again observed the same circuit active when a social superior was viewed, we now isolated neurostructures that were exclusively active during unstable hierarchies; the amygdala (a key node of emotional processing), thalamus, and cortical regions regulating amygdala. When participants performed worse than an inferior player, areas lower in the brain associated with emotional pain and frustration, such as the insula, were activated. Performing better than the superior player activated areas higher and toward the front of the brain controlling action planning. The more positive the mood experienced by participants while at the top of an unstable hierarchy, the stronger was activity in emotional pain circuitry when they viewed an outcome that threatened to move them down in status. This was the same emotional pain circuitry, including the insula, that was activated when losing to the inferior player. In other words, people who felt more joy when they won also felt more pain when they lost. In this initial inquiry, we used incidental differences in skill and accompanying rank symbols to create a hierarchy; many other aspects governing social rank relationships in humans remain to be studied. Even so, our findings demonstrate that brain responses to superiority and inferiority are dissociable, even in the absence of explicit competition, both when encountering an individual of a particular status and when faced with an outcome that can affect one's current position in the hierarchy. These results thus form a tentative confirmation of the research strategy idea that the identification of neural mechanisms for environmental risk is feasible.

These circuits, and in particular regulatory circuits with amygdala or the extended limbic system in general, form a point of departure for examining G × E related to social status. Independent evidence for the relevance of these systems for G × E comes from the fact that the same amygdala regulatory circuitry has been previously implicated in the effects for candidate genes in which G × E has been shown, although not for schizophrenia: the 5-HTTLPR has been implicated in amygdala regulation, harm avoidance/neuroticism, and risk for affective disorders (Pezawas et al., 2005) in the context of environmental adversity, and a variable number of tandem repeats polymorphism in MAOA has been nominated as a risk factor for impulsively violent behavior (Meyer-Lindenberg, Buckholtz, et al., 2006). Also, human neuroimaging studies implicated amygdala and functionally and structurally linked regions as targets of the prosocial neuropeptide oxytocin (Kirsch et al., 2005), a central mediator of attachment and maternal behavior, suggesting neural entry points for epigenetic mechanisms as well.

In summary, we have presented beginning evidence for neuromechanisms mediating G × E, taking schizophrenia as a paradigmatic example. Further work will explicitly study quantified environmental risk factors in the field in large samples and relate them to genetic and, in the future, also epigenetic variations. Risk factors and risk genes identified through such approaches can then be related back to neurosystems using the imaging genetics methods outlined in this chapter. This is necessary because hypothesis-free approaches to identifying G × E are limited by the strongly high dimensional nature of the data. It is to be hoped that a consortium-driven approach to G × E, such as the one pursued by the EU-GEI Consortium (2008), will be useful in further delineating the mechanisms mediating genetic and environmental risk factors and their interaction, thereby further defining the pathophysiology of the disease and pointing the way to evidence-based environmental protective interventions and novel biological therapies.

REFERENCES

Apud, J. A., Mattay, V., Chen, J., Kolachana, B. S., Callicott, J. H., Rasetti, R., et al. (2007). Tolcapone improves cognition and cortical information processing in normal human subjects. *Neuropsychopharmacology, 32,* 1011–1020.

Arnsten, A. F., & Goldman-Rakic, P. S. (1998). Noise stress impairs prefrontal cortical cognitive function in monkeys: Evidence for a hyperdopaminergic mechanism. *Archives of General Psychiatry, 55,* 362–368.

Bertolino, A., Blasi, G., Latorre, V., Rubino, V., Rampino, A., Sinibaldi, L., et al. (2006). Additive effects of genetic variation in dopamine regulating genes on working memory cortical activity in human brain. *Journal of Neurosciences, 26,* 3918–3922.

Brunelin, J., d'Amato, T., van Os, J., Cochet, A., Suaud-Chagny, M. F., & Saoud, M.

(2008). Effects of acute metabolic stress on the dopaminergic and pituitary–adrenal axis activity in patients with schizophrenia, their unaffected siblings and controls. *Schizophrenia Research, 100,* 206–211.

Buckholtz, J. W., Sust, S., Tan, H. Y., Mattay, V. S., Straub, R. E., Meyer-Lindenberg, A., et al. (2007). fMRI evidence for functional epistasis between COMT and RGS4. *Molecular Psychiatry, 12,* 893–895, 885.

Callicott, J. H., Bertolino, A., Mattay, V. S., Langheim, F. J., Duyn, J., Coppola, R., et al. (2000). Physiological dysfunction of the dorsolateral prefrontal cortex in schizophrenia revisited. *Cerebral Cortex, 10,* 1078–1092.

Callicott, J. H., Egan, M. F., Mattay, V. S., Bertolino, A., Bone, A. D., Verchinksi, B., et al. (2003). Abnormal fMRI response of the dorsolateral prefrontal cortex in cognitively intact siblings of patients with schizophrenia. *American Journal of Psychiatry, 160,* 709–719.

Caspi, A., Moffitt, T. E., Cannon, M., McClay, J., Murray, R., Harrington, H., et al. (2005). Moderation of the effect of adolescent-onset cannabis use on adult psychosis by a functional polymorphism in the catechol-O-methyltransferase gene: Longitudinal evidence of a gene × environment interaction. *Biological Psychiatry, 57,* 1117–1127.

Chen, J., Lipska, B. K., Halim, N., Ma, Q. D., Matsumoto, M., Melhem, S., et al. (2004). Functional analysis of genetic variation in catechol-O-methyltransferase (COMT): Effects on mRNA, protein, and enzyme activity in postmortem human brain. *American Journal of Human Genetics, 75,* 807–821.

Dreher, J. C., Meyer-Lindenberg, A., Kohn, P., & Berman, K. F. (2008). Age-related changes in midbrain dopaminergic regulation of the human reward system. *Proceedings of the National Academies of Science USA, 105,* 15106–15111.

Durstewitz, D., Seamans, J. K., & Sejnowski, T. J. (2000). Dopamine-mediated stabilization of delay-period activity in a network model of prefrontal cortex. *Journal of Neurophysiology, 83,* 1733–1750.

EU GEI Consortium. (2008). Schizophrenia aetiology: Do gene–environment interactions hold the key? *Schizophrenia Research, 102,* 21–26.

Fan, J. B., Zhang, C. S., Gu, N. F., Li, X. W., Sun, W. W., Wang, H. Y., et al. (2005). Catechol-O-methyltransferase gene Val/Met functional polymorphism and risk of schizophrenia: A large-scale association study plus meta-analysis. *Biological Psychiatry, 57,* 139–144.

Featherstone, R. E., Kapur, S., & Fletcher, P. J. (2007). The amphetamine-induced sensitized state as a model of schizophrenia. *Progress in Neuropsychopharmacology and Biological Psychiatry, 31,* 1556–1571.

Flint, J., & Munafò, M. R. (2007). The endophenotype concept in psychiatric genetics. *Psychological Medicine, 37,* 163–180.

Goldman, A., Pezawas, L., Mattay, V., Fischl, B., Verchinski, B., Chenk, Q., et al. (2009). Widespread reductions of cortical thickness in schizophrenia and spectrum disorders and evidence for heritability. *Archives of General Psychiatry, 66*(5), 467–477.

Goldman, A. L., Pezawas, L., Mattay, V. S., Fischl, B., Verchinski, B. A., Zoltick, B., et al. (2007). Heritability of brain morphology related to schizophrenia: A large-scale automated magnetic resonance imaging segmentation study. *Biological Psychiatry, 63*(5), 475–483.

Goldman-Rakic, P. S., Muly, E. C., III, & Williams, G. V. (2000). D(1) receptors in prefrontal cells and circuits. *Brain Research Review, 31*, 295–301.

Honea, R. A., Meyer-Lindenberg, A., Hobbs, K. B., Pezawas, L., Mattay, V. S., Egan, M. F., et al. (2007). Is gray matter volume an intermediate phenotype for schizophrenia?: A voxel-based morphometry study of patients with schizophrenia and their healthy siblings. *Biological Psychiatry, 63*(5), 465–474.

Huttunen, J., Heinimaa, M., Svirskis, T., Nyman, M., Kajander, J., Forsback, S., et al. (2008). Striatal dopamine synthesis in first-degree relatives of patients with schizophrenia. *Biological Psychiatry, 63*, 114–117.

Kirsch, P., Esslinger, C., Chen, Q., Mier, D., Lis, S., Siddhanti, S,, et al. (2005). Oxytocin modulates neural circuitry for social cognition and fear in humans. *Journal of Neurosciences, 25*, 11489–11493.

Laruelle, M., & Abi-Dargham, A. (1999). Dopamine as the wind of the psychotic fire: New evidence from brain imaging studies. *Journal of Psychopharmacology, 13*, 358–371.

Lewis, D. A., Melchitzky, D. S., Sesack, S. R., Whitehead, R. E., Auh, S., & Sampson, A. (2001). Dopamine transporter immunoreactivity in monkey cerebral cortex: Regional, laminar, and ultrastructural localization. *Journal of Comparative Neurology, 432*, 119–136.

Mattay, V. S., Goldberg, T. E., Fera, F., Hariri, A. R., Tessitore, A., Egan, M. F., et al. (2003). Catechol O-methyltransferase val158-met genotype and individual variation in the brain response to amphetamine. *Proceedings of the National Academy of Sciences USA, 100*, 6186–6191.

Meyer-Lindenberg, A., Buckholtz, J. W., Kolachana, B., Hariri, A. R., Pezawas, L., Blasi, G., et al. (2006). Neural mechanisms of genetic risk for impulsivity and violence in humans. *Proceedings of the National Academy of Sciences USA, 103*, 6269–6274.

Meyer-Lindenberg, A., Kohn, P. D., Kolachana, B., Kippenhan, S., McInerney-Leo, A., Nussbaum, R., et al. (2005). Midbrain dopamine and prefrontal function in humans: Interaction and modulation by COMT genotype. *Nature Neuroscience, 8*, 594–596.

Meyer-Lindenberg, A., Miletich, R. S., Kohn, P. D., Esposito, G., Carson, R. E., Quarantelli, M., et al. (2002). Reduced prefrontal activity predicts exaggerated striatal dopaminergic function in schizophrenia. *Nature Neuroscience, 5*, 267–271.

Meyer-Lindenberg, A., Nichols, T., Callicott, J. H., Ding, J., Kolachana, B., Buckholtz, J., et al. (2006). Impact of complex genetic variation in COMT on human brain function. *Molecular Psychiatry, 11*, 797, 867–877.

Meyer-Lindenberg, A., Straub, R. E., Lipska, B. K., Verchinski, B. A., Goldberg, T., Callicott, J. H., et al. (2007). Genetic evidence implicating DARPP-32 in human frontostriatal structure, function, and cognition. *Journal of Clinical Investigation, 117*, 672–682.

Meyer-Lindenberg, A., & Weinberger, D. R. (2006). Intermediate phenotypes and genetic mechanisms of psychiatric disorders. *Nature Reviews in Neuroscience, 7*, 818–827.

Mier, D., Kirsch, P., & Meyer-Lindenberg, A. (2010). Neural substrates of pleiotropic action of genetic variation in COMT: A meta-analysis. *Molecular Psychiatry, 15*(9), 918–927.

Munafò, M. R., Brown, S. M., & Hariri, A. R. (2008). Serotonin transporter (5-HTTLPR) genotype and amygdala activation: A meta-analysis. *Biological Psychiatry, 63,* 852–857.

Murphy, K. C. (2002). Schizophrenia and velo–cardio–facial syndrome. *Lancet, 359,* 426–430.

Murray, G. K., Corlett, P. R., Clark, L., Pessiglione, M., Blackwell, A. D., Honey, G., et al. (2008). How dopamine dysregulation leads to psychotic symptoms?: Abnormal mesolimbic and mesostriatal prediction error signalling in psychosis. *Molecular Psychiatry, 13,* 239.

Owen, M. J., Williams, N. M., & O'Donovan, M. C. (2004). The molecular genetics of schizophrenia: New findings promise new insights. *Molecular Psychiatry, 9,* 14–27.

Pezawas, L., Meyer-Lindenberg, A., Drabant, E. M., Verchinski, B. A., Munoz, K. E., Kolachana, B. S., et al. (2005). 5-HTTLPR polymorphism impacts human cingulate–amygdala interactions: A genetic susceptibility mechanism for depression. *Nature Neuroscience, 8,* 828–834.

Purcell, S. M., Wray, N. R., Stone, J. L., Visscher, P. M., O'Donovan, M. C., Sullivan, P. F., et al. (2009). Common polygenic variation contributes to risk of schizophrenia and bipolar disorder. *Nature, 460,* 748–752.

Rasetti, R., Mattay, V. S., Wiedholz, L. M., Kolachana, B. S., Hariri, A. R., Callicott, J. H., et al. (2009). Evidence that altered amygdala activity in schizophrenia is related to clinical state and not genetic risk. *American Journal of Psychiatry, 166,* 216–225.

Sapolsky, R. M. (2004). Social status and health in humans and other animals. *Annual Review of Anthropology, 33,* 393–418.

Schultz, W. (1998). Predictive reward signal of dopamine neurons. *Journal of Neurophysiology, 80,* 1–27.

Sesack, S. R., Carr, D. B., Omelchenko, N., & Pinto, A. (2003). Anatomical substrates for glutamate–dopamine interactions: Evidence for specificity of connections and extrasynaptic actions. *Annals of the New York Academy of Sciences, 1003,* 36–52.

Shi, J., Levinson, D. F., Duan, J., Sanders, A. R., Zheng, Y., Pe'er, I., et al. (2009). Common variants on chromosome 6p22.1 are associated with schizophrenia. *Nature, 460,* 753–757.

Shifman, S., Bronstein, M., Sternfeld, M., Pisante-Shalom, A., Lev-Lehman, E., Weizman, A., et al. (2002). A highly significant association between a COMT haplotype and schizophrenia. *American Journal of Human Genetics, 71,* 1296–1302.

Stefansson, H., Ophoff, R. A., Steinberg, S., Andreassen, O. A., Cichon, S., Rujescu, D., et al. (2009). Common variants conferring risk of schizophrenia. *Nature, 460,* 744–747.

Svenningsson, P., Nishi, A., Fisone, G., Girault, J. A., Nairn, A. C., & Greengard, P. (2004). DARPP-32: An integrator of neurotransmission. *Annual Review of Pharmacological Toxicology, 44,* 269–296.

Swerdlow, N. R., Geyer, M. A., & Braff, D. L. (2001). Neural circuit regulation of prepulse inhibition of startle in the rat: Current knowledge and future challenges. *Psychopharmacology (Berlin), 156,* 194–215.

Talkowski, M. E., Kirov, G., Bamne, M., Georgieva, L., Torres, G., Mansour, H., et al. (2008). A network of dopaminergic gene variations implicated as risk factors for schizophrenia. *Human Molecular Genetics, 17,* 747–758.

Tan, H. Y., Chen, Q., Sust, S., Buckholtz, J. W., Meyers, J. D., Egan, M. F., et al. (2007). Epistasis between catechol-O-methyltransferase and type II metabotropic glutamate receptor 3 genes on working memory brain function. *Proceedings of the National Academy of Sciences USA, 104,* 12536–12541.

Tan, H. Y., Nicodemus, K. K., Chen, Q., Li, Z., Brooke, J. K., Honea, R., et al. (2008). Genetic variation in AKT1 is linked to dopamine-associated prefrontal cortical structure and function in humans. *Journal of Clinical Investigations, 118,* 2200–2208.

van Os, J., & Poulton, R. (2008). Environmental vulnerability and genetic–environmental interactions. In H. J. Jackson & P. D. McGorry (Eds.), *The recognition and management of early psychosis: A preventive approach* (2nd ed., pp. 47–60). Cambridge, UK: Cambridge University Press.

Zink, C. F., Tong, Y., Chen, Q., Bassett, D. S., Stein, J. L., & Meyer-Lindenberg, A. (2008). Know your place: Neural processing of social hierarchy in humans. *Neuron, 58,* 273–283.

CHAPTER 5

Gene–Environment Interactions

State of the Science

Michael Rutter *and* Kenneth A. Dodge

Although some biometricians wish to dismiss gene–environment interactions (G × E) as a purely statistical phenomenon (see Munafò, Durrant, Lewis, & Flint, 2009; Risch et al., 2009), the concept of G × E is essentially a biological one. As Rutter (Chapter 1, this volume; see also Rutter, 2010) has argued, there are strong theoretical reasons for expecting G × E. Genetic influences on environmental susceptibility are basic for evolutionary theory; it would seem implausible that environmental susceptibility could be the one trait outside of genetic influence; and it is equally unlikely that genes would not be involved in the observed wide variations in individuals' responses to stress and adversity. Furthermore, as shown by Caspi, Hariri, Holmes, Uher, and Moffitt (Chapter 2, this volume), there is an abundance of empirical data documenting its existence. If evidence of G × E is to be of value in influencing policy or practice in the field of prevention or care of mental disorders, it is essential that it be based on an adequate understanding of the biology (see also Dodge & Rutter, Chapter 13, this volume).

The biological bases of G × E are clearly documented in this volume by Caspi and colleagues (Chapter 2), Hariri (Chapter 3), and Meyer-Lindenberg (Chapter 4), with findings accruing from basic science, human experimental research, and animal models, as well as human epidemiological investigations. In addition, it is crucial to take note of the strong expectations of G × E deriving from evolutionary considerations, genetic findings, and the heterogeneity in response to environmental hazards (see Rutter, Thapar, & Pickles, 2009). The failure to take these considerations into account in the Risch and colleagues (2009) meta-analysis, the exclusive focus on G × E as a particular kind of statistical concept, and the biases involved in the sampling for the meta-analyses (Uher & McGuffin, 2010) suggest that we do not need to discuss this destructive critique further. Instead, we focus on several further challenging issues that remain: (1) conceptualization and measurement of the environment, (2) intermediate phenotypes, (3) issues arising from advances in genetic research, (4) definition of phenotypes, and (5) selected analytic issues.

CONCEPTUALIZATION AND MEASUREMENT OF THE ENVIRONMENT

If the environment is to be taken seriously, its conceptualization and measurement must improve. Although innovative in its time, Bronfenbrenner's (1979) ecological model of the microsystem (e.g., *family, school, peer group, neighborhood*, and *child care* environments), mesosystem (a system comprising connections between immediate environments), exosystem (e.g., external environmental settings that indirectly affect development, such as parent's workplace), and macrosystem (e.g., culture) provides at best a crude model of how we might conceptualize and classify human environments. Furthermore, too many studies of G × E have relied on rather crude questionnaire measures of environment that lack good measurement of the timing of its occurrence. The time lag between measurements of the environment in longitudinal studies has often been chosen out of convenience (e.g., annual data collection) rather than due to a theoretical rationale for the noticeable time period in which behavioral change is hypothesized to occur. In many cases, the environment being investigated has not been subjected to rigorous tests of the postulate that the observed statistical associations with the outcome being investigated truly reflect environmentally mediated causation.

The causal influence of environments has been most effectively tested through the use of "natural experiments" of one kind or another (see Academy of Medical Sciences, 2007; Rutter, 2007, in press). Examples come from sexual abuse (Kendler & Prescott, 2006), physical abuse/maltreatment (Jaffee et al., 2004), bullying (Arseneault et al., 2008), a high number of negative life events (Kendler, Karkowski, & Prescott, 1999), and parent–child conflict (Pike, McGuire, Hetherington, Reiss, & Plomin, 1996). Five main features stand out with all of these types of environments. First, they can be measured as acute and discrete events. Although environments have also been measured as general contexts, such as being born into a family of poverty or living in a dangerous neighborhood, contexts typically operate through their impact on discrete events. For example, the context of family poverty exerts its effects on a child's externalizing behaviors through its impact on parental discipline and childrearing strategies (Dodge, Pettit, & Bates, 1994). Identifying the acute environmental mechanisms through which context variables such as socioeconomic status operate is an ongoing challenge. Although environmental impact can be measured through acute events, typically these events are actually recurrent or chronic. Whatever biological mechanism underlies G × E, the pathway is likely to be one that operates over a substantial period of time and not just during a brief moment of crisis. This feature means that it may be particularly important to time the occurrence of environment to check whether it precedes the outset of the mental disorder, and attention will need to be paid to which aspect of the environment constitutes the key risk factor. For example, are multiple negative life events the crucial stressors or, rather, do they index or reflect more lasting psychological hazards that constitute the main causal mechanism? At least with child psychopathology the limited available evidence suggests that chronic adversity is more important then acute events (Sandberg, McGuinness, Hillary, & Rutter, 1998).

Second, all of these environments involve interactions with other people, making it difficult, but crucial, to separate cause and consequence in relation to the individual's own role. What appears to be G × E in some circumstances might actually derive from gene–environment correlations (rGE), namely the correlation between some genetic polymorphism and some specific environment. Statistical analyses must examine that possibility when testing G × E. This test is reasonably straightforward with respect to the gene in question but is challenging with respect to some other, unmeasured, gene. It cannot be assumed that the only genetic effect on the environment stems from the one specific identified gene under investigation. Of course, it is not only gene causal effects on environment that matter. In studies of environmental risks for disease, it is very easy to mistake the features providing the origin of a postulated environment risk for the proximal risk itself (see Academy of Medical Sciences, 2007). That distinction must be appreciated and dealt with for any adequate measurement of environment.

Third, a distinction must be made between distal and proximal environmental risk factors. Sometimes, distal factors operate through proximal factors, and sometimes the distal factor is the direct causal factor, with the proximal variable being a noncausal by-product of the distal factor. For example, early research into the possible risk effects for children stemming from family dissolution showed that the main direct risk did not come from the breakup as such but rather from the poor parenting to which it gave rise in some instances (Harris, Brown, & Bifulco, 1986). Thus, poor parenting leads to family breakup and to child maladjustment, with the family breakup per se having little direct impact. More recent research (Silberg,

Maes, & Eaves, 2010) has shown that the distal factor of parental depression has an environmentally mediated proximal risk effect for depression in the children, raising the issue of what aspect mediates the risk. G × E could operate on either distal or proximal environments, but if the biological pathways of gene and environment coincide or are closely related the interaction is more likely to apply to the proximal environment.

Fourth, it has been known that individuals process and conceptualize the meaning of their experiences (especially interpersonal ones; see Crick & Dodge, 1994). For example, provocations by others have an effect on aggressive behavioral responses only if they are perceived as maliciously intended and not if perceived as accidental (Dodge, 1980). Does the true causal effect derive from this effective environment as perceived (see Cole, 2009)? If so, how should this factor be conceptualized and measured? The possibility that the causal impact occurs through perceived environment, and not through objectively measured environment, raises questions about how a taxonomy of environments should be formulated. That is, objective features of an environment may not be as relevant as features that are important to the perceiver. Measurement of these nuances may be difficult, however. There is a general appreciation that the investigation of G × E will require rather large samples (although if the G × E effect is a strong one, probably not as large as sometime claimed). Inevitably, measures of environment suitable for large population implementation must be developed and tested—this is quite a challenge, but one that must be met.

Fifth, most interpersonal risk processes involve some degree of two-way interaction. How a person behaves toward others influences how those others respond to him or her (see the studies on the effects of adopted children's behavior on their adoptive parents—Ge et al., 1996; O'Connor, Deater-Deckard, Fulker, Rutter, & Plomin, 1998). It will not be easy to incorporate all these various considerations into measures of environment suitable for medium or large sample surveys. Nevertheless, we need to recognize that the finding of yet another example of G × E is of very little value unless the particular characteristic of any one G × E helps to shed light on the possible underlying biological mechanisms. That criterion necessarily means careful conceptualization and measurement of environment.

INTERMEDIATE PHENOTYPES

The experimental study of G × E in humans has largely involved the bringing together of imaging technology, molecular genetics, and the devising of "intermediate phenotypes" that provide an immediate window into one step on the biological pathways leading to psychopathology. One disadvantage of relying on epidemiological/longitudinal studies to examine G × E is that after a candidate environmental factor occurs, it may be necessary to wait a substantial time for the disorder under investigation to develop. During that intervening period, many other events are likely to occur, rendering the causal role of the environmental factor suspect. The experimental approach has the very important advantage of short-circuiting this waiting process by using an experimental environment to induce an immediate response that is relevant to the overall causal biological pathway. Thus Battaglia, Marino, Maziade, Molteni, and D'Amato (2008) used the inhalation of CO_2 to induce panic; Hariri (Chapter 3, this volume) used frightening pictures to induce a negative emotional response; and Meyer-Lindenberg (Chapter 4, this volume) used a rigged game to induce high and low social power relationships. Intermediate phenotypes have the additional important advantage over psychiatric diagnoses of focusing on a biological feature (Meyer-Lindenberg, 2010).

A related experimental approach to G × E is to implement short-term clinical intervention to examine impact on behavior under different genetic circumstances. Brody, Beach, Philibert, Chen, and Murry (2009) randomly assigned adolescents to preventive intervention involving parental training in heightened monitoring and supervision and found that this environmental variable moderated the impact of the gene *5-HTTLPR* on substance-use problems. There has been surprisingly little use of such approaches, and we suggest that there should be more.

GENETICS

Broadly similar issues apply to genetics. Currently, there is much enthusiasm for genomewide association studies (GWAS) on the grounds that, as the technology exists to scan the whole genome, new risk genes can be identified and control for chance factors in identifying a single candidate gene can be gained by large-sample testing of all genes. The argument has some force if only because the choice of candidate genes rests on such a narrow knowledge base. If the studies of G × E are to be confined to the handful of genes for which there is some evidence of their role in psychopathology, how are we to break really new ground? It is for these reasons that we favor the inclusion of GWAS as one element in the overall research strategy. The approach could result in the discovery of genes that warrant inclusion in studies of G × E because their actions seem to operate on environmental susceptibility. However, we emphasize that gene discovery (i.e., the identification of a susceptibility gene on a particular chromosome in a particular position) is of no immediate value. Its importance lies in the clues that it provides for the direction that biological research should take in order to delineate gene actions.

Moreover, we need to note that the limitations in GWAS have come to be increasingly recognized. To begin with, apart from the notable example of macular degeneration, the strategy has delivered remarkably few significant findings and the genes identified mostly have quite tiny effects. The contrast between the substantial heritabilities that are typically found in twin and adoptee studies and the miniscule effects of individual identified genes have led to the apparent paradox of a supposed "missing heritability" (McClellan & King, 2010). It should be added that GWAS are susceptible to population stratification (see Coop et al., 2009), and hence to contradictions between two GWAS studies (see Wang et al., 2009; Weiss, Arking, The Gene Discovery Project of Johns Hopkins & the Autism Consortium, 2009). Furthermore, it has been noted that few of the genes have known functional biological effects (see McClellan & King, 2010). Some are on introns and not on exons, and those with effects are often ones that do not connect with messenger RNA that codes for proteins. Rather, their effects operate through influences on gene transcription or expression. It is necessary that we broaden our concept of susceptibility/protective genes beyond those that produce proteins to include those DNA elements that influence gene effects through their impact on gene expression. Notably several of the genes involved in G × E are of this kind (e.g., the serotonin transporter promoter gene; see Caspi et al., 2003; Rutter, 2010). Finally, the very small effects of genes means that the initial high hopes that commercial gene sequencing would be of major value for predictive or diagnostic purposes need to be toned down (see, e.g., the results with respect to heart disease; Paynter et al., 2010).

At least for the time being, the focused candidate gene approach seems the most advantageous for G × E studies. Three key reasons stand out. First, the choice of genes has been (and should have been) based on scientific findings showing a possible biological pathway for the candidate gene and candidate environment to interact on a causal pathway leading to psychopathology. In other words, the start point is on a reasonable scientific footing. The negative flipside, of course, is that this requirement makes it less likely that an unexpected novel causal pathway will be discovered. The great need is not for more genes to be statistically associated with some diagnostic condition. Rather, the need is to identify genes that have already been shown to be associated with a brain system and to be relevant for the origins of psychopathology.

The second reason for candidate gene approaches is that, with respect to the most studied examples of G × E (namely, the serotonin transporter gene and depression with the interaction involving multiple life events of maltreatment; and the *MAOA* gene and antisocial behavior with the interaction involving maltreatment), the human experimental studies show the neural effects of G × E apply both to individuals *without* psychopathology and not just to those with a mental disorder. The implication is that it would have been utterly futile to screen the genome for genes showing a main effect on depression or on antisocial behavior. Not only did the Caspi and colleagues (2002, 2003) epidemiological studies show no statistical main effect, but the Hariri and Weinberger (2002, 2005) experimental studies showed that the effects of the G × E operated in the absence of depression and antisocial disorder. The G × E findings have important implications for the causal pathways leading to psychopathology, but such pathways operate in the general population and therefore are likely to predispose to mental disorder only indirectly.

The third reason for candidate gene approaches is that the genetic causal processes may not operate in relation to psychiatric conditions as we currently conceptualize them. For example, Caspi and colleagues (2008) found that the COMT gene had a significant effect on antisocial behavior in individuals with an attention-deficit/hyperactivity disorder (ADHD) without there being a main effect on either antisocial behavior itself or ADHD itself. That particular finding has been replicated in a quite different sample, so it is likely to be robust, but we do not yet know how common this sort of effect may be. Clearly, there is some degree of diagnostic specificity in genetic effects but there is more diagnostic overlap in genetic effects than used to be thought (see, e.g., the findings on schizophrenia and bipolar disorder) (Craddock, O'Donovan, & Owen, 2005), and it also clear that most genes have pleiotropic effects (e.g., COMT; Caspi et al., 2008). Inevitably, this circumstance much complicates the search for susceptibility genes in general and, by the same token, will complicate the study of G × E.

Because of the small number of replicated susceptibility genes in the field of psychopathology, it has been difficult to undertake any systematic study of synergistic interactions among genes or between different genetic alleles. Nevertheless, animal models suggest that such interactions may be more common than previously appreciated and therefore will complicate studies of G × E (Mackay, Stone, & Ayroels, 2009; Phillips, 2008; Wolf, Leamy, Routman, & Ceverud, 2005). However, there is the puzzle that behavioral genetic studies of mental disorders suggest that additive effects predominate over synergistic ones and it is not clear what to make of the rather different animal findings.

The best way forward is likely to lie in the study of genes that have been shown to affect environmental susceptibility or brain systems. We suggest that a continuing focus on candidate genes is likely to constitute the best strategy (Moffitt, Caspi, & Rutter, 2005) until we learn more about how genes work.

Finally, there is one other way in which genes may be important in G × E—through epigenetic effects (Meaney, 2010). Genes can only operate once they have been "expressed," and expression is influenced by background genes, stochastic chance effects, and environmental influences. It is possible that the environment effects involved in G × E operate through effects on gene expression (Tsuang et al., 2005), although this mechanism has yet to be demonstrated. What is evident, however, is that the study of E effects on gene expression constitutes a possible avenue by which to investigate G × E. The underlying message of all these gene and environment considerations is that the investigation of G × E constitutes the starting point (and certainly not the end point) of an important means of elucidating the various possible biological pathways involved in the understanding of psychopathology.

With respect to epigenetic effects, although there is no doubt that this constitutes a field of study of great importance, several challenges have yet to be overcome. Most basically, it is known that such effects are usually tissue-specific, making their study in living humans extremely problematic. The proposed solution has been to use lymphocytes as a proxy for the brain on the grounds that levels of gene expression tend to be particularly high in the brain. Nevertheless, animal studies to test the extent to which they are a valid proxy remain incomplete. Moreover, it is known that all types of lymphocytes are not the same with respect to gene expression. In addition, basic data on the temporal stability of expression patterns are largely lacking (although it has been shown that they vary with age) (Fraga et al., 2005). In addition, it is evident that epigenesis is influenced by genes as well as the environment and chance, and that these genetic influences will need to be factored into our understanding. While it is quite possible that epigenesis may be crucial in G × E, it is important that we do not claim too much too soon. Finally, if all experiences have epigenetic effects, they are useless for explaining individual phenotypic differences unless *variations* in epigenesis can be shown to account for individual heterogeneity in environmental effects on the phenotypes being studied. This is yet another task for the future.

Rare structural mutations and copy number variations (CNVs) have recently been shown to be important in autism (Bucan et al., 2009; Guilmatre et al., 2009; Sebat et al., 2007), schizophrenia (International Schizophrenia Consortium, 2008; Stefansson et al., 2008; Walsh et al., 2008; Xu et al., 2008), and ADHD (Williams et al., 2010). The findings have cast doubt on the usual previous assumption that multifactorial disorders arise on the basis of combinations of common genetic variants that in themselves are not necessarily pathogenic or deleterious. Each rare mutation is associated with only a tiny proportion of cases of autism or schizophrenia, but it has been argued that the findings argue for a high degree of genetic heterogeneity and that a large number of rare genes could account for a substantial proportion of cases. The findings have several attractions: they provide a possible explanation for why neither autism nor schizophrenia have died out (as a result of low fecundity and hence low transgenerational transmission); and many of the rare genes (or genes disrupted by CNVs) are concerned with signaling, neurodevelopment, and other possible causal biological pathways. Nevertheless, serious queries remain. First, many of the mutations arise de novo and these may represent a genetic cause but they cannot account for the demonstrated familiality of both autism and schizophrenia. Second, the same mutation has usually been implicated in more than one psychiatric or developmental disorder or even normality (Chubb, Bradshaw, Soares, Porteous, & Millar, 2008; Cook & Scherer, 2008). While it is known that many genetic effects are pleiotropic, the degree of heterogeneity poses the question of whether the findings cast much light on the neural basis of the disorder. Third, the most recent large-scale collaborative study of CNVs in autism (Pinto et al., 2010) adds the further complication that many of the findings are specific to individual families. Fourth, the raised rate of CNVs in autism and schizophrenia prompts the need to ask what leads to this raised rate. For example, might the association with being born to an older father (Durkin et al., 2008; Reichenberg et al., 2006) constitute part of the explanation (because of the increased rate of mutations; see Walter, Intano, McCarrey, McMahan, & Walter, 1998)?

Finally, it is necessary to appreciate that the empirical findings indicate that autism and schizophrenia arise on the basis of both common and rare genes. Also, G × E findings may apply to important risk pathways rather than to the disorder itself. For example, this would seem to be the case with respect to the role of particular *COMT* polymorphisms in moderating the risk effect of cannabis in predisposing to schizophrenia (Caspi et al., 2005; Henquet et al., 2008). Even more crucially, the human experimental studies (Meyer-Lindenberg & Weinberg, 2006) show that the neural effects associated with G × E (at least in the case of depression and antisocial disorder) are found in individuals free of psychopathology. We conclude that any adequate understanding of genetic influences on mental disorder must take on board the findings on rare structural mutations and CNVs, but neither in any way invalidate the studies of G × E.

DEFINITION OF PHENOTYPES

While it has long been accepted that genes do not code for psychiatric categories, the complexities involved in the definition of phenotypes have become increasingly apparent. To begin with, it has become evident that not only do the genetic influences on anxiety and depressive disorders overlap greatly (as had been expected for a long time), but more surprisingly there is also overlap between the genetic influences on autism and schizophrenia, on schizophrenia and bipolar disorder, and on Tourette disorder and obsessive–compulsive disorder—to mention but a few examples. Inevitably, this poses problems in defining "cases" in association studies. But the difficulties do not stop there. Thus, a COMT polymorphism is associated with antisocial behavior in individuals with ADHD but not with antisocial disorder or ADHD as such (Caspi et al., 2008). Ideally, it may be preferable to define phenotypes on the basis of pathophysiology or biological pathways, but the evidence to do that is not yet available. In addition, as already noted, the G × E findings may operate on biological pathways operating in the normal population. None of this should be interpreted as an argument to abandon psychiatric diagnoses but we do suggest caution in interpreting GWAS findings—positive or negative.

SOME STATISTICAL CONSIDERATIONS

It has long been known that variations in scaling can readily create artificial interactions or disguise valid ones. Thus, it ought to be a matter of routine (as it was in the Dunedin studies) to check whether apparent G × E had been created by scaling artifacts (with respect to measurement of the gene or environment or the phenotype being investigated).

As in the whole of science, replications are essential in order to determine the robustness of any finding. Conceptual replication should be tested within a study by checking whether the G × E effect is found when the outcome phenotype is measured dimensionally rather then categorically or is focused somewhat differently (e.g., violent crime rather than any other serious crime). This internal replication was completed in the Dunedin studies, but it has been rather inconsistent across other studies. When replicating a biological finding, it is usually better to vary the samples and vary the measures so long as the relevant constructs remain the same (see Rutter et al., 2009). It has become popular to bring studies together in the form of data pooling in order to conduct a meta-analysis (Risch et al., 2009), which is a sound approach when there is sufficient commonality in the approach taken and a discrete outcome is measured in the same way in all studies. Unfortunately, this commonality is more easily claimed than found, and misleading findings are all too easily obtained (Uher & McGuffin, 2010).

The final point is that heterogeneity in G × E, as in genetic findings generally, needs to be expected. This phenomenon implies either heterogeneity in the outcome variable of interest or a G × E × E or G × G × E effect, which has been found in medicine generally and has been demonstrated also in several mental disorders. This phenomenon is not just a quality of genes but also of environments because multiple nongenetic causal pathways have been found for several medical conditions (Rutter, 1997). Obviously, that possibility greatly complicates the study of G × E, but the rule to be followed is straightforward. That is, it is never acceptable to be content with invoking heterogeneity as explanation of nonreplication. Rather, if the heterogeneity is valid, it too will be replicable once the relevant factors are understood (e.g., like is being compared with like with respect to features such as age, ethnicity, culture, or meaning of environment).

Given all these difficulties, it may seem surprising that the G × E findings have stood up to replication as well as they have. However, findings are also clear in showing that many puzzles and inconstancies remain. In this chapter, we have simply sought to outline the conceptual and methodological issues that need attention in order to undertake the high-quality research that, hopefully, will bring greater clarity in the years ahead. In the meanwhile, what has been established is a valid biological phenomenon that carries the potential of increasing our understanding of causal biological processes implicated on the cause and course of developmental psychopathology.

REFERENCES

Academy of Medical Sciences. (2007). *Identifying the environmental causes of disease: How should we decide what to believe and when to take action?* London: Author.

Arseneault, L., Milne, B. J., Taylor, A., Adams, F., Delgado, K., Caspi, A., et al. (2008). Being bullied as an environmentally mediated contributing factor to children's internalizing problems: A study of twins discordant for victimization. *Archives of Pediatrics and Adolescent Medicine, 162,* 145–150.

Battaglia, M., Marino, C., Maziade, M., Molteni, M., & D'Amato, F. (2008). Gene–environment interaction and behavioural disorders: A developmental perspective based on endophenotypes. In M. Rutter (Ed.), *Genetic effects on environmental vulnerability to disease* (pp. 103–119). Chichester, UK: Wiley.

Brody, G. H., Beach, S. R., Philibert, R. A., Chen, Y., & Murry, V. (2009). Prevention effects moderate the association of 5-HTTLPR and youth risk behavior initiation: Gene × environment hypotheses tested via a randomized prevention trial. *Child Development, 80,* 645–661.

Bronfenbrenner, U. (1979). *The ecology of human development: Experiments by nature and design.* Cambridge, MA: Harvard University Press.

Bucan, M., Abrahams, B. S., Wang, K., Glessner, J. T., Herman, E. I., Sonnenblick, L. I., et al. (2009). Genome-wide analyses of exonic copy number variants in a family-based study point to novel autism susceptibility genes. *PLoS Genetics, 5,* e1000536.

Caspi, A., Langley, K., Milne, B., Moffitt, T., O'Donovan, M., Owen, M., et al. (2008). A replicated molecular genetic basis for subtyping antisocial behavior in children with attention-deficit/hyperactivity disorder. *Archives of General Psychiatry, 65,* 203–210.

Caspi, A., McClay, J., Moffitt, T. E., Mill, J., Martin, J., Craig, I. W., et al. (2002). Role of genotype in the cycle of violence in maltreated children. *Science, 297,* 851–854.

Caspi, A., Moffitt, T. E., Cannon, M., McClay, J., Murray, B., Harrington, H., et al. (2005). Moderation of the effect of adolescent-onset cannabis use on adult psychosis by a functional polymorphism in the catechol-o methyltransferase gene: Longitudinal evidence of a gene–environment interaction. *Biological Psychiatry, 57,* 1117–1127.

Caspi, A., Sugden, K., Moffitt, T. E., Taylor, A., Craig, I. W., Harrington, H., et al. (2003). Influence of life stress on depression: Moderation by a polymorphism in the 5-HTT gene. *Science, 301,* 386–389.

Chubb, J. E., Bradshaw, N. J., Soares, D. C., Porteous, D. J., & Millar, J. K. (2008). The DISC locus in psychiatric illness. *Molecular Psychiatry, 13,* 36–64.

Cole, S. W. (2009). Social regulation of human gene expression. *Current Directions in Psychological Science, 18,* 132–137.

Cook, E. H., & Scherer, S. W. (2008). Copy-number variations associated with neuropsychiatric conditions. *Nature, 455,* 919–923.

Coop, G., Pickrell, J. K., Novembre, J., Kudaravalli, S., Li, J., Absher, D., et al. (2009). The role of geography in human adaptation. *PLoS Genetics, 5,* e1000500.

Craddock, N., O'Donovan, M. C., & Owen, M. J. (2005). Genes for schizophrenia and bipolar disorder?: Implications for psychiatric nosology. *Schizophrenia Bulletin, 32,* 9–16.

Crick, N. R., & Dodge, K. A. (1994). A review and reformulation of social information-processing mechanisms in children's social adjustment. *Psychological Bulletin, 115,* 74–101.

Dodge, K. A. (1980). Social cognition and children's aggressive behavior. *Child Development, 51,* 162–170.

Dodge, K. A., Pettit, G. S., & Bates, J. E. (1994). Socialization mediators of the relation between socioeconomic status and child conduct problems. *Child Development, 65,* 649–665.

Durkin, M. S., Maenner, M. J., Newschaffer, C. J., Lee, L. C., Cunniff, C. M., Daniels J. L., et al. (2008). Advanced parental age and the risk of autism spectrum disorder. *American Journal of Epidemiology, 168,* 1268–1276.

Fraga, M. F., Ballestar, E., Paz, M. F., Ropero, S., Setien, F., Ballestar, M. L., et al. (2005). Epigenetic differences arise during the lifetime of monozygotic twins. *Proceedings of the National Academy of Sciences USA, 102,* 10604–10609.

Ge, X., Conger, R. D., Cadoret, R. J., Neiderhiser, J. M., Yates, W., Troughton, E., et al. (1996). The developmental interface between nature and nurture: A mutual influence model of child antisocial behavior and parent behaviors. *Developmental Psychology, 32,* 574–589.

Guilmatre, A., Dubourg, C., Mosca, A.-L., Legallic, S., Goldenberg, A., Drouin-Garraud, V., et al. (2009). Recurrent rearrangements in synaptic and neurodevelopmental genes and shared biologic pathways in schizophrenia, autism, and mental retardation. *Archives of General Psychiatry, 66,* 947–956.

Hariri, A. R., Drabant, E. M., Munoz, K. E., Kolachana, B. S., Mattay, V. S., Egan, M. F., et al. (2005). A susceptibility gene for affective disorders and the response of the human amygdala. *Archives of General Psychiatry, 62,* 146–152.

Hariri, A. R., Mattay, V. S., Tessitore, A., Kolachana, B., Fera, F., Goldman, D., et al. (2002). Serotonin transporter genetic variation and the response of the human amygdala. *Science, 297,* 400–403.

Harris, T., Brown, G. W., & Bifulco, A. (1986). Loss of parent in childhood and adult psychiatric disorder: The role of lack of adequate parental care. *Psychological Medicine, 16,* 641–659.

Henquet, C., Rosa, A., Delespaul, P., Papiol, S., Fananás, L., van Os, J., et al. (2009). COMT ValMet moderation of cannabis-induced psychosis: A momentary assessment study of "switching on" hallucinations in the flow of daily life. *Acta Psychiatrica Scandanavia, 119,* 156–160.

International Schizophrenia Consortium. (2008). Rare chromosomal deletions and duplications increase risk of schizophrenia. *Nature, 455,* 237–241.

Jaffee, S. R., Caspi, A., Moffitt, T. E., Polo-Tomas, M., Price, T. S., & Taylor, A. (2004). The limits of child effects: Evidence for genetically mediated child effects on corporal punishment but not on physical maltreatment. *Developmental Psychology, 40,* 1047–1058.

Kendler, K. S., Karkowski, L. M., & Prescott, C. A. (1999). Causal relationship between stressful life events and the onset of major depression. *American Journal of Psychiatry 156,* 837–841.

Kendler, K. S., & Prescott, C. A. (2006). *Genes, environment, and psychopathology: Understanding the causes of psychiatric and substance use disorders.* New York: Guilford Press.

Mackay, T. F. C., Stone, E. A., & Ayroels, J. F. (2009). The genetics of quantitative traits: Challenges and prospects. *Nature Reviews Genetics, 10,* 565–577.

McClellan, J., & King, M.-C. (2010). Genetic heterogeneity in human disease. *Cell, 141,* 210–217.

Meaney, M. J. (2010). Epigenetics and the biological definition of gene × environment interactions. *Child Development, 81,* 47–79.

Meyer-Lindenberg, A. (2010). Intermediate or brainless phenotypes for psychiatric research? *Psychological Medicine, 40,* 1057–1062.

Meyer-Lindenberg, A., & Weinberger, D. R. (2006). Intermediate phenotypes and genetic mechanisms of psychiatric disorders. *Nature Reviews Neuroscience, 7,* 818–827.

Moffitt, T. E., Caspi, A., & Rutter, M. (2005). Strategy for investigating interactions between measured genes and measured environments. *Archives of General Psychiatry, 62,* 473–481.

Munafò, M. R., Durrant, C., Lewis, G., & Flint, J. (2009). Gene × environment interactions at the serotonin transporter locus. *Biological Psychiatry, 65,* 211–219.

O'Connor, T. G., Deater-Deckard, K., Fulker, D., Rutter, M., & Plomin, R. (1998). Genotype–environment correlations in late childhood and early adolescence: Antisocial behavioral problems and coercive parenting. *Developmental Psychology, 34,* 970–981.

Paynter, N. P., Chasman, D. I., Paré, G., Buring, J. E., Cook, N. R., Miletich, J. P., et al. (2010). Association between a literature-based genetic risk score and cardiovascular events in women. *Journal of the American Medical Association, 303*, 631–637.

Phillips, P. C. (2008). Epistasis—the essential role of gene interactions in the structure and evolution of genetic systems. *Nature Reviews Genetics, 9*, 855–867.

Pike, A., McGuire, S., Hetherington, E. M., Reiss, D., & Plomin, R. (1996). Family environment and adolescent depression and antisocial behavior: A multivariate genetic analysis. *Developmental Psychology, 32*, 590–603.

Pinto, D., Pagnamenta, A. T., Klei, L., Anney, R., Merico, D., Dregan, R., et al. (2010). Functional impact of global rare copy number variation in autism spectrum disorders. *Nature, 466*, 368–372.

Reichenberg, A., Gross, R., Weiser, M., Bresnahan, M., Silverman, J., Harlap, S., et al. (2006). Advancing paternal age and autism. *Archives of General Psychiatry, 63*, 1026–1032.

Risch, N., Herrell, R., Lehner, T., Liang, K. Y., Eaves, L., Hoh, J., et al. (2009). Interaction between the serotonin transporter gene (5-HTTLPR), stressful life events, and risk of depression: A meta-analysis. *Journal of the American Medical Association, 301*, 2462–2471.

Rutter, M. (1997). Comorbidity: Concepts, claims and choices. *Çriminal Behavior and Mental Health, 7*, 265–286.

Rutter, M. (2007). Proceeding from observed correlations to causal inference: The use of natural experiments. *Perspectives in Psychological Science, 2*, 377–395.

Rutter, M. (2010). Gene–environment interplay. *Depression and Anxiety, 27*, 1–4.

Rutter, M. (in press). "Natural experiments" as a means of testing causal inferences. In C. Barzini, P. Dawid, & L. Bernardinelli (Eds.), *Statistical methods in causal inference.*

Rutter, M., Thapar, A., & Pickles, A. (2009). Gene–environment interactions: Biologically valid pathway or artifact? *Archives of General Psychiatry, 66*, 1287–1289.

Sandberg, S., McGuinness, D., Hillary, C., & Rutter, M. (1998). Independence of childhood life events and chronic adversities: A comparison of two patient groups and controls. *Journal of the American Academy of Child and Adolescent Psychiatry, 37*, 728–735.

Sebat, J., Lakshmi, B., Malhotra, D., Troge, J., Lese-Martin, C., Walsh, T., et al. (2007). Strong association of de novo copy number mutations with autism. *Science, 316*, 445–449.

Silberg, J. L., Maes, H., & Eaves, L. J. (2010). Genetic and environmental influences on the transmission of parental depression to children's depression and conduct disturbance: An extended children of twins study. *Journal of Child Psychology and Psychiatry, 51*, 734–744.

Stefansson, H., Rjuescu, D., Cichon, S., Pietiläinen, O. P. H., Ingason, A., Steinberg, S., et al. (2008). Large recurrent microdeletions associated with schizophrenia. *Nature, 455*, 232–236.

Tsuang, M. T., Nossova, N., Yager, T., Tsuang, M.-M., Guo, S.-C., Shyu, K. G., et al. (2005). Assessing the validity of blood-based gene expression profiles for the classification of schizophrenia and bipolar disorder: A preliminary report. *American Journal of Medical Genetics (Neuropsychiatric Genetics),* *133b*(1), 1–5.

Uher, R., & McGuffin, P. (2010). The moderation by the serotonin transporter gene of environmental adversity in the etiology of depression: 2009 update. *Molecular Psychiatry, 15,* 18–22.

Walsh, T., McClellan, J. M., McCarthy, S. E., Addington, A. M., Pierce, S. B., Cooper, G. M., et al. (2008). Rare structural variants disrupt multiple genes in neurodevelopmental pathways in schizophrenia. *Science, 320,* 539–543.

Walter, C. A., Intano, G. W., McCarrey, J. R., McMahan, C. A., & Walter, R. B. (1998). Mutation frequency declines during spermatogenesis in young mice but increases in old mice. *Proceedings of the Natoinal Academy of Sciences USA, 95,* 10015–10019.

Wang, K., Zhang, H., Ma, D., Bucan, M., Glessner, J. T., Abrahams, B. S., et al. (2009). Common genetic variants on 5p14.1 associate with autism spectrum disorders. *Nature, 459,* 528–533.

Weiss, L. A., Arking, D. E., & The Gene Discovery Project of Johns Hopkins & the Autism Consortium. (2009). A genome-wide linkage and association scan reveals novel loci for autism. *Nature, 461,* 802–808.

Williams, N., Zaharieva, I., Martin, A., Langley, K., O'Donovan, M., Owen, M., et al. (2010). Rare chromosomal deletions and duplications are associated with attention deficit hyperactivity disorder and overlap with autism suscepti-bility loci. *Lancet, 376,* 1401–1408.

Wolf, J. B., Leamy, L. J., Routman, E. J., & Ceverud, J. M. (2005). Epistatic pleiotropy and the genetic architecture of covariation within early and late-developing skull trait complexes in mice. *Genetics, 171,* 683–694.

Xu, B., Roos, J. L., Levy, S., va Rensburg, S. L., Gogos, J. A., & Karayiorgou, M. (2008). Strong association of de novo copy number mutations with sporadic schizophrenia. *Nature Genetics, 40,* 880–885.

PART II

PRACTICE AND POLICY

CHAPTER 6

Marital Dynamics
and Child Proaction

Genetics Takes a Second Look
at Developmental Theory

David Reiss *and* Jenae M. Neiderhiser

There is little question that recent advances in genetics hold great promise for improving our understanding of psychopathology in children and for improving treatment of these disorders. Recent discoveries in identifying genes associated with disorders promise to illumine neurobiological mechanisms that shape both normal and pathological development. What is less widely appreciated is that current genetic studies are providing new data on the role of family systems in the development of psychopathology as well.

For example, in a seminal publication, Tully, Iacono, and McGue (2008) used a genetically informed design to provide the strongest evidence to date that maternal (but not paternal) depression is associated with child psychopathology through environmental transmission. Although studies linking maternal depression to child psychopathology are legion (e.g., (Coyne, Low, Miller, Seifer, & Dickstein, 2007; Foster, Garber, & Durlak, 2008; Maughan, Cicchetti, Toth, & Rogosch, 2007; NICHD Early Child Care Research Network, 1999), most had been conducted with mothers and their biological children with whom they share exactly 50% of their individual differences genes. Thus, the links between the depressed mother and her infant may reflect genetic rather than social processes. For example, variations among individuals in self-worth and in parenting practices have shown notable genetic influences (McGuire et al., 1999; Neiderhiser et al., 2004); hence, parents' self-concepts and parenting practices might be influenced by the same genes that, when passed on to their children, influence the child's psychopathology as well. Indeed, recent advances in genetic research have provided an important *counterfactual* to common interpretations of the impact of parental psychopathology and parental practices on child development. Thus, a study like that of Tully and colleagues is of critical importance. They report a strong association between maternal depression and child psychopathology in families of adoptive mothers and their adopted children *with whom, by definition, they share no individual-difference genes*. The association between maternal depression and child psychopathology was not significantly greater in a control group of parents rearing their biological children, adding weight to their finding.

In this study, the genetically informed findings provide a *frame* in which further research can be conducted. Genetically informed designs do not, of course, always support an exclusively *environmental frame*. For example, Harden and colleagues (2007) found that the marital conflict of the father's identical twin brother (the child's uncle) with his wife predicted the child's antisocial behavior as well as did the marital conflict of the child's own father, even when the father's marriage showed little conflict, strongly suggesting a genetic mechanism linking marital conflict and antisocial behavior.

The impact of genetics on our understanding of the family system makes the new genetic frontier of essential relevance to child clinicians. We have long passed the simple notion that genes account for some part of the development of psychopathology and environmental circumstances—such as parenting and the parental marriage—account for other parts. The new genetics requires us to rethink our concepts of the family and how it operates. To illustrate this new view, we consider two closely related themes in current work, marriage and the child's proactive influences on the parent–child and marital relationships. Both themes concern how three subsystems in the family are linked: the marital relationship, the parental relationship, and the developmental mechanisms within the children of these parents. We review evidence that, by adolescence, developmental systems within the child not only evoke but sustain parent–child conflict across the span of many years. Thus, new evidence strongly weights a genetic frame for examining parent–child relationships.

ADVANCES IN THE GENETICS OF FAMILY PROCESS

The new frontier in the genetics of family relationships is fueled by three advances in the basic science of genetics: the novel use of genetically informed research designs, the increasing importance of animal models of human families, and an increasing understanding of the structure and function of the human genome, particularly the cellular and neuroregulatory mechanisms that regulate gene expression. In this chapter, we draw mostly on the first two of these, but touch lightly on the third as well.

Innovative Genetically Informed Research Designs

Recent twin studies have been designed especially to throw light on family dynamics. One version of this design has extended the twin model to include half-siblings (a mother brings a child from a first marriage, remarries, and has a second child by her new husband with the children being reared together from early childhood) and genetically unrelated siblings (the remarried married parents each bring a child from a former marriage into the new household). These twin and sibling studies not only permit generalizing findings beyond twins but have included detailed measurements of social processes inside the family as well as in the family's context (most notably peer relationships of the developing children). One example of this genre is the Nonshared Environment in Adolescent Development (NEAD; Reiss et al., 2000) study. The major discoveries of this genre of studies are the pervasiveness of influence of the children's genetic differences on how they are treated by other family members, the types of peer groups in which they become engaged, and the trajectories of their school careers. These studies have also clarified that many of the genetic influences on these social processes are closely related to those that influence psychopathology in these developing young people, and that genetic, not environmental, mechanisms account for a substantial portion of the association between measures of the social environment and developing systems within the child. These studies have also documented environmental mechanisms linking parenting to developmental outcomes in children. For example, Fearon and colleagues (2006) have shown that genetic influences have little to do with the association between maternal sensitivity and the quality of her infant's attachment to her, and the quality of a mother's attachment to one sibling may be suppressed by the quality of her attachment to the other.

Comparable in importance has been the use of the prospective adoption design for the study of family dynamics. This design recruits and studies birth parents, the adopted child, and the adoptive families rearing the child. There have been only two fully-realized examples of this design. One, the Colorado Adoption Study, was begun in the mid-1970s (Dunn & Plomin, 1986). More recently, the Early Growth and Development Study (EGDS; Leve et al., 2007) has been designed specifically to examine reciprocal relations between inherited temperamental qualities of the child; the quality of parental responses to these temperaments; and the effects of the adoptive parents' marital quality, psychopathology, and economic distress on the parents' response to inherited characteristics of their child. These studies are likely to shed considerable light on the gene–environment mechanisms by which social process in the family modify the influence of the children's genes on their developing psychological systems. It is already well established, for example, that parental monitoring and warmth can reduce dramatically the expression of genetic influence on the development of conduct problems and antisocial behavior in children and adolescents (Dick et al., 2007; Feinberg, Button, Neiderhiser, Reiss, & Hetherington, 2007).

Animal Models of Family Subsystems

For some time, researchers have explored both adult pair bonding and parent offspring relationships in animal family systems. While intriguing, this research was of uncertain relevance to human families. Current genetic research has required a second look at these potential animal analogues to human family systems for at least two complementary reasons. First, genes that influence these social behaviors in animals often have close analogues in humans. Second, the use of animal models has suggested an unanticipated mechanism linking the early experience of infant animals to later development. The effects of early stress and incompetent parental care in animals leave lifelong impairments in the expression of genes that are critical for the competent response to later stressful circumstances (Liu et al., 1997; Meaney, 2001; Plotsky & Meaney, 1993; Weaver et al., 2001), whereas competent maternal care favors the expression of genes that promote the development of maternal competence in the offspring (Champagne et al., 2006). These studies suggest an unanticipated system of "gene-based memory" that may supplement or have priority over psychological mechanisms and thus are of great interest to researchers focused on human development.

MARITAL DYNAMICS

The formal study of marriage and its dynamics has been a preoccupation of researchers for over a half-century, playing a prominent role in Freud's first reported clinical case (Dora) and continuing to be of keen interest to clinicians since. In Dora's case, an important seed for her "hysteria" was an apparent estrangement between her mother and father, intensified by his several illnesses for which Dora was a principal caretaker. The links between marriage and parenting have been studied through a variety of means including careful inquiries of parents about their marriage and parenting and direct observation, using coded videotapes of both marital and parent–child interaction patterns. In general, research has examined a hypothesis consistent with Freud's Dora case, which might be called "compensatory" mechanisms, in which troubled marriages lead to unusual closeness and intimacy between a parent and a child. Although there is little doubt that extreme cases such as Dora's do occur, in most cases the evidence argues against these mechanisms. Indeed, it is most often the case that when marriages are warm and companionate, so too are the relationships between husband and children and wife and children, but where marriages are high in conflict or low in warmth, parent and child relationships are equally strained. For a comprehensive review of this literature, see Erel and Burman (1995).

Research is exploring mechanisms that might account for this spillover, focusing on affective spillover (conflict in marriage renders spouses more irritable with their children), stress models (including the hypothesis that the stress of a poor marriage diminishes the attentiveness and responsiveness of parents to their children), and the impact of disruptive children on relationships with their parents and on their marriages. There is some support for all three of these mechanisms (Cui, Donnellan, & Conger, 2007).

Using the children-of-twins design, our group has tackled this problem from a genetic perspective based on several past findings. First, parental personality and psychopathology are notable long-term predictors of marital status (Johnson, McGue, Krueger, & Bouchard, 2004; Roberts, Kuncel, Shiner, Caspi, & Goldberg, 2007).

Twin studies have shown that genetic influences play a notable role in whether individuals ever become married (Johnson et al., 2004), in their liability for divorce (Jocklin, McGue, & Lykken, 1996), and in overall marital satisfaction (Spotts et al., 2004). The twin method serves well here. In the case of marital satisfaction, we assembled a large sample of monozygotic (MZ) and dizygotic (DZ) twins who were married and whose spouses agreed to participate in the study. Then we asked each twin and each spouse about his or her level of marital satisfaction and his or her level of disagreement on parenting. MZ twins who are wives report greater levels of similarity than DZ twins who are wives for both satisfaction and level of agreement, suggesting genetic influence on wives' *reports* of marital satisfaction, which might merely be attributable to genetic effects on their style of responding to questionnaires. More persuasive is the similar finding for their *husbands'* satisfaction and level of agreement. It is the influence of the *wives'* genes that are assessed here since this is a sample of twin women, not twin men. It is in this sense that we can argue that there are substantial genetic influences on the marital *relationship*, not just the wives' report of it.

Genetic influences on personality probably account for much of these effects. Personality is also a notable predictor of parenting style. Predictions from childhood and adolescent personality difficulties to adult parenting have been reported by several investigators (Brook, Brook, Ning, Whiteman, & Finch, 2006; Caspi, Elder, & Bem, 1987; Johnson, Cohen, Kasen, & Brook, 2008; Trentacosta & Shaw, 2008). Common across reports are the adverse effects of early childhood impulsiveness and aggressiveness. Considerable progress has been made in documenting the heritable influences on impulsive and aggressive developmental trajectories, with emerging findings that specific genes might play a role in associated neuroregulatory mechanisms (Dick, 2007). Given these findings, it is not surprising that there are substantial genetic effects on parental style and parental reactions to their children. Our direct observations have shown that maternal warmth, in particular, showed strong genetic influence: over 40% of variation in mothers' report of her warmth toward her child was influenced by the mother's genetic factors, just under 20% in her child reports and 25% of observer reports. The observer reports were based on twin mothers who were observed interacting with their adolescent children for just 10 minutes in their homes (Neiderhiser et al., 2004).

Of special interest is that, to a large extent, the genetic factors that influence marriage also influence parenting. Thus, about 40% of the observed association between marital conflict and parent–child negativity is attributable to genetic influences common to both, with the personality factor of aggression playing a notable role in this association (Ganiban et al., 2009).

Taken together, these studies suggest that a genetic frame will be important for further investigations of mechanisms shaping marital quality and dissolution and how the marital relationship shapes and sustains competent parenting. We will, of course, advance work in this field once specific genes are identified that suggest critical neuroregulatory mechanisms that shape and sustain subsystems in the family and account, in part, for their linkage. Recently, our group has reported one example of this molecular analysis in humans, based on the neuroscience of social behavior in animals (Walum et al., 2008).

It is well established that prairie voles form enduring social pair bonds which often last their entire lifetime while montane voles are notably socially promiscuous. In males, the differences between these two species have been traced to differences in a single gene known as *avpr1* that regulates the distribution of brain receptors that are activated by the neuropeptide arginine vasopressin that is manufactured in the hypothalamus and secreted by the pituitary. There are at least two morphological distinctive features in the *avpr1* gene of the prairie vole, in comparison to the montane vole, that are associated with a dense distribution of receptors in areas of the brain associated with both pleasure and social relationships. The causal role of these genes in the animal models was confirmed by cloning the prairie vole gene, attaching it to a viral vector, and injecting the gene into brains of conspecific voles as well as rats (Clinton, Miller, Watson, & Akil, 2008; Landgraf et al., 2003; Pitkow et al., 2001), producing enhanced social affiliation in both (Nair & Young, 2006).

Given the enormous complexity of human marriage, we were astonished to find a notable effect of this single gene on men's reports of engagement with their wives, their expectations for the endurance of their relationship, and marital crises. More convincing was that the *wives* of men with the risk allele reported lower levels of marital quality. Of particular interest, 32% of men with both copies of the risk allele were unmarried versus 17% of those who had no copies.

There are important differences between our data and those from voles. Most important is that in humans the size of the effect of this single gene is quite small. Although the risk allele is fairly common (approximately 40% of our male sample had least one risk allele), the d statistic varies around 0.2 for most comparisons, meaning that the mean of the men with one or both risk alleles is only about 15% higher than the mean of men without the alleles. Even though the effects are small they are, if replicated, important because they suggest that some biological processes shaping good marriages may be gender-specific and they highlight the role of animal models in understanding human family process.

To summarize, the evidence suggests that not only do genetic influences extend *into* family relationships but, in all likelihood, extend *through* family subsystems, thereby influencing other family subsystems. Second, these findings draw attention to quasi-stable, heritable features of individual family members, known as personality. Third, these findings suggest a more precise tailoring of the environmental frame that has informed almost all research on family subsystems and the relationships among these subsystems.

In what way must we "tuck in" the environmental frame? Additional genetic data provide two important clues. First, genetic factors account for only a portion of the differences among individuals in their liability for unhappy marriages or divorce. Likewise, genetic factors account for no more than a third of the association between marital process and parenting.

Second, environmental experiences shared by siblings in their family of origin, or shared by them subsequently, have little effect on their liability for divorce. Rather, it is experiences unique to each sibling that play a central role. We draw this inference because the correlations between MZ twins in divorce liability or marital dissatisfaction rarely exceed .5. Thus, even identical twins can have very different marriages. Once the genetic basis of similarities between twins is controlled, the residual similarity between them in marital satisfaction or in divorce is very little or none. Thus, we must exclude social factors common to both siblings. These findings rule out shared effects such as parental social class, maternal depression (if experienced by the siblings in comparable ways), or current common experiences including variations among sibling pairs in mutual feelings of closeness. The environmental experiences that differ between siblings are the main source of their liability for difficult marriages, and of course a chief candidate is the person they marry. Here genetic data provide yet another clue. Findings from our group (Towers, 2003) and Lykken and Tellegen (1993) suggest that an individual's genotype plays no role in the selection of mate: husbands of MZ twins are no more like each other than are husbands of DZ twins. Indeed, husbands of MZ twins are, along many measures, not more like each other than two individuals picked at random.

CHILD PROACTION

It is still the case that when a behavior is shown to have substantial genetic influences many clinicians incline toward pessimism regarding psychological treatment. As we have shown, there is ample evidence that genetic influences are strong for both marital and parent–child relationships. Indeed, since much of our work as child clinicians focuses on both marital and parent–child relationship, the genetic data raise questions as to whether there are serious genetic limits on the efficacy of our psychotherapeutic work. However, another important line of evidence from genetic research yields a very different conclusion. It centers on the proactive characteristics of children from infancy through adolescence, particularly the capacity of children to provoke hostile and negative reactions from their parents (as well as siblings and peers). Next, we follow one line of evidence, concerning the development of antisocial behavior in children and adolescents, for three reasons. First, this line of development has been particularly well studied by genetically informed designs. Second, recent data suggest that variations among children along a continuum of behavior, from socially responsible to severely antisocial, are heavily influenced by genetic factors. Third, antisocial and aggressive behavior in the marital partner and parent-to-be is a substantial risk factor for highly problematic marital parent–child relationships.

Children invoke many other forms of reactions from caretakers and peers. However, it is the arena of the provoking child that we now have genetically informed data that give us a picture of how malleable genetic influences may be, using modifications of the psychological intervention that we already employ. Elsewhere, we have reviewed findings that some genetic influences may be more malleable than many of the corrosive psychosocial influences of neighborhood decay, grinding poverty, ethnic prejudice, severe early childhood deprivation, and sustained, unmitigated trauma (Reiss & Leve, 2007).

Heritable characteristics of children play an important role in evoking negative parental reactions. The NEAD study (Reiss, 2000) showed that parenting toward MZ twins was more similar than parenting toward DZ twins and full siblings, and parenting was less similar still for half-siblings and genetically unrelated siblings. Indeed, approximately 60% of the differences among families on measures of negative parenting could be accounted for by genetically influenced behavior of the children.

A surprising finding from this study was that the same genetic factors in the adolescent that influenced parent–child negative interaction also influenced antisocial behavior. As explained above, we know that because we were able to predict antisocial behavior in one sibling from the parent–child relationship of the other. We could make this prediction more effectively in MZ twins than in DZ twins (rDZ = .34) and even less effectively in genetically unrelated siblings (Pike, McGuire, Hetherington, Reiss, & Plomin, 1996; Reiss et al., 2000).

At first, this finding seemed like a refutation of the importance of family in the development of antisocial behavior. However, evidence is now suggesting that the genetic effects, in large measure, affect family process first, and subsequent to that effect the troubled family process leads to pathological outcomes (Neiderhiser, 1995). Findings of this kind suggest that a heritable characteristic of the child evokes a distinctive parental response which then amplifies the child's characteristic into a serious maladjustment. Two more recent studies, using different statistical models, suggest a more reciprocal process, with parent and child characteristics playing equal roles in provoking the other (Burt, McGue, Krueger, & Iacono, 2005; Larsson, Viding, Rijsdijk, & Plomin, 2008).

We are learning a lot about what aspects of children evoke these parental responses. So far the two most potent aspects are temperamental aggressiveness (Narusyte, Andershed, Neiderhiser, & Lichtenstein, 2007) and emotional volatility. Indeed, recent unpublished findings from our group suggest these characteristics are a provocative stimulus for harsh and critical parental response and make parents more sensitive to a full range of heritable and provocative features of their children above and beyond emotional volatility. In contrast, some parents maintain warmth with their volatile and aggressive children and do not react harshly. In a strong case of gene–environment interaction (G × E), such parental reactions almost completely blunt the genetic influence on antisocial behavior (Feinberg et al., 2007). Dick and colleagues (2007) found similarly G × E effects on the blunting of the heritability of antisocial behavior by effective parental monitoring

How do these findings relate to marital dynamics? They suggest that at least some of genetically influenced personality features that play havoc for marriage, and for the "spillover" of marital conflict into parent–child relationships, are not indicators of immutable, "hard-wired" biological processes. Indeed, the concept of "hard-wired" is vanishing from many areas of neurobiology as we learn more not only about the plasticity inherent in gene expression but in many of the neuroregulatory systems with which they are associated.

In summary, we suggest that genetic factors such as infant temperaments help shape the parent–infant relationship, which, through environmental pathways help shapes the child's behavioral development. Indeed, in children as young as 5 months of age these evocative process are quite noticeable (Forget-Dubois et al., 2007), accounting for as much as 30% of variance among mothers in their hostile and negative reactions to their infants. In our EGDS, unpublished findings suggest that a substantial portion of the genetic effects on child impulsive and uncooperative behavior at 18 months and on diminished executive function at 27 months go "through" parental response to child emotional volatility much earlier in development. In this case, the mediating parental response style is overprotection. The genetically influenced characteristic of emotional volatility evokes overreactive parenting in the adoptive parents, which, in turn, leads to impulsive and uncooperative behavior at 18 months and diminished executive function at 27 months. Indeed, evidence both from genetic and nongenetic research suggests that a central dynamic of child and adolescence is a series of evocative response cycles. Heritable features in children evoke the response of primary caretakers: these evoked responses influence not only parenting but marital conflict about the child (Reiss, 2000). Genetic factors also evoke reactions from siblings (Pike et al., 1996), teachers and best friends (Manke, McGuire, Reiss, Hetherington, & Plomin, 1995), and peer groups (Harakeh et al., 2008; Iervolino et al., 2002). The reactions from the environment then play a role in shaping the child's future behavioral development. Thus, the environment both mediates genetic pathways and moderates those pathways.

GENES, MARITAL DYNAMICS, AND CHILD PROACTION: RELEVANCE FOR CLINICAL RESEARCH AND PRACTICE?

Clinicians, when confronting any body of research on social and psychological mechanisms relevant to child development, will sift through it for threads that reframe their own thinking about their patients. We offer a few ideas, knowing that they may be very wide of the mark because of undeniable gaps between the procedures and measurements of research and the understanding that clinicians achieve with their patients and because the findings have many gaps. With these caveats, we offer three broad ideas for consideration.

The first idea restates the themes already treated in this chapter. Might the emerging links between genes and behavior suggest novel pharmacological treatments or help us better match patients with a specific drug (and hence realize "personalized medicine"). Second, genetic research on the family has already identified several dynamic systems that may, in the near future, offer novel points of entry for behavioral interventions that might reduce genetic risk. The first point of entry is an ongoing tension between child provocation and parental response. As noted, most parents of children who are high in temperamental aggressiveness or emotional volatility are tempted to respond with hostility, criticism, and undermining of the child. But some parents do not respond in this way, and the preliminary evidence is that in their resistance to provocation lies the potential for sharply reducing their children's genetic liability for clinical levels of antisocial behaviors. A second point of dynamic tension is in the marital relationship. Genes play little or no role in whom adults (at least, women) pick for a mate. There is much to be learned for prevention and intervention purposes here. Not only might we gain additional leverage on reducing the genetic risk for impaired parenting, much of which seems to "pass through" marriage, but we might gain leverage on the prevention of depression in women as some of the genetic risk for that disorder also appears to "pass through" their marital relationships (Spotts et al., 2004). Genetically informed studies of these critical, dynamic points of tension within the family provide two opportunities for novel therapeutics. First, they help clarify precisely what are the genetically influenced provocative behaviors: what do they look like, when do they appear in development, what factors in the parent lead them to be highly sensitive to these provocation and respond with a counterattack? Second, these designs provide an opportunity to test whether interventions designed to shore up parents in such situations (and perhaps moderate the child's provocation) actually reduce genetic risk.

Third, these findings call attention to the unsurprising but central role of individual differences in personality and G × E effects from the earliest phases of a child's development. For example, we have observed in infants of birth mothers with antisocial behavior distinctive attentional fixation on a desired but unobtainable object. Behavior of this kind presages development of aggression later in development (Crockenberg, Leerkes, & Bárrigjó, 2008). However, this effect occurs only in infants whose rearing (adoptive) mother had elevated depressive or anxious symptoms (Leve et al., 2010). We carefully rule out the possibility that this effect is due to intrauterine factors such as exposure to drugs and can conclude that the link between birth mother and her child placed at birth reflects both a genetic risk as well as its buffering by adoptive mothers free of affective symptoms. This is an example of G × E. One can think of the mechanism for this interaction as reflecting the differential reactivity of mothers to genetically influenced proactive behaviors of their infants. The cumulative findings we have reviewed provide a frame for exploring therapeutic strategies aimed at helping mothers moderate their heightened reactions to their child's behavior in order to fashion effective parental strategies.

Clinicians and clinical trials rarely evaluate directly the marital or parenting outcomes of their treatments. We have failed to find a single randomized controlled trial of pharmacotherapy for any adult disorder for which there was systematic evaluation of its impact on marriage or parenting. Recently, Weissman and colleagues (2006; Talati et al., 2007) reported the impact of successful pharmacotherapeutic treatment of maternal depression on the mental health of their children. However, the findings were drawn from an efficacy trial without randomization, and the results required comparing mothers who had improved versus those who did not, all of whom were assigned to a treatment condition. We hope that future randomized controlled trials will evaluate the impact on marital, parenting, and family processes.

ACKNOWLEDGMENT

The writing of this chapter, and some of the data analysis reported in it, was supported by Grant No. R01 HD042608 from the National Institute of Child Health and Human Development; the National Institute on Drug Abuse; and the Office of the Director, National Institutes of Health, U.S. Public Health Service Commissioned Corps.

REFERENCES

Brook, J. S., Brook, D. W., Ning, Y., Whiteman, M., & Finch, S. J. (2006). The relationship of personality and behavioral development from adolescence to young adulthood and subsequent parenting behavior. *Psychological Reports, 99*(1), 3–19.

Burt, S., McGue, M., Krueger, R. F., & Iacono, W. G. (2005). How are parent–child conflict and childhood externalizing symptoms related over time?: Results from a genetically informative cross-lagged study. *Development and Psychopathology, 17*(1), 145–165.

Caspi, A., Elder, G. H., Jr., & Bem, D. J. (1987). Moving against the world: Life-course patterns of explosive children. *Developmental Psychology, 23*(2), 308–313.

Champagne, F. A., Weaver, I. C. G., Diori, J., Dymov, S., Szyf, M., & Meaney, M. J. (2006). Maternal care associated with methylation of the estrogen receptor-alpha1b promoter and estrogen receptor-alpha expression in the medial pre-optic area of female offspring. *Endocrinology, 147*(6), 2909–2915.

Clinton, S., Miller, S., Watson, S. J., & Akil, H. (2008). Prenatal stress does not alter innate novelty-seeking behavioral traits, but differentially affects individual differences in neuroendocrine stress responsivity. *Psychoneuroendocrinology, 33*(2), 162–177.

Coyne, L. W., Low, C. M., Miller, A. L., Seifer, R., & Dickstein, S. (2007). Mothers' empathic understanding of their toddlers: Associations with maternal depression and sensitivity. *Journal of Child and Family Studies, 16*(4), 483–497.

Crockenberg, S. C., Leerkes, E. M., & Bárrigjó, P. S. (2008). Predicting aggressive behavior in the third year from infant reactivity and regulation as moderated by maternal behavior. *Development and Psychopathology, 20*(1), 37–54.

Cui, M., Donnellan, M. B., & Conger, R. D. (2007). Reciprocal influences between parents' marital problems and adolescent internalizing and externalizing behavior. *Developmental Psychology, 43*(6), 1544–1552.

Dick, D. M. (2007). Identification of genes influencing a spectrum of externalizing psychopathology. *Current Directions in Psychological Science, 16*(6), 331–335.

Dick, D. M., Viken, R., Purcell, S., Kaprio, J., Pulkkinen, L., & Rose, R. J. (2007). Parental monitoring moderates the importance of genetic and environmental influences on adolescent smoking. *Journal of Abnormal Psychology, 116*(1), 213–218.

Dunn, J., & Plomin, R. (1986). Determinants of maternal behaviour towards 3-year-old siblings. *British Journal of Developmental Psychology, 4*(2), 127–137.

Erel, O., & Burman, B. (1995). Interrelatedness of marital relations and parent–child relations: A meta-analytic review. *Psychological Bulletin, 118*(1), 108–132.

Fearon, R. M., van IJzendoorn, M. H., Fonagy, P., Bakermans-Kranenburg, M. J., Schuengel, G., & Bokhorst, C. L. (2006). In search of shared and nonshared environmental factors in security of attachment: A behavior–genetic study of the association between sensitivity and attachment security. *Developmental Psychology, 42*(6), 1026–1040.

Feinberg, M. E., Button, T. M., Neiderhiser, J. M., Reiss, D., & Hetherington, E. M. (2007). Parenting and adolescent antisocial behavior and depression: Evidence of genotype × parenting environment interaction. *Archives of General Psychiatry, 64*(4), 457–465.

Forget-Dubois, N., Boivin, M., Dionne, G., Pierce, T., Tremblay, R. E., & Pérusse, D. (2007). A longitudinal twin study of the genetic and environmental etiology of maternal hostile–reactive behavior during infancy and toddlerhood. *Infant Behavior and Development, 30*(3), 453–465.

Foster, C. J. E., Garber, J., & Durlak, J. A. (2008). Current and past maternal depression, maternal interaction behaviors, and children's externalizing and internalizing symptoms. *Journal of Abnormal Child Psychology, 36*(4), 527–537.

Ganiban, J. M., Ulbricht, J. A., Spotts, E. L., Lichtenstein, P., Reiss, D., Hansson, K., et al. (2009). Understanding the role of personality in explaining associations between marital quality and parenting. *Journal of Family Psychology, 23*(5), 646–660.

Harakeh, Z., Neiderhiser, J. M., Spotts, E. L., Engels, R. C., Scholte, R. H., & Reiss, D. (2008). Genetic factors contribute to the association between peers and young adults smoking: Univariate and multivariate behavioral genetic analyses. *Addictive Behaviors, 33*(9), 1113–1122.

Harden, K. P., Turkheimer, E., Emery, R. E., D'Onofrio, B. M., Slutske, W. S., Heath, A. C., et al. (2007). Marital conflict and conduct problems in children of twins. *Child Development, 78*(1), 1–18.

Iervolino, A. C., Pike, A., Manke, B., Reiss, D., Hetherington, E. M., & Plomin, R. (2002). Genetic and environmental influences in adolescent peer socialization: Evidence from two genetically sensitive designs. *Child Development, 73*(1), 162–174.

Jocklin, V., McGue, M., & Lykken, D. T. (1996). Personality and divorce: A genetic analysis. *Journal of Personality and Social Psychology, 71*(2), 288–299.

Johnson, J. G., Cohen, P., Kasen, S., & Brook, J. S. (2008). Psychiatric disorders in adolescence and early adulthood and risk for child-rearing difficulties during middle adulthood. *Journal of Family Issues, 29*(2), 210–233.

Johnson, W., McGue, M., Krueger, R. F., & Bouchard, T. J., Jr. (2004). Marriage and personality: A genetic analysis. *Journal of Personality and Social Psychology, 86*(2), 285–294.

Landgraf, R., Frank, E., Aldag, J. M., Neumann, I. D., Sharer, C. A., Ren, X., al. (2003). Viral vector-mediated gene transfer of the vole V1a vasopressin receptor in the rat septum: Improved social discrimination and active social behaviour. *European Journal of Neuroscience, 18*(2), 403–411.

Larsson, H., Viding, E., Rijsdijk, F. V., & Plomin, R. (2008). Relationships between parental negativity and childhood antisocial behavior over time: A bidirectional effects model in a longitudinal genetically informative design. *Journal of Abnormal Child Psychology, 36*(5), 633–645.

Leve, L. D., Kerr, D. C., Shaw, D., Ge, X., Neiderhiser, J. M., Scaramella, L. V., et al. (2010). Infant pathways to externalizing behavior: Evidence of genotype Ã—environment interaction. *Child Development, 81*(1), 340–356.

Leve, L. D., Neiderhiser, J. M., Ge, X., Scaramella, L. V., Conger, R. D., Reid, J. B., et al. (2007). The Early Growth and Development Study: A prospective adoption design. *Twin Research and Human Genetics, 10*(1), 84–95.

Liu, D., Diorio, J., Tannenbaum, B., Caldji, C., Francis, D., Freedman, A., et al. (1997). Maternal care, hippocampal glucocorticoid receptors, and hypothalamic–pituitary–adrenal responses to stress. *Science, 277*, 1659–1662.

Lykken, D. T., & Tellegen, A. (1993). Is human mating adventitious or the result of lawful choice?: A twin study of mate selection. *Journal of Personality and Social Psychology, 65*(1), 56–68.

Manke, B., McGuire, S., Reiss, D., Hetherington, E. M., & Plomin, R. (1995). Genetic contributions to adolescents' extrafamilial social interactions: Teachers, best friends, and peers. *Social Development, 4*(3), 238–256.

Maughan, A., Cicchetti, D., Toth, S. L., & Rogosch, F. A. (2007). Early-occurring maternal depression and maternal negativity in predicting young children's emotion regulation and socioemotional difficulties. *Journal of Abnormal Child Psychology, 35*(5), 685–703.

McGuire, S., Manke, B., Saudino, K. J., Reiss, D., Hetherington, E. M., & Plomin, R. (1999). Perceived competence and self-worth during adolescence: A longitudinal behavioral genetic study. *Child Development, 70*(6), 1283–1296.

Meaney, M. J. (2001). Maternal care, gene expression, and the transmission of individual differences in stress reactivity across generations. *Annual Review of Neuroscience, 24*, 1161–1192.

Nair, H. P., & Young, L. J. (2006). Vasopressin and pair-bond formation: Genes to brain to behavior. *Physiology, 21*(2), 146–152.

Narusyte, J., Andershed, A.-K., Neiderhiser, J. M., & Lichtenstein, P. (2007). Aggression as a mediator of genetic contributions to the association between negative parent–child relationships and adolescent antisocial behavior. *European Child and Adolescent Psychiatry, 16*(2), 128–137.

Neiderhiser, J. M. (1995). Family environment and adjustment in adolescence: Genetic and environmental influences over time. *Dissertation Abstracts International: Section B: The Sciences and Engineering, 55*(9-B), 4144.

Neiderhiser, J. M., Reiss, D., Pederson, N. L., Lichtenstein, P., Spotts, E. L., Hansson, K., et al. (2004). Genetic and environmental influences on mothering of adolescents: A comparison of two samples. *Developmental Psychology, 40*(3), 335–351.

NICHD Network Early Child Care Research. (1999). Chronicity of maternal depressive symptoms, maternal sensitivity, and child functioning at 36 months. *Developmental Psychology, 35*(5), 1297–1310.

Pike, A., McGuire, S., Hetherington, E. M., Reiss, D., & Plomin, R. (1996). Family environment and adolescent depression and antisocial behavior: A multivariate genetic analysis. *Developmental Psychology, 32*(4), 590–603.

Pitkow, L. J., Sharer, C. A., Ren, X., Insel, T. R., Terwilliger, E. F., & Young, L. J. (2001). Facilitation of affiliation and pair-bond formation by vasopressin receptor gene transfer into the ventral forebrain of a monogamous vole. *Journal of Neuroscience, 21*(18), 7392–7396.

Plotsky, P. M., & Meaney, M. J. (1993). Early, postnatal experience alters hypothalamic corticotropin-releasing factor (CRF) mRNA, median eminence CRF content and stress-induced release in adult rats. *Brain Research: Molecular Brain Research, 18*(3), 195–200.

Reiss, D., & Leve, L. D. (2007). Genetic expression outside the skin: Clues to mechanisms of genotype × environment interaction. *Development and Psychopathology, 19*(4), 1005–1027.

Reiss, D., with Neiderhiser, J., Hetherington, E. M., & Plomin, R. (2000). *The relationship code: Deciphering genetic and social patterns in adolescent development.* Cambridge, MA: Harvard University Press.

Roberts, B. W., Kuncel, N. R., Shiner, R., Caspi, A., & Goldberg, L. R. (2007). The power of personality: The comparative validity of personality traits, socioeconomic status, and cognitive ability for predicting important life outcomes. *Perspectives on Psychological Science, 2*(4), 313–345.

Spotts, E. L., Neiderhiser, J. M., Ganiban, J., Reiss, D., Lichtenstein, P., Hansson, K., et al. (2004). Accounting for depressive symptoms in women: A twin study of associations with interpersonal relationships. *Journal of Affective Disorders, 82*(1), 101–111.

Talati, A., Wickramaratne, P. J., Pilowsky, D. J., Alpert, J. E., Cerda, G., Garber, J., et al. (2007). Remission of maternal depression and child symptoms among single mothers: A STAR*D-Child report. *Social Psychiatry and Psychiatric Epidemiology, 42*(12), 962–971.

Towers, H. (2003). Contributions of current family factors and life events to women's adjustment: Nonshared environmental pathways. *Dissertation Abstracts International: Section B. Sciences and Engineering, 63,* 6123.

Trentacosta, C. J., & Shaw, D. S. (2008). Maternal predictors of rejecting parenting and early adolescent antisocial behavior. *Journal of Abnormal Child Psychology, 36*(2), 247–259.

Tully, E. C., Iacono, W. G., & McGue, M. (2008). An adoption study of parental depression as an environmental liability for adolescent depression and childhood disruptive disorders. *American Journal of Psychiatry, 165*(9), 1148–1154.

Walum, H., Westberg, L., Henningsson, S., Neiderhiser, J. M., Reiss, D., Igl, W., et al. (2008, September 16). Genetic variation in the vasopressin receptor 1a gene (AVPR1A) associates with pair-bonding behavior in humans. *Proceedings of the National Academies of Sciences, 105*(37), 14153–14156.

Weaver, I. C., La Plante, P., Weaver, S., Parent, A., Sharma, S., Diorio, J., et al. (2001). Early environmental regulation of hippocampal glucocorticoid receptor gene expression: Characterization of intracellular mediators and potential genomic target sites. *Molecular and Cellular Endocrinology, 185*(1–2), 205–218.

Weissman, M. M., Pilowsky, D. J., Wickramaratne, P. J., Talati, A., Wisniewski, S. R., Fava, M., et al. (2006). Remissions in maternal depression and child psychopathology: A STAR*D-Child report. *Journal of the American Medical Association, 295*(12), 1389–1398.

CHAPTER 7

Gene–Environment Interactions for Delinquency

Promises and Difficulties

Guang Guo

BACKGROUND

Until recently, while studying individual traits and behaviors such as cognitive development, educational achievement, occupational attainment, mental health, binge drinking, smoking, and illegal drug use, most social scientists either assumed that individuals are the same at birth or treat the differences across individuals at birth as a "black box." When treated as a black box, intrinsic individual differences are typically subsumed by unobserved heterogeneity. Though it is possible to exercise some control over it via statistical methods (e.g., fixed effect models), unobserved heterogeneity is considered generally impenetrable and incomprehensible.

Now the spectacular advances in molecular genetics over the past few decades have made it possible to begin to decipher the black box. Evidence is mounting that substantial genetic variation exists across individuals. The year 2007 saw an unparalleled succession of discoveries in the genomics of complex traits (e.g., Frayling et al., 2007; Scott et al., 2007; Sladek et al., 2007; Steinthorsdottir et al., 2007; Zeggini et al., 2007). These studies identified genetic variants associated with acute lymphoblastic leukemia, obesity, type 2 diabetes mellitus, prostate cancer, breast cancer, and coronary heart disease.

The newly acquired confidence in the scientific community in the genetic findings for complex human traits has developed so rapidly that the American Association for the Advancement of Science chose human genetic variation as *Science*'s breakthrough of the year of 2007 (Pennisi, 2007). If individuals do have different genetic propensities for disease, then they might well differ in genetic propensities for cognitive development, educational achievement, occupational attainment, mental health, binge drinking, smoking, and illegal drug use. Thus social scientists will be compelled to reevaluate their long-standing related assumptions and strategies.

Genetics-Informed Social Sciences

For much of social sciences in which the emphasis is on understanding the influences of social context, these developments are challenges as well as opportunities. Social scientists are challenged to reexamine relevant areas in light of the new developments, which have given rise to opportunities to enhance their respective fields. By whether they are primarily geneticists/ medical researchers or social scientists, the opportunities and challenges are of two types. The first type focuses on understanding the effects of genes. In this context, the focus of a gene–environment interaction (G × E) could still be on effects of genes, that is, on how environmental effects moderate genetic effects. The second type advances social science models of how genes moderate environmental effects. It is in the context of the second type of challenges and opportunities that we propound the approach of genetics-informed social sciences.

Geneticists and medical researchers have increasingly recognized that social scientists' expertise in social context is essential for understanding many complex human diseases. The success of the Human Genome Project (Collins, Morgan, & Patrinos, 2003) and the HapMap Project (International HapMap Consortium, 2005) are improving the design and effectiveness of genetic studies of complex outcomes. The International HapMap Project is a multicountry endeavor to identify and catalogue genetic similarities and differences in human beings. The project is a collaboration among scientists and funding agencies from Japan, the United Kingdom, Canada, China, Nigeria, and the United States. These advances, however, do not lessen the need for understanding the social/environmental component of the puzzles. On the contrary, inadequate understanding of social environments has increasingly become a bottleneck for the rapid technological advances in molecular genetics. Recently, the HapMap Project (International HapMap Consortium, 2005), the National Human Genome Research Institute (Collins et al., 2003), and the Committee on Gene–Environment Interactions for Health Outcomes at the Institute of Medicine in the National Academies of Sciences (Hernandez & Blazer, 2006) called for heavy investment in information on social and cultural exposures and in longitudinal studies of adequate size that could obtain such information.

Our theoretical proposition is closely related to "personalized medicine"—a new major health care approach that has been accumulating evidence rapidly and which may become a major component of health care in the next several decades (Bottinger, 2007; Guttmacher & Collins, 2003, 2005). Personalized medicine uses genetic tests to place individuals in subcategories of persons who share statistical likelihood of susceptibility to a disease, adverse reaction to drug dosage, and favorable response to a medical treatment. The information is then used to develop personalized strategies for disease prevention and "designer" drugs to reduce adverse reactions and increase efficacy.

So far, cancer research has produced the most evidence for personalized medicine. The best known genetic test for disease susceptibility on the market is a test for the *BRCA1* and *BRCA2* variants (Nelson, Huffman, Fu, & Harris, 2005). The test identifies increased susceptibility for breast cancer and provides a basis for preventive measures such as earlier and more frequent mammography, prophylactic surgery, and chemoprevention.

The following example of tests for drug efficacy is also from cancer research. A substantial proportion of breast cancers (25%) is marked by overexpression of a cell surface protein called *HER2*. The overexpression of the *HER2* gene leads to more rapid tumor growth, higher risk of recurrence after surgery, and poorer response to standard chemotherapy (Ross & Fletcher, 1998). The development of the trastuzumab (Herceptin) therapy specifically targeted for tumors overexpressing *HER2* protein has greatly improved the survival rate of women with this deadly form of cancer. To determine *HER2* status, molecular diagnostic tests have been developed to identify *HER2*-positive patients by measuring either *HER2* protein levels or gene copy numbers (Dendukuri, Khetani, McIsaac, & Brophy, 2007).

Although there seems to be little doubt that the scientific foundation of personalized medicine will accrue rapidly, pointing to its growing weight in heath care, many potential economic, ethical, legal, and social complications remain. For example, many individuals may be reluctant to take beneficial genetic tests because of potential genetic discrimination in health insurance and at the workplace.

Genetics-informed social sciences take advantage of the information on genetic propensity to advance the understanding of effects of social context. The primary motivation for the approach is that individuals with different genetic propensity may respond to the same social context differently. In such a case, a social model that assumes a uniform social influence on all individuals would be unable to model empirical data adequately. Genetics-informed social sciences model different social context effects under different genetic circumstances, without prejudice regarding the direction of effects. The direction depends on a particular genotype and/or a particular social influence.

There are at least two specific ways through which genetics can advance social sciences: (1) isolating purer effects of social context from genetic confounders and (2) understanding how effects of social context are conditioned by genetic propensities through G × E analysis. These studies have immediate impact on policies and practices that rely on empirical findings of environmental effects by refining our understanding of those effects.

Many presumed effects of social context yielded by conventionally sociological models may be overestimated because of genetic confounding. For example, conventionally estimated effects of parental education on children's educational attainment may not be "purely" environmental because parents and children share 50% of genes. "Purer" effects of parental education can be estimated, to the extent that genetic measures that are correlated with parental education are included in the analysis. The current difficulty with this strategy is that many of these genetic measures have not yet been discovered. For this reason, G × E analysis will likely remain the most fruitful vehicle for some time to come for social scientists whose primary interest is to understand effects of social context.

Gene–Social-Control Interactions

G × E refers to the principle that an environment may influence how sensitive we are to the effects of a genotype and vice versa (Hunter, 2005). A classic example is that of phenylketonuria (PKU), an autosomal recessive disease that could potentially cause hopeless mental and physical degeneration. However, only individuals who have recessive mutations in the phenylalanine hydroxylase gene and who are exposed to phenylalanine in the diet are susceptible to PKU (Khoury, Adams, & Flanders, 1988). The disease or the gene expression can be effectively controlled by restricting the dietary intake of phenylalanine starting within the first month after birth.

An influential social science example comes from recent work by Caspi and colleagues (2002). Their study found that a functional polymorphism in monoamine oxidase A (*MAOA*) modifies the effect of maltreatment. Only maltreated children with a genotype generating low levels of *MAOA* expression tended to develop a violent behavior problem. Maltreated children with a genotype that produces high levels of *MAOA* activity were less affected. Likewise, the adverse effect of maltreatment was exacerbated for children with the genotype for high *MAOA* activity and muted for children with the genotype for low *MAOA* activity.

Two recent studies using twins and siblings reported evidence for G × E for educational performance, showing that under circumstances of social disadvantage genetic influence is suppressed. Guo and Stearns (2002) showed that heritability for a cognitive measure is much lower among those growing up in disadvantaged social environments than those living in "normal" environments, suggesting genetic potential's dependence on social environments. Turkheimer and colleagues (2003) analyzed scores on the Wechsler Intelligence Scale in a sample of 7-year-old twins from the National Collaborative Perinatal Project. Results demonstrated that the proportions of IQ variance attributable to genes and environment vary with socioeconomic status. These models suggest that in impoverished families, 60% of the variance in IQ is accounted for by the shared environment and the contribution of genes is close to zero; in affluent families, the result is almost exactly the opposite.

Because environmental measures used in a G × E study may be genetically influenced, animal models can be used to create genuine environmental conditions by manipulation. Suomi (2004) assigned rhesus monkeys to one of two groups at birth: mother-reared (MR) and nursery- and peer-reared (NPR). MR infants were reared in the first 6 months in a group that consisted of 8–12 adult females including their mothers. NPR infants were separated from their mothers at birth and reared in a neonatal nursery. From the 37th day on, each NPR monkey was placed with three other monkeys of similar ages; no adult was included in the group. Using these experimental monkeys, a number of studies demonstrated interactions between the *5-HTTLPR* polymorphism in the serotonin transporter gene (*5-HTT*) and rearing type. Among nursery- and peer-reared monkeys, compared with the *5-HTT*l/l* genotype, the *5-HTT*l/s* genotype had lower cerebrospinal fluid concentrations, an indicator of central nervous system (CNS) function (Bennett et al., 2002); higher adrenocorticotropic hormone (ACTH) levels during a separation/stress experiment (interpreted as exaggerated limbic–hypothalamic–pituitary–adrenal [LHPA] responses to stress) (Barr et al., 2004); lower visual orientation scores assessed on days 7, 14, 21, and 30 of life (Bennett et al., 2002); and increased level of alcohol consumption among females (Barr et al., 2004).

The mechanisms of G × E are understood only in a few isolated cases. A particularly interesting case is the interplay between maternal behavior of mother rats and the glucorticoid receptor gene for offspring's responses to stress (Meaney, Szyf, & Seckl, 2007). Epigenetics promises to be the key to revealing the mechanisms of how gene expression is regulated in response to environment. Meaney and colleagues (Weaver et al., 2004) discovered that rats' maternal behavior alters the dynamics of methylation and demethylation of the promoter in offspring's glucorticoid receptor genes. In response to stress, this receptor protein helps bring about gene expression in the brain. Methylation is observed only in the gene promoter shortly after birth (not before birth) and among offspring of low LG-ABN mothers. It is hypothesized that low LG-ABN nursing causes the methylation, which leads to lowered levels of gene expression and produces more stressed animals. These biochemical and behavioral changes are stable and tend to last for the remainder of an animal's life.

G × E IN CRIME AND DELINQUENCY

We next present summaries of G × E findings in crime and delinquency from two papers from our research group (Guo, Cai, Guo, Wang, & Harris, 2010; Guo, Roettger, & Cai, 2008). Our genotypes focused on three polymorphisms that have been found to relate to crime and delinquency in past studies. Our measures of the environment ranged from completely exogenous influences such as being reared by two biological parents to influences that might be partially driven by the child, such as being retained at a grade level and interacting with delinquent peers. Furthermore, we examined the interaction between genotype and age, knowing that age represents both a biological variable and an environmental–cultural variable.

The first study by Guo and colleagues (2008) had two specific objectives. First, we investigated the main effects of genetic propensities on serious and violent delinquency by adding—both separately and jointly—three genetic polymorphisms to a social control model of delinquency. The three genetic polymorphisms were the 30-bp promoter-region variable number tandem repeat (VNTR) in the *MAOA* gene, the 40-bp VNTR in the *DAT1* gene, and the TaqI polymorphism in the *DRD2* gene. Second, we examined potential interactive effects on serious and violent delinquency between the three genetic polymorphisms and social controls that included family, school, and social network processes.

The objective of the second study (Guo et al., 2010) was twofold: to provide credible evidence for a protective effect regarding the dopamine transporter gene (*DAT1*) and to show how the legal and social context may influence the strength of such an effect. Our first objective was to test if the 9R/9R genotype in the VNTR of the dopamine transporter gene (*DAT1*) has a protective effect against a spectrum of risky behaviors relative to the 9R/10R or 10R/10R genotype. Although previous work had examined the links between the *DAT1* gene and tobacco and alcohol consumption (Munafò, Clark, Johnstone, Murphy, & Walton, 2004; Sieminska, Buczkowski, Jassem, Niedoszytko, & Tkacz, 2009), no work had yet examined the link with a large number of health behaviors simultaneously in one single study sample: delinquency (a collection of criminal behaviors), number of sexual partners, binge drinking, drinking quantity, smoking quantity, smoking frequency, marijuana use, cocaine use, other illegal drug use (LSD, PCP, ecstasy, mushrooms, speed, ice, heroin, or pills), and seatbelt nonwearing. Our second objective examined whether the strength of the protection effect interacts with the lifecourse in adolescence and adulthood in such a way that can be explained by the age-specific legal status of a behavior.

Data Source and Measures

The data source for our analysis was the DNA subsample in the National Longitudinal Study of Adolescent Health (Add Health), which started as a nationally representative sample of about 20,000 adolescents in grades 7–12 in 1994–1995 (Wave I) in the United States (Harris et al., 2003). Add Health is longitudinal; initial interviews with respondents were followed by two additional in-home interviews in 1996 (Wave II) and 2001–2002 (Wave III). Our analysis used the sibling sample of Add Health because DNA measures collected at Wave III in 2002 are available only for this subset of the respondents. The subset consists of about 2,500 MZ twins, DZ twins, full biological siblings, and singletons. This study is based on approximately 1,000 males whose DNA, behavior, and social contextual data are available in Add Health.

For the analysis in the first article (Guo et al., 2008), we constructed a serious delinquency scale and a violent delinquency scale using 12 questions asked of all the Add Health respondents at Waves I–III. These two scales are variations of a type of scale widely used in contemporary research on delinquency and criminal behavior (Thornberry & Krohn, 2000). Our scales are closely related to the scales used by Hagan and Foster (2003) and Haynie (2001, 2003) in analysis of Add Health data and by Hannon (2003) in analysis of data from the 1979 National Longitudinal Study of Youth.

Following the delinquency literature (Hagan & Foster, 2003; Hannon, 2003; Haynie 2001), we divided the 12 items into the nonviolent and violent categories. Nonviolent delinquency includes stealing amounts larger or smaller than $50, breaking and entering, and selling drugs. Violent delinquency includes serious physical fighting that resulted in injuries needing medical treatment, use of weapons to get something from someone, involvement in physical fighting between groups, shooting or stabbing someone, deliberately damaging property, and pulling a knife or gun on someone. The serious delinquency scale is based on the entire 12 items and the violence scale is based on a subset (eight) of the 12 items.

The second article whose findings are summarized in this chapter examined a spectrum of 10 risky behaviors: delinquency, number of sexual partners, binge drinking, drinking quantity, smoking quantity, smoking frequency, marijuana use, cocaine use, other illegal drug use (LSD, PCP, ecstasy, mushrooms, speed, ice, heroin, or pills), and seatbelt nonwearing.

At Wave III, in collaboration with the Institute for Behavioral Genetics in Boulder, Colorado, Add Health collected, extracted, and quantified

DNA samples from the sibling subsample. The articles report findings from three genetic polymorphisms in three genes: a 40-bp VNTR polymorphism in the 3' region of the *DAT1* gene; a polymorphic TaqIA restriction endonuclease site about 2500 bp downstream from the coding region of the *DRD2* gene; and the 30-bp VNTR in the promoter region of the *MAOA* gene. The additional details on these genetic polymorphisms can be found at the Add Health website.

G × E Effects for Serious Delinquency and Violent Behavior

Data analyses yielded myriad G × E effects that support the hypothesis that genetic effects on serious delinquency and violent behavior are moderated by life experiences. The *DRD2*178/304* genotype has an effect on these outcomes, but the effect is almost completely mitigated by having a regular meal with parents (Figure 7.1). The *MAOA*2R* genotype has an effect on these outcomes, but this effect is entirely mitigated under circumstances in which the child has never repeated a grade in school (Figure 7.2). The *DRD2*178/304* genotype has an effect on these outcomes, but this effect is sharply mitigated under circumstances in which both biological parents remain in the family home (Figure 7.3). Finally, the *DRD2*178/304* genotype has an effect, but this effect is mitigated in circumstances in which the youth's friends report engaging in relatively little delinquent behavior (Figure 7.4). In all of these effects, the effect of the risky genotype is muted when the child is reared in a favorable environment of having regular meals with parents or two biological parents or when the child is able to maintain a favorable environment through passing grades or avoiding delinquent peers.

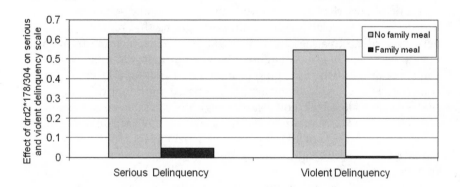

FIGURE 7.1. The effect of *DRD2*178/304* genotype depends on whether having regular meals with parents.

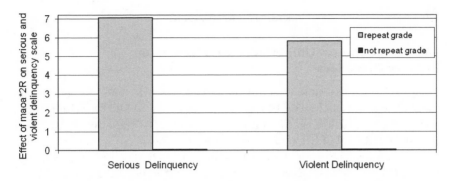

FIGURE 7.2. The effect of *MAOA*2R* genotype depends on whether having repeated a grade.

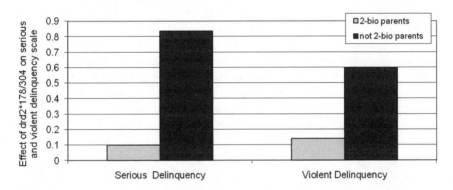

FIGURE 7.3. The effect of *DRD2*178/304* genotype depends on whether both biological parents are present.

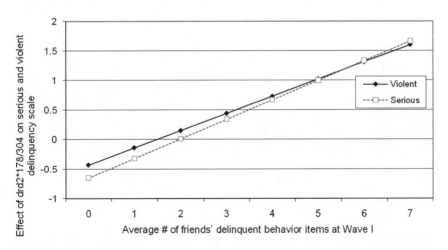

FIGURE 7.4. The effect of *DRD2*178/304* genotype depends on friends' delinquent behavior.

Gene–Age Interaction Effects for a Spectrum of Risky Behaviors

Figure 7.5 plots the main effect of the *DAT1 Any10R* genotype relative to the *9R/9R* genotype for the 10 risky behaviors. The results for delinquency and seatbelt usage are based on linear regression. For these two behaviors, the estimated level of behavior is plotted for the two genotypes. For the levels of delinquency, the indices are 1.02 and 1.02 + 0.58 = 1.60, respectively for the *9R/9R* and *Any10R* genotypes. The difference between 1.02 and 1.60 is statistically significant with a *p*-value of 0.03. For the other eight behaviors, count ratios are plotted, with the count of the *9R/9R* genotype set as one. For example, individuals with the *Any10R* genotype reported about 72% (1/0.58 = 1.72) more sexual partners than individuals with the *9R/9R* genotype, and the associated *p*-value is 0.0015.

The interaction model was not estimated for *number of sexual partners* because unlike the other behavior measures, number of partners measures the lifetime cumulative number of partners at each Add Health Wave and is thus inappropriate for gene–lifecourse analysis. The main effect analysis forces the protective effect to be constant over adolescence and young adulthood, estimating an average effect over the age range of 13–25. If the protective effect is only present in a portion of the age range and not in another, averaging over the effects in both portions may yield an effect that is weaker, less statistically significant, or statistically nonsignificant. Thus, a nonsignificant main effect does not necessarily indicate an absence of a protective effect. A gene–lifecourse interaction model tests if a protective effect is only present in a portion of the age range of 13–25.

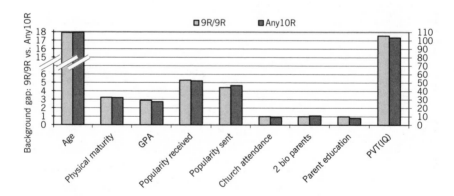

FIGURE 7.5. Behavior gap between the *DAT1*9R/9R* and the *DAT1*Any10R* genotypes among white males: Ten risky behaviors.

To interpret the findings of the interaction analysis, we graphed the protective effect of the *DAT1*9R/9R* genotype relative to the *DAT1*Any10R* genotype as a function of age over adolescence and young adulthood. Figure 7.6 has nine parts, one for each behavior measure. The lines indicate the predicted values from regression analysis. The lines in Parts 1 and 9, based on linear regression, represent the predicted levels of delinquency and seatbelt wearing, respectively. Parts 2 through 8, based on Poisson regression, present the predicted count of a particular behavior. For example, Parts 6–8 plot the number of times that study participants used an illicit drug over the previous 30 days. The prevalence is reflected by both the level of the lines and the unit on the vertical axis. For instance, the prevalence rate of marijuana use is about 10 times as high as cocaine use.

The nine graphs display patterns of the gene–lifecourse interaction. For four behaviors (binge drinking, drinking quantity, smoking quantity, and smoking frequency), the protective effect of *9R/9R* diminishes in young adulthood. In contrast, the protective effect remains large in both adolescence and young adulthood for marijuana use and other illegal drugs and increases sharply for cocaine use. For seatbelt wearing, the protective effect becomes prominent only after the ages of 17–18.

These findings are extremely important in showing that genetic effects vary not only with the environment as we traditionally construe it, but also with age. Age might be construed as a strictly biological variable, but age also represents changing culture and environmental treatment by authorities.

One intriguing insight from this analysis is that all of the patterns of gene–lifecourse interactions exhibited in Figure 7.6 can be explained by one single factor: the age-specific legal status of the behaviors or the age-specific social tolerance for the behaviors. The common pattern of lifecourse–gene interaction for binge drinking, drinking quantity, smoking quantity, and smoking frequency can be explained by the legal age for alcohol and smoking. In all of these cases, the protective effect is more prominent during adolescence when drinking and smoking are illegal than during young adulthood when drinking and smoking are becoming legal and more accepted.

The National Minimum Drinking Age Act of 1984 required all states to raise the legal age for purchase and public possession of alcohol to 21 and tied this to the highway funds (Mooney, Gramling, & Forsyth, 1992). All 50 states in the United States attempt to limit youth access to cigarettes by banning sales to individuals younger than 18 or 19 years old (Ahmad, 2005; Ahmad & Billimek, 2007). In spite of these alcohol and tobacco laws, underage drinking and smoking are common in the United States (Johnston, O'Malley, & Bachman, 2000). Our empirical evidence

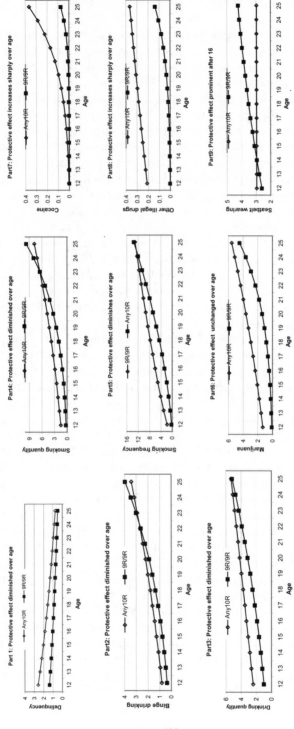

FIGURE 7.6. The protective effect of the *DAT1*9R/9R* genotype relative to the *DAT1*Any10R* genotype depends on age and legal status of the behavior in adolescence and young adulthood: Parts 1–9.

132

shows that underage drinking and smoking do not happen randomly. Individuals with the *9R/9R* genotype are less likely to engage in drinking and smoking; however, this protective effect tends to diminish and disappear when drinking and smoking are tolerated as these individuals grow from adolescence into young adulthood. In young adulthood, more legally and socially tolerated drinking and smoking are not considered as risky as in adolescence.

The pattern of gene–lifecourse interaction for illicit drug use (Parts 6–8) can also be explained by the same legal/social factor. Illegal drugs in this study are measured by three variables: *marijuana, cocaine*, and *other illegal drugs*. These illicit drugs differ from alcohol and tobacco in at least two important aspects (Goode, 2008). First, compared with the age-specific legal restrictions for the possession and sale of alcohol and tobacco, these drugs are decidedly illegal and illegal for all ages. Second, the prevalence rates of these drugs are much lower than those for alcohol and tobacco. Marijuana is by far the most commonly used illicit drug in the United States and worldwide; still, the possession and sale of any quantity of marijuana is prohibited by federal law in all but 12 states. In contrast to drinking and smoking, where the protective effect of *9R/9R* quickly diminishes beyond adolescence because of legal and social acceptance of drinking and smoking in young adulthood, the protective effect of *9R/9R* for illicit drug use continues beyond adolescence because illicit drug use in young adulthood is no more socially and legally tolerated than in adolescence.

Seatbelt wearing represents a third pattern of gene–lifecourse interaction. The much larger protective effect of *9R/9R* after the ages of 15–16 is not accidental; it can be explained by the legal driving age of 16 in the United States. The legal driving age is much more observed than the legal age for alcohol and/or tobacco probably because access to a car is much harder than access to alcohol/tobacco and because the perceived consequences of driving a car below the legal age are more severe than using alcohol and tobacco below the legal age. Before the legal driving age, an adolescent is not driving, and his or her friends are likely not driving. An adolescent under the legal driving age is much more likely to be under the supervision of an adult than when he or she is over 16 when he or she would have much greater freedom to decide whether to wear a seatbelt, hence the increased protective effect after age 16.

Delinquency represents a distinct case. The protective effect of *9R/9R* against delinquency is most pronounced during early and mid-adolescence; it declines thereafter (Part 1 in Figure 7.6). The delinquency scale is designed to capture a wide range of serious illegal behaviors that could result in state sanction of arrest, conviction, and incarceration. That delinquency is illegal at all ages suggests a constant protective effect across ages. However, unlike alcohol use, tobacco use, and illicit drug use, which peak in young adulthood, delinquency reaches the highest level in adolescence. The sharp decline of delinquency from adolescence to young adulthood has been observed and documented universally in different cultures and across historical time (Hirschi, 1969). Part 1 in Figure 7.6 shows that the level of delinquency declines sharply for both the *Any10R* genotype and the *9R/9R* genotype, more so for the former than the latter. Our interpretation of the gene–lifecourse interaction is the universal and dramatic reduction in delinquency beyond adolescence is itself an immense protective factor. The age protection is so large that it renders the protection of *9R/9R* less noteworthy.

CONCLUSION

We begin our more general assessment of the prospect of gene–environment research by examining the findings from a 1942 study on aggression using highly inbred strains of mice (Ginsburg & Allee, 1942). Contrasting these earlier findings with the current molecular genetic findings may enable us to illustrate some of the difficulties facing gene–environment studies.

Before the DNA era, genetic influences could be estimated from highly inbred strains of mice—mice that had been inbred for more than 10 generations of brother–sister mating. As a result, each stock of animals was nearly pure breeding. These animals were characterized by small genetic differences within a stock and large genetic differences between stocks. Different levels and patterns of aggressive behavior across stocks were attributed to genetic influences.

When assisted by researchers, mice of a pacific strain could be rendered aggressive through winning fights. Similarly, mice of an aggressive strain could be rendered pacific by experiencing defeats. Although social hierarchy was largely determined by fighting, the hierarchy was not fixed. Manipulation of winning or losing by researchers could move animals upward or downward. However, it was far easier to move a high-status mouse downward by engineered defeats than to move a low-status mouse upward. Mice lowest in social scale showed extreme subordination. Mice with middle positions were more easily moved in either direction.

These findings were essentially gene–experience interaction or G × E in contemporary terminology. They indicate that genetic influences were not deterministic and that there should be plenty of G × E effects on behaviors such as aggression, at least for mice. However, abundant estimates of G × E effects from animal experiments do not necessarily suggest similar G × E effects could be estimated from observational human studies. We discuss another major complicating factor for G × E research before attempting to link the mice findings to current G × E efforts.

Large-scale gene–environment studies of humans are possible today because single nucleotide polymorphism (SNP) genotyping technology has improved dramatically in the past several years (Kwok & Chen, 2003). Technology has been developed that allows many (>1,000) SNPs to be genotyped in the same reaction, or multiplexed (Fan et al., 2003; Hardenbol et al., 2003; Kennedy et al., 2003; Matsuzaki et al., 2004; Patil et al., 2001). As a result, genotype costs have been reduced more than 50-fold from $1–2/genotype down to about $.01–.05/genotype. This increased throughput has been coupled with improved genotype accuracy and completion rates. For example, the Infinium technology available from Illumina is highly cost-effective for large-scale genotyping and its genotypes are highly accurate (>99.9%) and successful (>99.8%) (Gunderson, Steemers, Lee, Mendoza, & Chee, 2005; Steemers et al., 2006). Many studies published over the past few years have genotyped 300,000–1,000,000 genetic markers for each individual. For social scientists who routinely work with 10, 20, or even 30 independent variables, the sheer numbers of genetic markers present a huge methodological challenge. So far, genomewide association studies (GWAS) have focused on estimating genetic main effects, which is typically done by including one SNP in a regression at a time. The resulting multiple testing for the initial analysis was addressed by setting p at an extremely low value of 5×10^{-8}.

Two major difficulties are facing research on G × E in the current era of GWAs, both of which are related to statistical power: (1) the issue of multiple testing for G × E analysis is many times more daunting than main effect analysis and (2) observational data tend not to have a lot of statistical power for estimating gene–environmental effects.

In a GWAS with 1 million SNPs, an investigation of G × E effects could easily involve another several millions tests. Does this mean the p-values need to be dramatically reduced further? This difficulty is likely why no serious attempt has been made in GWAS in estimating G × E effects. While the 1942 mice study showed abundant G × E effects, it may not bode well for G × E analysis with observational data. The mice study has a much better control for genetic background, and for environmental influences. The researchers in the mice experiment could implement one factor and only one factor at a time. In contrast, the phenotypes captured in human observational studies are results of a large number of factors in real life. Even if we could identify factors we are interested in studying, individuals who are subject to those factors and other potential confounders are likely to be quite small.

Thus, although the general consensus is that G × E are part of the links between genetic heritage and complex human traits—especially human behaviors—the work that takes into account multiple genes, epigenetic markers, environmental factors, and the interactions among these sources remains enormously complicated.

ACKNOWLEDGMENTS

This research uses data from Add Health, a program project designed by J. Richard Udry, Peter S. Bearman, and Kathleen Mullan Harris, and funded by Grant No. P01-HD31921 from the National Institute of Child Health and Human Development, with cooperative funding from 17 other agencies (*www.cpc.unc.edu/ addhealth/contract.html*). Special acknowledgment is due to Andrew Smolen and John K. Hewitt of the Institute for Behavior Genetics, University of Colorado, for DNA isolation and genotyping. We gratefully acknowledge support from the National Institutes of Health: Grant Nos. P01-HD31921 to Add Health, and R03 HD042490-02 to Guang Guo, R03 HD053385-01 to Guang Guo; and support from the National Science Foundation: Grant No. SES-0210389 to Guang Guo.

REFERENCES

Ahmad, S. (2005). Closing the youth access gap: The projected health benefits and cost savings of a national policy to raise the legal smoking age to 21 in the United States. *Health Policy, 75*(1), 74–84.

Ahmad, S., & Billimek, J. (2007). Limiting youth access to tobacco: Comparing the long-term health impacts of increasing cigarette excise taxes and raising the legal smoking age to 21. *Health Policy, 80*, 378–391.

Barr, C. S., Newman, T. K., Lindell, S., Shannon, C. Champoux, M., Lesch, K. P., et al. (2004). Interaction between serotonin transporter gene variation and rearing condition in alcohol preference and consumption in female primates. *Archives of General Psychiatry, 61*, 1146–1152.

Barr, C. S., Newman, T. K., Shannon, C., Parker, C., Dvoskin, R. L., Becker, M. L., et al. (2004). Rearing condition and rh5-HTTLPR interact to influence limbic–hypothalamic–pituitary–adrenal axis response to stress in infant macaques. *Biological Psychiatry, 55*, 733–738.

Bennett, A. J., Lesch, K. P., Heils, A., Long, J. C., Lorenz, J. G., Shoaf, S. E., et al. (2002). Early experience and serotonin transporter gene variation interact to influence primate CNS function. *Molecular Psychiatry, 7*, 118–122.

Bottinger, E. P. (2007). Foundations, promises and uncertainties of personalized medicine. *Mount Sinai Journal of Medicine, 74*, 15–21.

Caspi, A., McClay, J., Moffitt, T. E., Mill, J., Martin, J., Craig, I. W., et al. (2002). Role of genotype in the cycle of violence in maltreated children. *Science, 297*, 851–854.

Collins, F. S., Morgan, M., & Patrinos, A. (2003). The Human Genome Project: Lessons from large-scale biology. *Science, 300*, 286–290.

Dendukuri, N., Khetani, K., McIsaac, M., & Brophy, J. (2007). Testing for HER2-positive breast cancer: A systematic review and cost-effectiveness analysis. *Canadian Medical Association Journal, 176*, 1429–1434.

Fan, J. B., Oliphant, A., Shen, R., Kermani, B. G., Garcia, F., Gunderson, K. L., et al. (2003). Highly parallel SNP genotyping. *Cold Spring Harbor Symposium in Quantitative Biology, 68*, 69–78.

Frayling, T. M., Timpson, N. J., Weedon, M. N., Zeggini, E., Freathy, R. M.,

Lindgren, C. M., et al. (2007). A common variant in the FTO gene is associated with body mass index and predisposes to childhood and adult obesity. *Science, 316*, 889–894.

Ginsburg, B. E., & Allee, W. C. (1942). Some effects of conditioning on social dominance and subordination in inbred strains of mice. *Physiology and Zoology, 15*, 485–506.

Goode, E. (2008). *Drugs in American society*. New York: McGraw-Hill.

Gunderson, K. L., Steemers, F. J., Lee, G., Mendoza, L. G., & Chee, M. S. (2005). A genome-wide scalable SNP genotyping assay using microarray technology. *Nature Genetics, 37*, 549–554.

Guo, G., Cai, T., Guo, R., Wang, H., & Harris, K. M. (2010). The dopamine transporter gene, a spectrum of most common risky behaviors, and the legal status of the behaviors. *PLoS ONE, 5*(2), e9352.

Guo, G., Roettger, E. M., & Cai, T. (2008). The integration of genetic propensities into social control models of delinquency and violence among male youths. *American Sociological Review, 73*, 543–568.

Guo, G., & Stearns, E. (2002). The social influences on the realization of genetic potential for intellectual development. *Social Forces, 80*, 881–910.

Guttmacher, A. E., & Collins, F. S. (2003). Welcome to the genomic era. *New England Journal of Medicine, 349*, 996–998.

Guttmacher, A. E., & Collins, F. S. (2005). Realizing the promise of genomics in biomedical research. *Journal of the American Medical Association, 294*, 1399–1402.

Hagan, J., & Foster, H. (2003). S/he's a rebel: Toward a sequential stress theory of delinquency and gendered pathways to disadvantage in emerging adulthood. *Social Forces, 82*, 53–86.

Hannon, L. (2003). Poverty, delinquency, and educational attainment: Cumulative disadvantage or disadvantage saturation? *Sociological Inquiry, 73*, 575–594.

Hardenbol, P., Baner, J., Jain, M., Nilsson, M., Namsaraev, E. A., Karlin-Neumann, G. A., et al. (2003). Multiplexed genotyping with sequence-tagged molecular inversion probes. *Nature Biotechnology, 21*, 673–678.

Harris, K. M., Florey, F., Tabor, J., Bearman, P. S., Jones, J., & Udry, J. R. (2003). The National Longitudinal Study of Adolescent Health: Research design. Available at *www.cpc.unc.edu/projects/addhealth/design*.

Haynie, D. L. (2001). Delinquent peers revisited: Does network structure matter? *American Journal of Sociology, 106*, 1013–1057.

Haynie, D. L. (2003). Contexts of risk?: Explaining the link between girls' pubertal development and their delinquency involvement. *Social Forces, 82*, 355–397.

Hernandez, L. M., & Blazer, D. G. (2006). *Genes, behavior, and the social environment: Moving beyond the nature/nurture debate*. Washington, DC: National Academies Press.

Hirschi, T. (1969). *Causes of delinquency*. Los Angeles: University of California Press.

Hunter, D. J. (2005). Gene–environment interactions in human diseases. *Nature Reviews Genetics, 6*, 287–298.

International HapMap Consortium. (2005). A haplotype map of the human genome. *Nature, 437,* 1299–1320.

Johnston, L. D., O'Malley, P. M., & Bachman, J. G. (2000). *Monitoring the Future national survey results on adolescence drug use, 1975-2002: Vol. 1. Secondary school students* (NIH Pub. No. 03-5375). Bethesda, MD: National Institute of Drug Abuse.

Kennedy, G. C., Matsuzaki, H., Dong, S., Liu, W. M., Huang, J., Liu, G., et al. (2003). Large-scale genotyping of complex DNA. *Nature Biotechnology, 21,* 1233–1237.

Khoury, M. J., Adams, M. J., & Flanders, W. D. (1988). An epidemiologic approach to ecogenetics. *American Journal of Human Genetics, 42,* 89–95.

Kwok, P. Y., & Chen, X. (2003). Detection of single nucleotide polymorphisms. *Current Issues in Molecular Biology, 5,* 43–60.

Matsuzaki, H., Loi, H., Dong, S., Tsai, Y. Y., Fang, J., Law, J., et al. (2004). Parallel genotyping of over 10,000 SNPs using a one-primer assay on a high-density oligonucleotide array. *Genome Research, 14,* 414–425.

Meaney, M. J., Szyf, M., & Seckl, J. R. (2007). Epigenetic mechanisms of perinatal programming of hypothalamic–pituitary–adrenal function and health. *Trends in Molecular Medicine, 13,* 269–277.

Mooney, L. A., Gramling, R., & Forsyth, C. (1992). Legal drinking age and alcohol-consumption. *Deviant Behavior, 13,* 59–71.

Munafò, M. R., Clark, T. G., Johnstone, E. C., Murphy, M. F. G., & Walton, R. T. (2004). The genetic basis for smoking behavior: A systematic review and meta-analysis. *Nicotine and Tobacco Research, 6,* 583–597.

Nelson, H. D., Huffman, L. H., Fu, R. W., & Harris, E. L. (2005). Genetic risk assessment and BRCA mutation testing for breast and ovarian cancer susceptibility: Systematic evidence review for the U.S. Preventive Services Task Force. *Annals of Internal Medicine, 143,* 362–379.

Patil, N., Berno, A. J., Hinds, D. A., Barrett, W. A., Doshi, J. M., Hacker, C. R., et al. (2001). Blocks of limited haplotype diversity revealed by high-resolution scanning of human chromosome 21. *Science, 294,* 1719–1723.

Pennisi, E. (2007). Breakthrough of the year: Human genetic variation. *Science, 318,* 1842–1843.

Ross, J. S., & Fletcher, J. A. (1998). The HER-2/neu oncogene in breast cancer: Prognostic factor, predictive factor, and target for therapy. *Stem Cells, 16,* 413–428.

Scott, L. J., Mohlke, K. L., Bonnycastle, L. L., Willer, C. J., Li, Y., Duren, W. L., et al. (2007). A genome-wide association study of type 2 diabetes in Finns detects multiple susceptibility variants. *Science, 316,* 1341–1345.

Sieminska, A., Buczkowski, K., Jassem, E., Niedoszytko, M., & Tkacz, E. (2009). Influences of polymorphic variants of DRD2 and SLC6A3 genes, and their combinations on smoking in Polish population. *BMC Medical Genetics, 10.*

Sladek, R., Rocheleau, G., Rung, J., Dina, C., Shen, L., Serre, D., et al. (2007). A genome-wide association study identifies novel risk loci for type 2 diabetes. *Nature, 445,* 881–885.

Steemers, F. J., Chang, W., Lee, G., Barker, D. L., Shen, R., & Gunderson, K.

L. (2006). Whole-genome genotyping with the single-base extension assay. *Nature Methods, 3*, 31–33.

Steinthorsdottir, V., Thorleifsson, G., Reynisdottir, I., Benediktsson, R., Jonsdottir, T., Walters, G. B., et al. (2007). A variant in CDKAL1 influences insulin response and risk of type 2 diabetes. *Nature Genetics, 39*, 770–775.

Suomi, S. J. (2004). Genetic and environmental factors influencing the expression of impulsive aggression and serotonergic functioning in rhesus monkeys. In R. E. Tremblay, W. W. H. Hartup, & J. Archer (Eds.), *Developmental origins of aggression* (pp. 63–82). New York: Guilford Press.

Thornberry, T. P., & Krohn, M. D. (2000). The self-report method for measuring delinquency and crime. In *Criminal Justice 2000* (Vol. 4, pp. 33–38). Washington, DC: National Institute of Justice.

Turkheimer, E., Haley, A., Waldron, M., D'Onofrio, B., & Gottesman, I. I. (2003). Socioeconomic status modifies heritability of IQ in young children. *Psychological Science, 14*, 623–628.

Weaver, I. C. G., Cervoni, N., Champagne, F. A., D'Alessio, A. C., Sharma, S., Seckl, J. R., et al. (2004). Epigenetic programming by maternal behavior. *Nature Neuroscience, 7*, 847–854.

Zeggini, E., Weedon, N., Lindgren, C. M., Frayling, T. M., Elliott, K. S., Lango, H., et al. (2007). Replication of genome-wide association signals in UK samples reveals risk loci for type 2 diabetes. *Science, 316*, 1336–1341.

CHAPTER 8

Genes, Environment,
and Personalized Treatment
for Depression

Rudolf Uher

The last three decades have seen an expansion of knowledge on the occurrence and causation of various types of mental illness, including anxiety, depression, and schizophrenia. We know that most of these conditions start early in life, and that interplay between genetic predisposition and environmental adversity has a major role in their development. Large longitudinal studies of well-characterized cohorts in conjunction with molecular genetic technology have enabled the detection of specific causal mechanisms including measured genetic variants and environmental exposures. A substantial body of evidence has been accumulated over a relatively short period of time, providing a sketch of some general principles underlying the development of mental illness (Caspi, Hariri, Holmes, Uher, & Moffitt, Chapter 2, this volume). However, this rapidly advancing knowledge has so far not been applied to improve prevention and treatment of mental illness. Indeed, it has been suggested that in spite of progress in research and the wide availability of multiple treatment options, the burden of mental illness in the population remains undiminished (Lopez & Murray, 1998). This chapter explores the possibility that knowledge of causes of mental illness might inform its prevention and cure. The primary focus is on depression, a common disorder for which a substantial body of knowledge is available, but evidence on other disorders will be included where relevant. The aim is to provide a framework that may generalize to most types of mental illness.

DEPRESSION

Depression is a common and disabling condition characterized by protracted periods of low mood, lack of energy and enjoyment, pessimism, and disturbance of sleep and appetite. It may affect up to one in two individuals at some point of their life (Moffitt et al., 2009). In about half the cases, depression becomes a recurrent or chronic condition (Eaton et al., 2008) associated with substantial impairment, disability, and poor physical health (Lopez & Murray, 1998; ten Doesschate, Koeter, Bockting, & Schene, 2010). Depression doubles the risk of premature death (Cuijpers & Smit, 2002) and is responsible for the majority of suicides (Cavanagh, Carson, Sharpe, & Lawrie, 2003).

The presently used classifications of depression make no reference to causes or risk factors that contributed to its pathogenesis. Depression is diagnosed if a person has a specified number of symptoms (e.g., five out of 10) for at least 2 weeks. It is further classified as unipolar or bipolar based on the history of manic episodes. A number of treatment options are available for depression, including 30 different antidepressant drugs with proven efficacy in placebo-controlled trials (Lam et al., 2009; Thase & Denko, 2008), and an array of structured psychological treatments, which appear to have similar efficacy as antidepressant medication (DeRubeis, Siegle, & Hollon, 2008). While each of these treatments is, on average, more effective than no treatment or placebo, the differences between placebo and active treatment are small, therapeutic effects vary substantially from person to person, and it is presently impossible to predict who will respond to which treatment (Ghaemi, 2008; Kirsch et al., 2008; Parker, 2009). As a result, many individuals with depression have to undergo repeated treatment trials, prolonging disability, causing frustration, and risking adverse outcomes, including suicide (Perroud et al., 2009; Rush et al., 2006). Such a state of affairs is unsatisfactory and there have been calls for a shift from a one-treatment-fits-all approach to personalized treatment for depression (Holsboer, 2008; Parker, 2005).

GENE–ENVIRONMENT INTERACTIONS AND CAUSAL HETEROGENEITY

Converging evidence from multiple genetic association and gene–environment studies suggests several preliminary conclusions about the causation of mental illness. First, there are no common genetic variants that would have strong direct effects on the development of mental illness irrespective of environmental factors (Muglia et al., 2008; Need et al., 2009;

Stefansson et al., 2009; Sullivan et al., 2009; Wellcome Trust Case Control Consortium, 2007). Second, aspects of environmental adversity, including poverty, child neglect and abuse, bullying, and traumatic experiences, strongly contribute to the incidence of mental illness, but their impact is highly individually variable (Collishaw et al., 2007; Luthar, Sawyer, & Brown, 2006; Masten & Obradovic, 2006; Rutter, 2006; Vanderbilt-Adriance & Shaw, 2008). Third, in a number of cases it has been shown that common variants in functional candidate genes substantially moderate the impact of known environmental pathogens on individuals (Caspi et al., Chapter 2, this volume).

Although these gene–environment interactions (G × E) are regularly accompanied by strong overall effects of environmental exposures, there are no direct associations between the genetic variants and outcomes (Uher & McGuffin, 2008). This lack of genetic main effect is due to the fact that individuals carrying the "sensitive" genotype are often better off in the absence of adversity, suggesting that vulnerability is accompanied by adaptive advantages (Belsky et al., 2009; Uher, 2008b). Importantly, this pattern of risks indicates the presence of multiple causative pathways to mental illness: if a proportion of cases is caused by an interaction between genotype A and environmental exposure E but the alternative genotype B is associated with a higher risk of illness in the absence of E, then these excess cases must be caused by a mechanism distinct from the interaction between A and E (Uher, 2008b). In other words, individuals carrying the "resilient" genotype become ill just as often, but for different reasons. Thus, the presence of G × E not accompanied by a direct gene–outcome association is indicative of etiological heterogeneity within a disorder. In the specific case of the serotonin transporter length polymorphism (5-HTTLPR) and depression, there are indications that different environmental exposures may be pathogenic in carriers of the alternative genotypes: while individuals carrying the short alleles are more vulnerable to develop depression following childhood abuse and stressful life events (Caspi et al., 2003; Uher & McGuffin, 2008), those carrying the long alleles of 5-HTTLPR may be more likely to develop depressive symptoms in response to other challenges, such as hormonal changes associated with pregnancy (Doornbos et al., 2009; Sanjuan et al., 2008). It is plausible that subgroups of depression caused by such different mechanisms may respond to different types of treatment and that combined information on genotype and environmental history may inform treatment selection. In the following paragraphs I will summarize the evidence that genetic variation and environmental history can predict response to specific treatments and then explore ways of combining genetic and environmental data to inform personalized treatment selection.

BEYOND ONSET: GENES, ENVIRONMENTS, AND THE COURSE OF DEPRESSION

Most etiological research, including that presented in earlier chapters of this book, focuses on factors leading to the development of mental disorder in previously healthy individuals. Results of such research can be translated into preventive interventions that address causal risk factors. However, causal factors determining first onsets may be distinct from maintenance factors that shape the course of the disorder to be recurrent or chronic, rather than transient and self-limiting. Most burden and disability is related to chronicity and recurrence of depression and chronic forms of the disorder are more likely to present for treatment (Spijker et al., 2002). Therapeutic approaches have to interrupt the complex vicious cycles involved in the persistence of mental illness. Therefore, good understanding of the maintenance mechanisms is needed to inform treatment.

Longitudinal research on a cohort of U.K. women from disadvantaged backgrounds exemplifies the distinction between causation and perpetuation of depression (Brown et al., 2008). It found that the effect of childhood abuse and neglect on new onsets of depression is indirect and mediated by more proximal factors including quality of intimate relationship, self-esteem, and generation of stressful life events through putting oneself in situations where one is more likely to come to harm. However, childhood abuse and neglect have strong direct effects on perpetuation of depression into chronicity that are not explained by any measured proximal factors (Figure 8.1). These results suggest that early childhood experiences may be even more important for treatment than for etiological research. Numerous other studies confirm the strong association between early factors, such as child abuse and neglect, and chronic forms of depression (Brown & Moran, 1994; Hayden & Klein, 2001; Klein et al., 2009; Wiersma et al., 2009).

Any treatment aimed at restoring health in a depressed individual must act on the background of genetic predisposition and psychosocial history, which is written down in long-term memory traces that mediate the relation between early environmental factors and outcome of depression in adulthood. Research on animal models of depression suggests that these long-term memory traces could take the form of epigenetic modifications and that pharmacological and psychosocial treatment in adulthood may be able to counteract such changes through additional modifications rather than reverting them (Tsankova et al., 2006; Uher, 2008b). Figure 8.2 shows how long-term memory traces in the form of epigenetic modifications may build upon a genetic disposition in the genesis of a mental disorder and how treatment acts on the background of these layered traces of past experience. While both pharmacological and psychosocial interventions have the

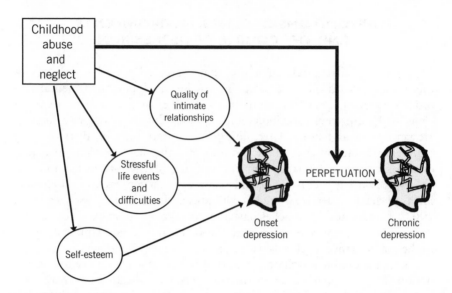

FIGURE 8.1. The role of child abuse and neglect in the onset and maintenance of depression. Most of the association between child abuse and neglect and new depression onsets can be explained by measured proximal factors, including stressful life events, quality of intimate relationship, and low self-esteem. The bold arrow shows a strong direct effect of childhood abuse and neglect on the maintenance of depression, which can not be explained by any measured proximal factors. Data from Brown, Craig, and Harris (2008).

potential to modify such long-standing vulnerabilities, detailed knowledge of specific genetic variants and a history of adversity over the stages of individual development would be needed to design interventions that target the maintenance mechanism of mental illness in a specific individual.

GENETICS AND TREATMENT OUTCOME

An important role of genes in determining individual differences in treatment response has long been suspected based on the clinical observation that good or poor response to a specific drug tends to run in families. The knowledge of molecular characteristics of psychotropic drugs and their action allowed an informed guess on which genes may be involved in drug response, facilitating a first wave of candidate gene pharmacogenetic studies. Several findings have emerged from these investigations.

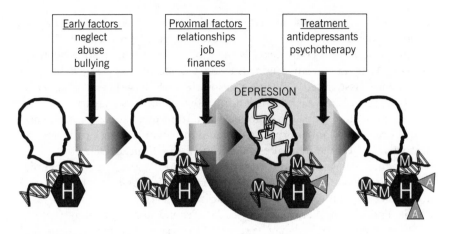

FIGURE 8.2. Developmental model of depression aetiology and treatment. Genetic script is modified with long-lasting epigenetic stamps (e.g., DNA methylation, "M") under the influence of early environmental factors. Proximal exposures in adolescence and adulthood lead to further modifications (e.g., histone [H] modifications, "A") and trigger the onset of mental illness. Pharmacological and psychosocial treatments act on the background of genetic information modified by previous environmental factors, which is likely to be counterbalanced rather than reversed by these treatments.

Early pharmacogenetic studies have focused on variants in genes coding the liver enzymes responsible for breaking down psychotropic drugs, known as cytochromes, and have found that functional variants in these genes determine the relation between medication dose and blood levels of active medication, that is, the pharmacokinetics of antidepressants (Zanger, Turpeinen, Klein, & Schwab, 2008). These findings may be useful to determine individual dosing regimens and avoid unwanted effects of medication (de Leon, Susce, & Murray-Carmichael, 2006; Kirchheiner et al., 2001). However, these pharmacokinetic associations do not explain why different people respond to different drugs, even when the dose is individually optimized, and variations in the cytochrome genes do not appear to be associated with treatment outcome (Peters et al., 2008; Serretti et al., 2009).

Genes encoding proteins that are involved in the antidepressants' mechanism of action on mood, that is, the pharmacodynamics of antidepressants, need to be explored and identified to establish qualitative individual differences in response to various psychotropic drugs. The most consistent finding in this respect has been an association between a functional length polymorphism of the serotonin transporter gene (*5-HTTLPR*) and response to the serotonin reuptake inhibiting antidepressants (SSRIs), for which the serotonin transporter is the molecular target. Among depressed individuals of European origin, the short allele of *5-HTTLPR* has been consistently associated with poor response to SSRIs (Huezo-Diaz et al., 2009; Serretti, Kato, De, & Kinoshita, 2007). This association appears to be specific to the serotonin reuptake inhibiting mechanism of antidepressant action, as the polymorphism does not influence response to antidepressants that inhibit the reuptake of norepinephrine (Huezo-Diaz et al., 2009; Kim et al., 2006). However, this finding is unlikely to influence clinical practice for two reasons. First, the effect of this single genetic variant is not strong enough to inform individualized selection of an antidepressant (Perlis, Patrick, Smoller, & Wang, 2009). Second, the effect of *5-HTTLPR* varies with ethnicity and may be reversed in Asians, among whom the short allele is more frequent than the long allele at the *5-HTTLPR* locus (Kim et al., 2006; Mrazek et al., 2008; Serretti et al., 2007).

Pharmacogenetic investigations of several other candidate genes have brought some intriguing results. There is a degree of specificity between the function of candidate genes and the type of antidepressant that is moderated by sequence variations in these genes. For example, in a large European study, variants in serotonin-related genes influenced outcome of treatment with the serotonin reuptake inhibiting antidepressant escitalopram and variants in norepinephrine-related genes moderated the action of the norepinephrine reuptake inhibiting antidepressant nortriptyline, but not vice versa (Uher, Huezo-Diaz, et al., 2009; Figure 8.3). However, exact replication of the same genetic variant influencing outcome in the same direction in different samples remains elusive. For example, the *HTR2A* gene encoding a serotonin receptor has shown the strongest pharmacogenetic associations in each of the three largest studies that reported a systematic investigation of a number of candidate genes (Horstmann & Binder, 2009; McMahon et al., 2006; Uher, Huezo-Diaz, et al., 2009). However, a different polymorphism has been associated with response in each of these studies. All three polymorphisms are located in the same intron of this gene, but there are no strong links between them that would point to a common causal variant (i.e., they are in weak or no linkage disequilibrium). While these findings provide a strong indication for a role of the *HTR2A* gene in the response to antidepressants, the heterogeneity between studies precludes a direct translation of this knowledge into a clinically useful test (Perlis et al., 2009). Nonexact replications appear to be a rule in candidate gene pharmacogenetic studies (Lekman et al., 2008; Menke et al., 2008; Uher, Huezo-Diaz, et al., 2009), and further research is needed to understand the source of these inconsistencies.

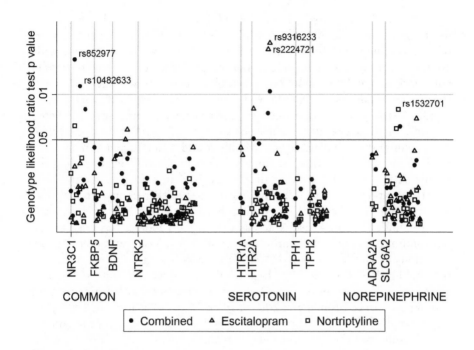

FIGURE 8.3. Pharmacogenetic effects of genetic variants in 10 candidate genes on outcome of treatment with serotonergic and norepinephrinergic antidepressants. On the x axis, genes are ordered according to hypothesis (common pathway, serotonergic, norepinephrinergic), and markers within a gene are ordered according to chromosomal position. The y axis represents the p-value of single marker association, based on likelihood-ratio tests of mixed linear models with and without additive genetic term, plotted on a log scale. Variants in the serotonin-related genes (mainly the serotonin receptor gene *HTR2A*) predicted response to the serotonin-reuptake-inhibiting antidepressant escitalopram, variants in the norepinephrine-related genes (mainly the norepinephrine transporter gene *SLC6A2*) predicted response to the norepinephrine reuptake–inhibiting antidepressant nortriptyline, and common pathway genes (mainly the glucocorticoid receptor gene *NR3C1*) predicted response irrespective of which antidepressant was used. From Uher, Huezo-Diaz, et al. (2009). Copyright 2009 by Nature Publishing Group. Reprinted by permission.

Meanwhile, the first genomewide pharmacogenetic studies are starting to give a more comprehensive picture of the genetic variants underlying individual differences in antidepressant response. A genomewide analysis of a German naturalistic sample of depressed inpatients treated with various antidepressants has not found unequivocal evidence for any specific candidate gene, but showed that a score composed from several hundred strongest pharmacogenetic associations significantly predicted response in an independent sample (Ising et al., 2009). A multicenter European comparative pharmacogenetic study found different genes involved in the response to two antidepressants: variants in the *UST* gene, coding the uronyl-sulfotransferase enzyme that is involved in neurogenesis and neuronal migration, were significantly associated with response to the norepinephrine reuptake blocking antidepressant nortriptyline after controlling for multiple comparisons across the whole genome; response to the serotonin reuptake blocking antidepressant escitalopram was predicted by variations in the interleukin 11 (*IL11*) gene at a more modest statistical threshold (Uher et al., 2010). These results are consistent with the neurogenesis and immune system involvement in depression and antidepressant action (Duman & Monteggia, 2006; Miller, Maletic, & Raison, 2009), but require replication before they can be considered for applications in clinical care. Results of other genomewide pharmacogenetic studies are expected in the near future. A systematic synthesis of findings from these studies will be needed to establish to what extent are pharmacogenetic associations detected in genomewide studies generalizable to independent samples and if a genetic test can be constructed that would enable individually tailored prescription of antidepressants.

While pharmacogenetics is a rapidly evolving field, the impact of genetic variation on outcomes of psychological treatments has been underresearched. An extrapolation of knowledge from gene–environment interactions (G × E), conceptualizing psychological treatment as a positive/protective environmental exposure, allows some predictions about environmental sensitivity genes predisposing to beneficial outcomes of psychological therapies (Uher, 2008b). A study evaluating the moderation by the *5-HTTLPR* of a complex psychosocial intervention effect on risk behavior initiation in adolescents appears to support this prediction (Brody, Beach, Philibert, Chen, & Murry, 2009). Another study showed a moderation by a polymorphism in the *DRD4* dopamine receptor gene of a parenting intervention effect on cortisol secretion in toddlers (Bakermans-Kranenburg, van IJzendoorn, Mesman, Alink, & Juffer, 2008). However, there has been no study on genetic moderation of the effect of psychosocial intervention in depression and a lack of genetic data in most clinical trials of psychological treatment limits progress in this field.

ENVIRONMENTAL EXPOSURE HISTORY
AND TREATMENT OUTCOME

For decades, experienced clinicians have felt that in cases where a mental illness had developed in response to environmental adversity, the psychosocial approach should be an important part of its treatment. This clinical intuition found its research application in the distinction between reactive and endogenous depression (Kiloh & Garside, 1963). However, this stream of research focused on relatively proximal environmental risk factors, such as life events preceding the onset of a depressive episode, or even attempted to infer the reactive or endogenous character of depression from the composition of symptoms. The resulting definitions of reactive and endogenous depression failed to provide consistent predictors of response to antidepressants (Garvey, Schaffer, & Tuason, 1984; Sotsky et al., 1991). While life events preceding the onset of a depressive episode do not seem to predict outcome of treatment in most studies (Bock, Bukh, Vinberg, Gether, & Kessing, 2009; Garvey, Hollon, & Derubeis, 1994), stressful life events and continuing difficulties during the course of treatment are consistently associated with a poor treatment outcome (Brown et al., 2009; Enns & Cox, 2005). The latter observation suggests that antidepressants do not act independently of environment, and their mechanism of action may involve a restoration of the ability to benefit from salubrious environmental conditions (Harmer, Goodwin, & Cowen, 2009; Wichers et al., 2009).

Studies of the natural course of depression indicate a strong role of early environmental factors in the perpetuation of depression into chronicity (see "Beyond Onset," above), suggesting that research on the environmental determinants of treatment outcome should refocus from proximal triggering factors to early exposures, including inadequate parental care and child abuse. While there has been some resistance to collecting retrospective data on child abuse and neglect in treatment studies (Becker-Blease & Freyd, 2006), the available evidence gives strong indications that the early factors are important and consistent predictors of treatment outcome. Moreover, there is some evidence that childhood abuse and neglect may differentially predict outcome of different treatment modalities. While reported history of childhood abuse and neglect predicted poor response to pharmacological treatment with antidepressant medication in a number of studies (Enns & Cox, 2005; Johnstone et al., 2009; Kaplan & Klinetob, 2000; Klein et al., 2009; Nemeroff et al., 2003; Wichers et al., 2009), it was associated with good response to psychological treatments for depression (Nemeroff et al., 2003), irritable bowel syndrome (Creed et al., 2005), and deliberate self-harm (Spinhoven, Slee, Garnefski, & Arensman, 2009). The study by Nemeroff and colleagues (2003) is especially compelling, as it found that a history of childhood trauma predicted better response to structured psychological treatment and worse response to an antidepressant in a large randomized study that was designed to compare the two types of treatment in individuals with chronic depression. If this finding replicates, retrospectively reported history of child abuse and neglect collected before the start of treatment could support clinical decisions on treatment choice in individual patients. Unfortunately, as a history of childhood abuse and neglect has not been collected in other large comparisons of psychological and pharmacological treatment of depression, this important finding is still awaiting independent validation.

INTERPLAY OF GENES AND ENVIRONMENT IN TREATMENT OUTCOMES

Although there is evidence that both genes and environmental exposures influence outcome of treatment for depression, the two influences are unlikely to be independent. Pharmacological and psychosocial interventions act on the script of genetic information annotated by history of exposures over the individual development (Figure 8.2). Therefore, it is likely that a combination of genetic information with environmental exposure history could provide the strongest predictors of outcomes and the best tools for personalizing treatment. However, joint evaluation of multiple nonindependent genetic and environmental predictors and interactions between them in their effects on treatment outcome presents formidable methodological challenges. On the one hand, statistical tests of higher order effects such as interactions between multiple factors have limited power to detect anything but very strong effects (McClelland & Judd, 1993; Uher, 2008a). On the other hand, the large number of possible combinations of multiple factors in prediction models increases the risk of overfitting with the ensuing poor generalizability and replicability of prediction. As a result, there are almost no data on individualized treatment outcome prediction from a combination of genetic and environment variables to date.

The only published study reported an interaction between *5-HTTLPR* and stressful life events preceding onset in their effects on response to fluvoxamine among 159 depressed individuals (Mandelli et al., 2009). This study shows that individuals carrying the short alleles at the *5-HTTLPR* and exposed to severe stressful life events prior to onset of their first depressive episode had the worst response to fluvoxamine. It provides an indication that genetic effects on treatment outcome are contextualized by environmental exposure history. However, it is likely that multiple genetic variants and multiple early and proximal environmental exposures all contribute in a nonindependent way to the individual differences in treatment response. Establishing such complex mechanisms will require advanced methodology in large well-characterized samples.

Two different approaches can be advocated to overcome the challenges associated with multiple interacting predictors and advance this important field of knowledge. First, a simple hypothesis-driven approach can be taken, where a single predictive score can be constructed as an arithmetic combination of multiple known predictors. This approach has been applied to genomewide pharmacogenetic data, in which a single score reflecting a number of risk alleles derived from a discovery sample predicted response in an independent replication sample, even though no specific pharmacogenetic association could be replicated (Ising et al., 2009). A similar approach has been suggested for probing the effects of etiological G × E on treatment outcome in depression, in which a score composed of a number of sensitive genetic variants and relevant environmental exposures could be used to summarize probability of G × E playing a role in the development of depression for a specific individual (Uher, 2008b). However, such simple approaches will have limited explanatory power, as they include substantial data reduction and are of approximative nature.

Eventually, intensive approaches that reflect the complexity of the predictive variables, such as machine learning methods, are likely to make better use of multiple predictors and enable the use of all available information without unnecessary data reduction (Larder, Wang, & Revell, 2008). These methods have the potential to use the available mega-variate data to construct an algorithm that maximizes the accuracy of prediction of a desired outcome (e.g., response to a specific treatment), taking into account both additive and conditional effects of multiple genetic and clinical variables. Applications of machine learning methodology as support tools for clinical decision making have been emerging in other medical specialties (Connor, Symons, Feeney, Young, & Wiles, 2007; Wang, Hershman, & Neugut, 2006; Yang et al., 2008) and are likely to be tested in individualized treatment selection for mental illness in the near future. However, the eventual success of this rapidly advancing methodology will crucially depend on the availability of good quality genetic and environmental history data in large samples of individuals treated with various approaches. At present, there is a striking asymmetry, with genetic data being available for trials involving pharmacological but not psychosocial treatments and good quality data on early and proximal environmental exposure history being collected in studies on psychosocial but not pharmacological interventions. This imbalance will have to be redressed to fulfill the potential of genetic and environmental predictors for personalized medicine.

CONCLUSIONS

Large individual differences in response to various treatments for depression reveal the inadequacy of the current one-size-fits-all approach and highlight the need for personalized medicine. G × E in the etiology of depression point to a heterogeneity with putative subtypes of depression as possible targets for personalized treatment. However, recent advances in etiological research have not been translated to clinical applications and etiology is not considered in diagnosis and clinical decisions. A review of the available literature shows important influences of genetic variants and early environmental factors on treatment outcome. However, each factor is individually weak or requires extension and replication. The predictive power needed for personalized medicine could be achieved by a combination of multiple genetic and environmental factors. Comprehensive assessment of environmental history and genetic variation in large studies on pharmacological and psychosocial interventions together with methodological advances in using complex information are needed to finally answer the question of whether the cause can inform cure for mental illness.

REFERENCES

Bakermans-Kranenburg, M. J., van IJzendoorn, M. H., Mesman, J., Alink, L. R., & Juffer, F. (2008). Effects of an attachment-based intervention on daily cortisol moderated by dopamine receptor D4: A randomized control trial on 1- to 3-year-olds screened for externalizing behavior. *Development and Psychopathology, 20*, 805–820.

Becker-Blease, K. A., & Freyd, J. J. (2006). Research participants telling the truth about their lives: The ethics of asking and not asking about abuse. *American Psychologist, 61*, 218–226.

Belsky, J., Jonassaint, C., Pluess, M., Stanton, M., Brummett, B., & Williams, R. (2009). Vulnerability genes or plasticity genes? *Molecular Psychiatry, 14*, 746–754.

Bock, C., Bukh, J. D., Vinberg, M., Gether, U., & Kessing, L. V. (2009). Do stressful life events predict medical treatment outcome in first episode of depression? *Social Psychiatry in Psychiatric Epidemiology, 44*, 752–760.

Brody, G. H., Beach, S. R., Philibert, R. A., Chen, Y. F., & Murry, V. M. (2009). Prevention effects moderate the association of 5-HTTLPR and youth risk behavior initiation: Gene × environment hypotheses tested via a randomized prevention design. *Child Development, 80*, 645–661.

Brown, G. W., Craig, T. K., & Harris, T. O. (2008). Parental maltreatment and proximal risk factors using the Childhood Experience of Care & Abuse (CECA) instrument: A life-course study of adult chronic depression—5. *Journal of Affective Disorders, 110*, 222–233.

Brown, G. W., Harris, T. O., Kendrick, T., Chatwin, J., Craig, T. K., Kelly, V., et al. (2009). Antidepressants, social adversity and outcome of depression in general practice. *Journal of Affective Disorders, 121,* 239–246.

Brown, G. W., & Moran, P. (1994). Clinical and psychosocial origins of chronic depressive episodes: I. A community survey. *British Journal of Psychiatry, 165,* 447–456.

Caspi, A., Sugden, K., Moffitt, T. E., Taylor, A., Craig, I. W., Harrington, H., et al. (2003). Influence of life stress on depression: Moderation by a polymorphism in the 5-HTT gene. *Science, 301,* 386–389.

Cavanagh, J. T., Carson, A. J., Sharpe, M., & Lawrie, S. M. (2003). Psychological autopsy studies of suicide: A systematic review. *Psychological Medicine, 33,* 395–405.

Collishaw, S., Pickles, A., Messer, J., Rutter, M., Shearer, C., & Maughan, B. (2007). Resilience to adult psychopathology following childhood maltreatment: Evidence from a community sample. *Child Abuse and Neglect, 31,* 211–229.

Connor, J. P., Symons, M., Feeney, G. F., Young, R. M., & Wiles, J. (2007). The application of machine learning techniques as an adjunct to clinical decision making in alcohol dependence treatment. *Substance Use and Misuse, 42,* 2193–2206.

Creed, F., Guthrie, E., Ratcliffe, J., Fernandes, L., Rigby, C., Tomenson, B., et al. (2005). Reported sexual abuse predicts impaired functioning but a good response to psychological treatments in patients with severe irritable bowel syndrome. *Psychosomatic Medicine, 67,* 490–499.

Cuijpers, P., & Smit, F. (2002). Excess mortality in depression: A meta-analysis of community studies. *Journal of Affective Disorders, 72,* 227–236.

de Leon, J., Susce, M. T., & Murray-Carmichael, E. (2006). The AmpliChip CYP450 genotyping test: Integrating a new clinical tool. *Molecular Diagnostics and Therapy, 10,* 135–151.

DeRubeis, R. J., Siegle, G. J., & Hollon, S. D. (2008). Cognitive therapy versus medication for depression: Treatment outcomes and neural mechanisms. *Nature Reviews of Neuroscience, 9,* 788–796.

Doornbos, B., Dijck-Brouwer, D. A., Kema, I. P., Tanke, M. A., van Goor, S. A., Muskiet, F. A., et al. (2009). The development of peripartum depressive symptoms is associated with gene polymorphisms of MAOA, 5-HTT and COMT. *Progress in Neuropsychopharmacology and Biological Psychiatry, 33,* 1250–1254.

Duman, R. S., & Monteggia, L. M. (2006). A neurotrophic model for stress-related mood disorders. *Biological Psychiatry, 59,* 1116–1127.

Eaton, W. W., Shao, H., Nestadt, G., Lee, H. B., Bienvenu, O. J., & Zandi, P. (2008). Population-based study of first onset and chronicity in major depressive disorder. *Archives of General Psychiatry, 65,* 513–520.

Enns, M. W., & Cox, B. J. (2005). Psychosocial and clinical predictors of symptom persistence vs. remission in major depressive disorder. *Canadian Journal of Psychiatry, 50,* 769–777.

Garvey, M. J., Hollon, S. D., & Derubeis, R. J. (1994). Do depressed patients with higher pretreatment stress levels respond better to cognitive therapy than imipramine? *Journal of Affective Disorders, 32*, 45–50.

Garvey, M. J., Schaffer, C. B., & Tuason, V. B. (1984). Comparison of pharmacological treatment response between situational and non-situational depressions. *British Journal of Psychiatry, 145*, 363–365.

Ghaemi, S. N. (2008). Why antidepressants are not antidepressants: STEP-BD, STAR*D, and the return of neurotic depression. *Bipolar Disorders, 10*, 957–968.

Harmer, C. J., Goodwin, G. M., & Cowen, P. J. (2009). Why do antidepressants take so long to work?: A cognitive neuropsychological model of antidepressant drug action. *British Journal of Psychiatry, 195*, 102–108.

Hayden, E. P., & Klein, D. N. (2001). Outcome of dysthymic disorder at 5-year follow-up: The effect of familial psychopathology, early adversity, personality, comorbidity, and chronic stress. *American Journal of Psychiatry, 158*, 1864–1870.

Holsboer, F. (2008). How can we realize the promise of personalized antidepressant medicines? *Nature Reviews in Neuroscience, 9*, 638–646.

Horstmann, S., & Binder, E. B. (2009). Pharmacogenomics of antidepressant drugs. *Pharmacological Therapeutics, 124*, 57–73.

Huezo-Diaz, P., Uher, R., Smith, R., Rietschel, M., Henigsberg, N., Marusic, A., et al. (2009). Moderation of antidepressant response by the serotonin transporter gene. *British Journal of Psychiatry, 195*, 30–38.

Ising, M., Lucae, S., Binder, E. B., Bettecken, T., Uhr, M., Ripke, S., et al. (2009). A genome-wide association study points to multiple loci predicting treatment outcome in depression. *Archives of General Psychiatry, 66*, 966–975.

Johnstone, J. M., Luty, S. E., Carter, J. D., Mulder, R. T., Frampton, C. M., & Joyce, P. R. (2009). Childhood neglect and abuse as predictors of antidepressant response in adult depression. *Depression and Anxiety, 26*, 711–717.

Kaplan, M. J., & Klinetob, N. A. (2000). Childhood emotional trauma and chronic posttraumatic stress disorder in adult outpatients with treatment-resistant depression. *Journal of Nervous and Mental Disease, 188*, 596–601.

Kiloh, L. G., & Garside, R. F. (1963). The independence of neurotic depression and endogenous depression. *British Journal of Psychiatry, 109*, 451–463.

Kim, H., Lim, S. W., Kim, S., Kim, J. W., Chang, Y. H., Carroll, B. J., et al. (2006). Monoamine transporter gene polymorphisms and antidepressant response in koreans with late-life depression. *Journal of the American Medical Association, 296*, 1609–1618.

Kirchheiner, J., Brosen, K., Dahl, M. L., Gram, L. F., Kasper, S., Roots, I., et al. (2001). CYP2D6 and CYP2C19 genotype-based dose recommendations for antidepressants: A first step towards subpopulation-specific dosages. *Acta Psychiatrica Scandinavia, 104*, 173–192.

Kirsch, I., Deacon, B. J., Huedo-Medina, T. B., Scoboria, A., Moore, T. J., & Johnson, B. T. (2008). Initial severity and antidepressant benefits: A meta-analysis of data submitted to the Food and Drug Administration. *PLoS Medicine, 5*, e45.

Klein, D. N., Arnow, B. A., Barkin, J. L., Dowling, F., Kocsis, J. H., Leon, A. C., et al. (2009). Early adversity in chronic depression: Clinical correlates and response to pharmacotherapy. *Depression and Anxiety, 26*, 701–710.

Lam, R. W., Kennedy, S. H., Grigoriadis, S., McIntyre, R. S., Milev, R., Ramasubbu, R., et al. (2009). Canadian Network for Mood and Anxiety Treatments (CANMAT) clinical guidelines for the management of major depressive disorder in adults: III. Pharmacotherapy. *Journal of Affective Disorders, 117*(Suppl. 1), S26–S43.

Larder, B., Wang, D., & Revell, A. (2008). Application of artificial neural networks for decision support in medicine. *Methods in Molecular Biology, 458*, 123–136.

Lekman, M., Laje, G., Charney, D., Rush, A. J., Wilson, A. F., Sorant, A. J., et al. (2008). The FKBP5-gene in depression and treatment response—An association study in the Sequenced Treatment Alternatives to Relieve Depression (STAR*D) Cohort. *Biological Psychiatry, 63*, 1103–1110.

Lopez, A. D., & Murray, C. C. (1998). The global burden of disease, 1990–2020. *Nature Medicine, 4*, 1241–1243.

Luthar, S. S., Sawyer, J. A., & Brown, P. J. (2006). Conceptual issues in studies of resilience: Past, present, and future research. *Annals of the New York Academy of Sciences, 1094*, 105–115.

Mandelli, L., Marino, E., Pirovano, A., Calati, R., Zanardi, R., Colombo, C., et al. (2009). Interaction between SERTPR and stressful life events on response to antidepressant treatment. *European Neuropsychopharmacology, 19*, 64–67.

Masten, A. S., & Obradovic, J. (2006). Competence and resilience in development. *Annals of the New Academy of Sciences, 1094*, 13–27.

McClelland, G. H., & Judd, C. M. (1993). Statistical difficulties of detecting interactions and moderator effects. *Psychological Bulletin, 114*, 376–390.

McMahon, F. J., Buervenich, S., Charney, D., Lipsky, R., Rush, A. J., Wilson, A. F., et al. (2006). Variation in the gene encoding the serotonin 2A receptor is associated with outcome of antidepressant treatment. *American Journal of Human Genetics, 78*, 804–814.

Menke, A., Lucae, S., Kloiber, S., Horstmann, S., Bettecken, T., Uhr, M., et al. (2008). Genetic markers within glutamate receptors associated with antidepressant treatment-emergent suicidal ideation. *American Journal of Psychiatry, 165*, 917–918.

Miller, A. H., Maletic, V., & Raison, C. L. (2009). Inflammation and its discontents: The role of cytokines in the pathophysiology of major depression. *Biological Psychiatry, 165*, 732–741.

Moffitt, T. E., Caspi, A., Taylor, A., Kokaua, J., Milne, B. J., Polanczyk, G., et al. (2009). How common are common mental disorders?: Evidence that lifetime prevalence rates are doubled by prospective versus retrospective ascertainment. *Psychological Medicine, 40*, 899–909.

Mrazek, D. A., Rush, A. J., Biernacka, J. M., O'Kane, D. J., Cunningham, J. M., Wieben, E. D., et al. (2008). SLC6A4 variation and citalopram response. *American Journal of Medical Genetics: Neuropsychiatric Genetics, 150B*, 341–351.

Muglia, P., Tozzi, F., Galwey, N. W., Francks, C., Upmanyu, R., Kong, X. Q., et al. (2008). Genome-wide association study of recurrent major depressive disorder in two European case–control cohorts. *Molecular Psychiatry, 16,* 589–601.

Need, A. C., Ge, D., Weale, M. E., Maia, J., Feng, S., Heinzen, E. L., et al. (2009). A genome-wide investigation of SNPs and CNVs in schizophrenia. *PLoS Genetics, 5,* e1000373.

Nemeroff, C. B., Heim, C. M., Thase, M. E., Klein, D. N., Rush, A. J., Schatzberg, A. F., et al. (2003). Differential responses to psychotherapy versus pharmacotherapy in patients with chronic forms of major depression and childhood trauma. *Proceedings of the National Academy of Sciences USA, 100,* 14293–14296.

Parker, G. (2005). Beyond major depression. *Psychological Medicine, 35,* 467–474.

Parker, G. (2009). Antidepressants on trial: How valid is the evidence? *British Journal of Psychiatry, 194,* 1–3.

Perlis, R. H., Patrick, A., Smoller, J. W., & Wang, P. S. (2009). When is pharmacogenetic testing for antidepressant response ready for the clinic?: A cost-effectiveness analysis based on data from the STAR*D study. *Neuropsychopharmacology, 34,* 2227–2236.

Perroud, N., Uher, R., Marusic, A., Rietschel, M., Mors, O., Henigsberg, N., et al. (2009). Suicidal ideation during treatment of depression with escitalopram and nortriptyline in GENDEP: A clinical trial. *BMC Medicine, 7,* 60.

Peters, E. J., Slager, S. L., Kraft, J. B., Jenkins, G. D., Reinalda, M. S., McGrath, P. J., et al. (2008). Pharmacokinetic genes do not influence response or tolerance to citalopram in the STAR*D sample. *PLoS ONE, 3,* e1872.

Rush, A. J., Trivedi, M. H., Wisniewski, S. R., Nierenberg, A. A., Stewart, J. W., Warden, D., et al. (2006). Acute and longer-term outcomes in depressed outpatients requiring one or several treatment steps: A STAR*D report. *American Journal of Psychiatry, 163,* 1905–1917.

Rutter, M. (2006). Implications of resilience concepts for scientific understanding. *Annals of the New York Academy of Sciences, 1094,* 1–12.

Sanjuan, J., Martin-Santos, R., Garcia-Esteve, L., Carot, J. M., Guillamat, R., Gutierrez-Zotes, A., et al. (2008). Mood changes after delivery: role of the serotonin transporter gene. *British Journal of Psychiatry, 193,* 383–388.

Serretti, A., Calati, R., Massat, I., Linotte, S., Kasper, S., Lecrubier, Y., et al. (2009). Cytochrome P450 CYP1A2, CYP2C9, CYP2C19 and CYP2D6 genes are not associated with response and remission in a sample of depressive patients. *International Clinical Psychopharmacology, 24,* 250–256.

Serretti, A., Kato, M., De, R. D., & Kinoshita, T. (2007). Meta-analysis of serotonin transporter gene promoter polymorphism (5-HTTLPR) association with selective serotonin reuptake inhibitor efficacy in depressed patients. *Molecular Psychiatry, 12,* 247–257.

Sotsky, S. M., Glass, D. R., Shea, M. T., Pilkonis, P. A., Collins, J. F., Elkin, I., et al. (1991). Patient predictors of response to psychotherapy and pharmacotherapy: Findings in the NIMH Treatment of Depression Collaborative Research Program. *American Journal of Psychiatry, 148,* 997–1008.

Spijker, J., de Graff, R., Bijl, R. V., Beekman, A. T., Ormel, J., & Nolen, W. A.

(2002). Duration of major depressive episodes in the general population: Results from The Netherlands Mental Health Survey and Incidence Study (NEMESIS). *British Journal of Psychiatry, 181*, 208–213.

Spinhoven, P., Slee, N., Garnefski, N., & Arensman, E. (2009). Childhood sexual abuse differentially predicts outcome of cognitive-behavioral therapy for deliberate self-harm. *Journal of Nervous and Mental Disease, 197*, 455–457.

Stefansson, H., Ophoff, R. A., Steinberg, S., Andreassen, O. A., Cichon, S., Rujescu, D., et al. (2009). Common variants conferring risk of schizophrenia. *Nature, 460*, 744–747.

Sullivan, P. F., de Geus, E. J., Willemsen, G., James, M. R., Smit, J. H., Zandbelt, T., et al. (2009). Genome-wide association for major depressive disorder: A possible role for the presynaptic protein piccolo. *Molecular Psychiatry, 14*(4), 359–375.

ten Doesschate, M. C., Koeter, M. W., Bockting, C. L., & Schene, A. H. (2010). Health related quality of life in recurrent depression: A comparison with a general population sample. *Journal of Affective Disorders, 120*(1–3), 126–132.

Thase, M. E., & Denko, T. (2008). Pharmacotherapy of mood disorders. *Annual Review of Clinical Psychology, 4*, 53–91.

Tsankova, N. M., Berton, O., Renthal, W., Kumar, A., Neve, R. L., & Nestler, E. J. (2006). Sustained hippocampal chromatin regulation in a mouse model of depression and antidepressant action. *Nature Neuroscience, 9*, 519–525.

Uher, R. (2008a). Gene–environment interaction: Overcoming methodological challenges. *Novartis Foundation Symposium, 293*, 13–26.

Uher, R. (2008b). The implications of gene–environment interactions in depression: Will cause inform cure? *Molecular Psychiatry, 13*, 1070–1078.

Uher, R., Huezo-Diaz, P., Perroud, N., Smith, R., Rietschel, M., Mors, O., et al. (2009). Genetic predictors of response to antidepressants in the GENDEP project. *Pharmacogenomics Journal, 9*, 225–233.

Uher, R., & McGuffin, P. (2008). The moderation by the serotonin transporter gene of environmental adversity in the aetiology of mental illness: Review and methodological analysis. *Molecular Psychiatry, 13*, 131–146.

Uher, R., Perroud, N., Ng, M. Y., Hauser, J., Henigsberg, N., Maier, W., et al. (2010). Genome-wide pharmacogenetics of antidepressant response in the GENDEP project. *American Journal of Psychiatry, 167*, 555–564.

Vanderbilt-Adriance, E., & Shaw, D. S. (2008). Conceptualizing and re-evaluating resilience across levels of risk, time, and domains of competence. *Clinical Child and Family Psychology Review, 11*, 30–58.

Wang, X., Hershman, D. L., & Neugut, A. I. (2006). Using machine learning, general regression, and Cox proportional hazards regression to predict the effectiveness of treatment in patients with breast cancer. *AMIA Annual Symposium Proceedings, 1133*.

Wellcome Trust Case Control Consortium. (2007). Genome-wide association study of 14,000 cases of seven common diseases and 3,000 shared controls. *Nature, 447*, 661–678.

Wichers, M. C., Barge-Schaapveld, D. Q., Nicolson, N. A., Peeters, F., de Vries, M.,

Mengelers, R., et al. (2009). Reduced stress-sensitivity or increased reward experience: The psychological mechanism of response to antidepressant medication. *Neuropsychopharmacology, 34*, 923–931.

Wiersma, J. E., Hovens, J. G., van Oppen, P., Giltay, E. J., van Schaik, D. J., Beekman, A. T., et al. (2009). The importance of childhood trauma and childhood life events for chronicity of depression in adults. *Journal of Clinical Psychiatry, 70*, 983–989.

Yang, J. Y., Yang, M. Q., Luo, Z., Ma, Y., Li, J., Deng, Y., et al. (2008). A hybrid machine learning-based method for classifying the Cushing's syndrome with comorbid adrenocortical lesions. *BMC Genomics, 9*(Suppl. 1), S23.

Zanger, U. M., Turpeinen, M., Klein, K., & Schwab, M. (2008). Functional pharmacogenetics/genomics of human cytochromes P450 involved in drug biotransformation. *Analytical and Bioanalytical Chemistry, 392*, 1093–1108.

CHAPTER 9

Promoting Resilience
in Maltreated Children

Joan Kaufman *and* Francheska Perepletchikova

This chapter highlights seminal gene–environment interaction (G × E) studies, summarizes our related research, and discusses the potential influence of this work on interventions with children involved with the child welfare system. Children within the child protective services system are at particularly high risk for developing psychiatric and substance use disorders (Kaufman, 2007; Landsverk, Burns, Stambaugh, & Reutz, 2009). These children typically come from families with high family loading for these problems, they have experienced abuse and neglect of sufficient severity to warrant out-of-home placement, and once in the system they frequently encounter additional traumatic experiences and losses that further increase risk for deleterious outcomes (De Bellis et al., 2001; Kaufman, 2007; Young, Boles, & Otero, 2007).

A central tenet of G × E research in psychiatry is the hypothesis that identifying susceptibility genes and how environmental factors interact with them will increase our capacity to identify those at greatest risk, identify targets for developing interventions to preempt illness onset, and guide efforts to tailor and personalize treatments for individuals with stress-related mental health problems (T. R. Insel, personal communication, October 3, 2007). Biological therapies will not be the only types of treatments suggested by this research, as in many areas of medicine understanding risk has led to nonmedical interventions to prevent disease onset. Phenylketonuria (PKU) is a good illustration of this point. PKU is a genetic disorder caused by an enzyme deficiency that affects the metabolism of the amino acid phenylalanine, causing toxic by-products to build up, damage to the infant brain, and mental retardation. Mental retardation in PKU can be prevented by controlling the environment by restricting phenylalanine intake in the diet. Stress-related psychiatric disorders, unlike PKU, are not caused by a single gene, and there is not one environmental factor that can eliminate risk for these problems. It is our firm belief, however, that a G × E framework can help to identify novel psychosocial and biological targets for future intervention efforts to help optimize the outcomes of this vulnerable population.

This tenet, however, has been subject to critique. A highly publicized meta-analysis of studies examining G × E predictors of depression, or more specifically, the association between the serotonin transporter gene (*5-HTTLPR*), stressful life events (SLE), and depression, was recently published in the *Journal of the American Medical Association* (*JAMA*) calling into the question the utility of G × E candidate gene studies in psychiatry (Risch et al., 2009). The authors of this article concluded that "this meta-analysis yielded no evidence that the serotonin transporter genotype alone or in interaction with stressful life events is associated with an elevated risk of depression in men alone, women alone, or in both sexes combined" (p. 2462). A smaller scale meta-analysis published earlier in the year was less noticed, but similarly concluded that "the literature leads us to suggest that the positive results for the *5-HTTLPR* × SLE interactions in logistic regression models are compatible with chance findings" (Munafò, Durrant, Lewis, & Flint, 2009, p. 211). These conclusions, however, were based on assumptions in the simulation model that are inconsistent with prior research findings and a bias in sampling strategy that call into question the authors' conclusions.

We have published a correspondence in *Biological Psychiatry* that delineates our concerns with the two meta-analyses (Kaufman, Gelernter, Kaffman, Caspi, & Moffitt, 2010). The nonrepresentative nature of the sample of studies included in both meta-analyses is a significant limitation of the reports. In the first published meta-analysis (Munafò et al., 2009), 14 studies out of 33 reports met the criteria for inclusion in the meta-analysis, but the authors were only able to get data from five of the 14 studies. The meta-analysis was conducted with data from less than half the studies that met the stated inclusion criteria, with a trend for negative studies to be overrepresented. Of the 14 studies meeting the inclusion criteria for the meta-analysis, 75% (3/4) of the negative studies and only 20% (2/10) of the positive studies were included in the analysis (Fisher's exact test: $p <$ .10). A similar problem exists with the second larger scale meta-analysis (Risch et al., 2009). Although a larger number of studies was included in the second meta-analysis, 12 studies were published after the data set for this second meta-analysis was closed and analyses were initiated, with only three of the 12 studies including adequate data in the published reports to be examined in the second meta-analysis (K. R. Merikangas, personal communication, July 6, 2009). Seven of the nine studies excluded because they were published after the data set was closed were full or partial replications, as were four other earlier studies that were not included in the second meta-analysis because the data were either not received or received in an incompatible format (Kaufman et al., 2010). Like the first meta-analysis, the second meta-analysis also included an excess representation of nonreplications. It was conducted with data from half of the 26 studies that met inclusion criteria for the meta-analysis (Risch et al., 2009), with a trend again for negative studies to be overrepresented. Of the 26 studies meeting the inclusion criteria for the second meta-analysis, 78% (7/9) of the negative studies and only 35% (6/17) of the positive studies were included in the analysis (Fisher's exact test: $p < .10$). In the 6 months following the publication of the *JAMA* meta-analysis, 12 additional papers were published that examined $5\text{-}HTTLPR \times SLE$ interactions.

A comprehensive meta-analysis that includes the majority of completed studies will be published in the *Archives of General Psychiatry* (Karg, Shedden, Burmeister, & Sen, in press). In order to perform a more inclusive meta-analysis, the authors used the Liptak–Stouffer Z-score method to combine findings of primary studies at the level of significance tests rather than the level of raw data. A total of 54 studies were included in the meta-analysis, and the $5\text{-}HTTLPR$ gene was found to confer a significant increased risk of developing depression in individuals with histories of significant life stress ($p = 0.00002$). When analyses were conducted using only the studies included in the previously published meta-analyses, there was no evidence of this association (Munafò studies, $p = 0.16$; Risch studies, $p = 0.11$). This suggests that the difference in results between meta-analyses was due to the different set of included studies, not the techniques used to conduct the meta-analyses. Contrary to the results of the smaller earlier published meta-analyses, this new comprehensive meta-analysis found strong evidence in support of the hypothesis that $5\text{-}HTTLPR$ moderates the relationship between stress and depression.

This chapter is organized into three sections. The first section provides relevant background information and an overview of the population and methods utilized in our G × E studies. The second section reviews relevant G × E and related research. The third section delineates future directions from a science, clinical practice, and public policy perspective, with a focus on the implications of emerging G × E research findings on designing interventions to promote resilience in maltreated children.

PROGRAM DESCRIPTION

The Child and Adolescent Research and Education (CARE) Program at Yale University is dedicated to work with maltreated children and their families. Child abuse occurs at epidemic rates, with victims of abuse comprising a significant proportion of all child psychiatric admissions. The lifetime incidence of physical and sexual abuse is estimated at 30% among child and adolescent outpatients (Lanktree, Briere, & Zaidi, 1991), and approximately 55% among psychiatric inpatients (McClellan, Adams, Douglas, McCurry, & Storck, 1995). In the state of Connecticut in the United States, wards of the state with a history of maltreatment comprise 1% of the child population, but 65% of psychiatric inpatients (Schaefer, 2007).

Although not all abused children develop difficulties, many experience a chronic course of psychopathology (Molnar, Buka, & Kessler, 2001). Compared to community controls, maltreated children have elevated rates of externalizing and internalizing psychiatric diagnoses, including conduct and antisocial personality disorders (Garland et al., 2001; Kolko, 2002; Rutter, Giller, & Hagell, 1998; Widom, 1989; Widom & Ames, 1994), posttraumatic stress disorder (Famularo, Fenton, Kinscherff, & Augustyn, 1996; Famularo, Kinscherff, & Fenton, 1992; Kilpatrick et al., 2003; Ruggiero, McLeer, & Dixon, 2000), major depression (Kaufman, 1991; Pelcovitz, Kaplan, DeRosa, Mandel, & Salzinger, 2000), and drug and alcohol problems (Molnar, et al., 2001; Schuck & Widom, 2003; Widom, Ireland, & Glynn, 1995). Maltreatment is also strongly associated with suicidal ideation, suicide attempts, and nonsuicidal self-injury in children and adolescents (e.g., Glassman, Weierich, Hooley, Deliberto, & Nock, 2007).

A goal of our G × E research has been to better understand why some maltreated children develop significant difficulties and others do not. Participants in our G × E research studies were drawn from a larger study examining the efficacy of a state intervention for maltreated children removed from their parents' care due to allegations of abuse or neglect (Permanency Planning: Service Use and Child Outcomes; Principal Investigator, Joan Kaufman, PhD). The maltreated children were recruited within 6 months of their initial out-of-home placement. Approximately equal numbers of maltreated and demographically matched community controls with no history of maltreatment or exposure to intrafamilial violence were recruited for the research.

In terms of maltreatment experiences, over 80% of the maltreated children experienced two or more types of maltreatment. Sixty-one percent of the sample had a history of physical abuse; 23% sexual abuse; 81% neglect; 64% emotional maltreatment; and 69% had a history of exposure to domestic violence. Problems with parental substance abuse were a presenting complaint in 83% of the families involved with protective services.

Children ranged in age from 5 to 15 years, with a mean age of 9.2. The sample was also approximately evenly divided by sex, and of mixed ethnic origin. Although the maltreated and comparison groups were comparable in terms of racial composition, to prevent spurious associations that can result from variation in allele frequency and prevalence of trait by population, ancestry proportion scores were generated and included as covariates in all analyses. A set of informative markers were used to generate ancestral proportion scores to estimate the ancestry of the children in the study, providing a more sensitive measure than categorical classifications of race to control for subpopulation differences in allele frequency that can confound the results of genetic analyses (Pritchard, Stephens, & Donnelly, 2000).

Participants underwent baseline interviews at their place of residence. The baseline data were collected in one session with the child and two sessions with the parent or guardian. Approximately 1 month following the baseline interview, all children attended a 1-week summer day camp program established specifically for our research purposes. The camp, free of charge to all participants, included 1–2 hours of research assessments per day. In the remaining time children engaged in recreational activities including art, sports, music, and outdoor water games. This data collection procedure allows for naturalistic observation and comprehensive assessments without overburdening children. The camps are fun for the children, cost-effective, and promote strong collaboration with birth parents and protective service workers. DNA specimens were collected from buccal (i.e., spit) cell specimens, and a range of standard and well-validated research instruments were completed while the children were at camp. At time of the baseline assessments, 67% of the maltreated children met criteria for one or more diagnoses, compared to 18% of the controls. Posttraumatic stress disorder (PTSD) was the most common diagnosis (55%), with a large proportion of the maltreated children also meeting criteria for a depressive (34%) or a behavioral (25%) disorder. Annual follow-ups were conducted in the 2 years following attendance in the research camp program to assess child well-being, service use, reabuse, and placement outcomes.

It is the goal of the CARE program to better understand risk and resiliency in children, and to utilize what we learn to develop effective interventions and social policies to help each child involved with the protective service system to reach his or her potential. The focus of our research is broad and spans from neurobiology to social policy. The focus on neurobiology derives from preclinical (e.g., animal) and clinical studies that suggest that stress early in life can promote long-term changes in stress reactivity and brain development. The focus on social policy comes from (1) preclinical studies demonstrating that the neurobiological effects of early stress can be altered by the quality of the subsequent caregiving environment; (2) clinical studies that suggest that the availability of a positive supportive relationship is the most important factor in promoting resiliency in maltreated children; and (3) knowledge of the problems that can occur once maltreated children enter the system to increase the likelihood of the development of long-term mental health problems (e.g., separation from siblings, multiple changes in foster care placements, reabuse).

THE ROLE OF GENETICS IN MODIFYING THE OUTCOMES OF MALTREATED CHILDREN

This section reviews studies examining predictors of sociopathy and aggression, depression, and substance use disorders. G × E and gene–gene–environment interaction (G × G × E) models are explored. Preliminary imaging genomics and translational studies of the effects of early stress that incorporate a G × E framework are also presented.

MAOA × Maltreatment Predictors of Sociopathy

As noted in other chapters of this book, Caspi, Moffitt, and colleagues (Caspi et al., 2002) were the first to examine the role of genetic factors in moderating the outcome of individuals with a history of child maltreatment. They studied a large epidemiological sample of 1,037 males from birth to adulthood. They used the data set to examine why some children who are maltreated grow up to develop antisocial behavior and others do not. A functional polymorphism in the gene encoding the neurotransmitter-metabolizing enzyme monoamine oxidase A (*MAOA*) was found to moderate the relation between maltreatment and later sociopathy. *MAOA* is an X-linked gene encoding an enzyme responsible for metabolizing neurotransmitters such as serotonin and norepinephrine. The absence of a functional *MAOA* gene has been associated with aggression in mice (Cases et al., 1995) and humans (Brunner, Nelen, Breakefield, Ropers, & van Oost, 1993). The number of copies in this variable number of tandem repeats (VNTR) *MAOA* polymorphism affects gene expression and efficiency of gene transcription (Deckert et al., 1999; Sabol, Hu, & Hamer, 1998). Caspi and colleagues (2002) found that adults who were maltreated as children with "low-activity" *MAOA* alleles were more likely to develop conduct disorder, antisocial personality symptoms, and violent behavior than adults maltreated as children with "high-activity" *MAOA* alleles, with this latter group having rates of these problems that were low and comparable to non-maltreated individuals with high-activity *MAOA*. Since the initial publication of this finding, multiple investigators have replicated this association (Kim-Cohen et al., 2006).

In our studies of extremely traumatized children (Weder et al., 2009), when using the categorical classification for maltreatment group status, we did not observe a G × E in predicting children's aggression scores. As described elsewhere (Weder et al., 2009), an index of total trauma exposure was then created for all subjects. Experiences assessed in the trauma index were physical abuse, sexual abuse, domestic violence exposure, out-of-home placements, and community violence exposure. Each adversity was rated on a scale of 0–2 and summed to create the continuous trauma index. In general, scores of 0 indicate the child was not exposed to this experience, scores of 1 indicate mild or subthreshold experiences (e.g., excessive physical discipline without bruising), and scores of 2 indicate clinically significant experiences—experiences of sufficient severity to warrant state intervention. Among controls, 30% had no exposure to trauma, 44% met criterion for one subthreshold experience of trauma, 24% met criteria for two subthreshold experiences of trauma, and 2% met criteria for three subthreshold experiences of trauma. As expected, the mean trauma exposure score for the maltreated children was significantly greater than the mean for controls (maltreated children: 5.2 ± 1.8, range: 2–9; community controls: 1.1 ± 0.8 ; range: 0–3). As is depicted in Figure 9.1, aggressive behavior was modified by *MAOA* genotype and trauma exposure, but only up to moderate levels of trauma exposure. Extreme levels of trauma appeared to overshadow the effects of *MAOA* genotype in our cohort.

5-HTTLPR × Maltreatment Predictors of Depression

Caspi, Moffitt, and colleagues (2003) were also the first to examine G × E in the development of depression—the *5-HTTLPR*–SLE association discussed at the beginning of this chapter. They were the first to report that the functional polymorphism in the promoter region of *5-HTTLPR* moderated the influence of early child maltreatment and SLE on the development of depression. The serotonin transporter is a protein critical to the regulation of serotonin function in the brain because it terminates the action of serotonin in the synapse via reuptake. This gene has a well-studied functional variable number of tandem repeats (VNTR) polymorphism in the promoter region. There are two common functional alleles of *5-HTTLPR*, the short ("s") allele and the long ("l") allele. The "s" allele encodes an attenuated promoter segment, and is associated with *in vitro* reduced transcription and functional capacity of the serotonin transporter relative to the "l" allele (Lesch et al., 1995). Caspi and colleagues reported that individuals with a history of recent SLE or childhood abuse and one or two copies of the short allele of *5-HTTLPR* exhibited more depressive symptoms and diagnosable

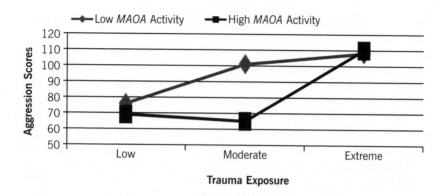

FIGURE 9.1. *MAOA* genotype and aggressive behavior: The changing impact of genotype at varying levels of stress. The low-activity *MAOA* gene was associated with increased aggression in the moderate range of scores on the trauma exposure index. With trauma exposure scores greater than this, genotype made no difference in children's aggression scores. Analyses were conducted using rank-transformed aggression scores because the data were not normal and standard transformations failed to normalize the distribution. For illustrative purposes, children were grouped into low, moderate, and extreme categories, but analyses were conducted using the full trauma exposure scale (0–9). From Weder et al. (2009). Copyright 2009 by the Society of Biological Psychiatry. Adapted by permission.

depression than individuals homozygous for the long allele. This is a finding that was replicated in children (*N* = 101) by our group (Kaufman et al., 2004), and in numerous other investigations.

5-HTTLPR × BDNF × Maltreatment Predictors of Depression

Given that gene by gene interactions have been theorized to contribute to the etiology of depression (Holmans et al., 2004; Kendler & Karkowski-Shuman, 1997), we hypothesized that a polymorphism in the brain-derived neurotrophic factor gene (*BDNF*) might interact with the *5-HTTLPR* gene to further increase the risk for depression in maltreated children. *BDNF* genetic variation has recently been associated with child-onset depression in two independent samples (Strauss, Barr, George, et al., 2004; Strauss, Barr, Vetro, et al., 2004). In addition, both BDNF (e.g., the protein product of the *BDNF* gene) and serotonin have been implicated in the etiology of depression, and they are also known to interact at multiple intra- and intercellular levels (Duman, Heninger, & Nestler, 1997; Malberg, Eisch, Nestler, & Duman, 2000). We were able to document in an enlarged sample (N = 196) a significant three-way interaction between *BDNF* geno-type, *5-HTTLPR*, and maltreatment history in predicting depression. As depicted in Figure 9.2, children with the met allele of the *BDNF* gene and two short alleles of *5-HTTLPR* had the highest depression scores, but the vulnerability associated with these two genotypes was only evident in the maltreated children (Kaufman et al., 2006). Since the publication of our original report, this three-way association has likewise been reported by other investigators (Wichers et al., 2008).

5-HTTLPR × **BDNF** × **Maltreatment** × **Social Supports** **Predictors of Depression**

As noted previously, clinical studies of individuals with a history of abuse suggest that the availability of a caring and stable parent or alternate guard-ian is one of the most important factors that distinguish abused individu-als with good developmental outcomes from those with more deleterious

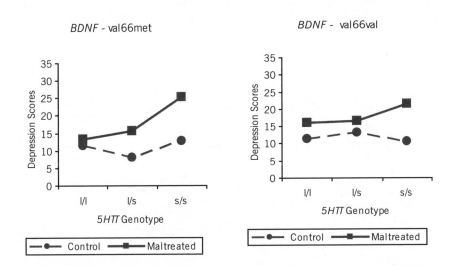

FIGURE 9.2. Three-way interaction between maltreatment history, *BDNF*, and *5-HTTLPR* genotype. These graphs depict the data of the maltreated and control children. There was a significant three-way interaction between *BDNF* genotype, *5-HTTLPR* genotype, and maltreatment history in predicting children's depres-sion scores. Children with the *BDNF* gene Val66Met polymorphism and the "s/s" *5-HTTLPR* genotype had the highest depression scores, with the vulnerability associated with these two genotypes only elevated in the maltreated children. From Kaufman et al. (2006). Copyright 2006 by the Society of Biological Psychiatry. Reprinted by permission.

outcomes (Kaufman & Henrich, 2000). Consequently, we examined the effect of social supports in the two reports discussed above (Kaufman et al., 2004, 2006). Children were asked to name people they (1) talk to about personal things, (2) count on to buy the things they need, (3) share good news with, (4) get together with to have fun, and (5) go to if they need advice. The summary social support measure used was the number of positive support categories listed for the child's top support. The children were most likely to name an adult as their primary support. Sixty-one percent of the maltreated children and 83% of the controls listed their mothers as their top support, and 30% of the maltreated children and 10% of the controls listed alternative parental figures (e.g., father, stepfather, foster mother), grandparents, or other adult relatives as their primary support.

Figure 9.3 illustrates the G × G × E × E finding. Maltreated children with positive supports had depression scores that were only slightly greater than controls, regardless of genotype. The quality and availability of social supports was extremely potent in reducing risk for depression in maltreated children—with the effect greatest for those maltreated children with the most vulnerable genotypes. Negative sequelae associated with abuse are not inevitable; they can be modified by both genetic and environmental

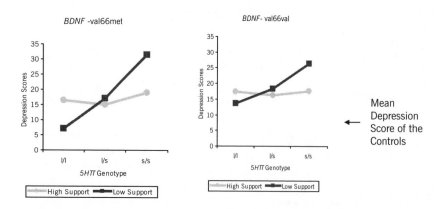

FIGURE 9.3. Four-way interaction between maltreatment history, *BDNF* genotype, *5-HTTLPR* genotype, and social supports: Maltreated children's data. These graphs depict only the data of the maltreated children. The mean score of the controls is indicated on the right as a frame of reference. The depression scores of the maltreated children with high social supports were close to the mean depression score of the controls, regardless of genotype. The "s/s" genotype was associated with an increase in maltreated children's depression scores, which was greatest for the children without positive supports and the additional presence of the met allele of the *BDNF* polymorphism. Reprinted from Kaufman et al. (2006). Copyright 2006 by the Society of Biological Psychiatry. Reprinted by permission.

factors. The ability of social supports to modify genetic and environmental risk for depression has likewise been replicated in several independent studies (Kilpatrick et al., 2007; Koenen et al., 2009).

There are probably multiple mechanisms by which social supports may ameliorate risk for depression. Data from preclinical (e.g., animal) studies suggest that maternal behavior can produce stable changes in DNA methylation and chromatin structure of the glucocorticoid receptor gene promoter in the hippocampus (Weaver et al., 2004). These epigenetic changes and the subsequent alteration in gene expression and hypothalamic–pituitary–adrenal (HPA) axis response to stress may be one important mechanism by which variations in maternal behavior/social supports alter risk for stress-related disorders. Support for this hypothesis is derived from a recent study of postmortem hippocampus tissue obtained from suicide victims with a history of childhood abuse, suicide victims with no childhood abuse, and nonabused nonpsychiatric controls (McGowan et al., 2009). Consistent with preclinical studies, samples from abused suicide victims showed increased cytosine methylation of the glucocorticoid receptor promoter, decreased transcription factor binding, and decreased gene transcription compared to nonabused suicide victims and nonsuicide controls.

5-HTTLPR × Maltreatment Predictors of Early Alcohol Use

We have also followed a subset of our cohort for 2 years and examined predictors of early alcohol use, including maltreatment, family loading for alcohol/substance use disorders, and 5-HTTLPR (Kaufman et al., 2007). Alcohol use before the age of 14 is a potent predictor of later alcohol problems and is associated with a 40% risk for the development of alcohol dependence (Grant & Dawson, 1997). Participants were 127 subjects: 76 maltreated children and 51 demographically matched community controls. At follow-up, 29% of the maltreated children reported alcohol use, a rate more than seven times the rate observed in controls. Maltreated children also started drinking, on average, more than 2 years earlier than controls (11.2 vs. 13.5 years). We chose to examine the impact of 5-HTTLPR variation in the development of alcohol problems as serotonin is a critical modulator of the stress response (Oroszi & Goldman, 2004). It is also one of the main neurotransmitter systems involved in brain reward circuitry (Koob et al., 1997), it is released in response to alcohol (Yoshimoto, McBride, Lumeng, & Li, 1992), and alcohol dependence is associated with serotonergic system dysregulation (Koob, 2003). In addition, in studies with nonhuman primates, polymorphic variation in 5-HTTLPR has been found to moderate the effects of early stress on alcohol consumption later in life (Barr et al., 2004), and there were two preliminary reports of 5-HTTLPR G × E in predicting alcohol use in older adolescents and young adults (Covault et al., 2007; Nilsson et al., 2005). Consistent with these other reports, after controlling for family loading of alcohol and substance use disorders, early alcohol use was predicted by maltreatment, *5-HTTLPR*, and a G × E, with increased risk for early alcohol use associated with the "s" allele. Psychopathology at baseline, severity of maltreatment, and poor mother–child relations also predicted early alcohol use (Kaufman et al., 2007).

Imaging Genomics

As detailed in the chapters by Hariri (Chapter 3) and Meyer-Lindenberg (Chapter 4) in this volume, there is growing interest in imaging genomics in clinical and nonclinical samples—examining the relationship between genetic variants and alterations in brain structure and function. Hariri and colleagues (2002) were the first to use functional magnetic resonance imaging (fMRI) to show that the "s" allele of *5-HTTLPR* is associated with increased amygdala activation in response to aversive stimuli. The amygdala is a key structure involved in the brain's orchestrated response to stress (Kaufman, Plotsky, Nemeroff, & Charney, 2000), and is a critical component of the emotion and reward-processing circuits in the brain, interconnected neural circuits implicated in the etiology of stress-related psychiatric disorders (Drevets, Price, & Furey, 2008; Krishnan & Nestler, 2008). Since Hariri and colleagues' initial publication there have been 17 studies investigating this association, and results of a recent meta-analysis supports the conclusion that *5-HTTLPR* variation moderates amygdala activation in response to a range of negative stimuli (Munafò, Brown, & Hariri, 2008).

In our imaging genomics work we chose to use a dichotic listening prosody task developed by Vuilleumier and colleagues (Grandjean et al., 2005; Sander et al., 2005). Male and female actors created the stimuli for the prosody task using nonsense words which were spoken in either an angry or a neutral tone of voice (e.g., "goster" and "niuvenci"). Participants simultaneously heard two stimuli, one spoken by a male in one ear, and one spoken by a female in the other ear. Children were asked to attend to either the left or right ear and indicate whether a man or woman spoke the word in that ear. Across blocks of trials, the to-be-attended-to ear was indicated via the presentation of the letters L and R, for left and right ear, respectively.

This implicit emotion-processing task, like other emotion-processing tasks used in previous studies, elicits amygdala activation when attention is focused on the angry prosody (Grandjean et al., 2005; Sander et al., 2005). In addition, performance of the dichotic listening task requires interhemispheric transfer through the posterior portion of the corpus callosum (Westerhausen et al., 2006), a region that has been shown in several independent samples to be altered in maltreated children and adolescents (De Bellis et al., 1999, 2002; Jackowski et al., 2008; Teicher, Andersen, Polcari, Anderson, & Navalta, 2002).

The children (N = 18) for this pilot project were recruited from our prior G × E studies. Participants were stratified in a 2 × 2 factorial design according to maltreatment history (e.g., maltreated vs. control) and genetic risk (e.g., "s/s" vs. "l/l") (Herrington et al., 2007). To test for differences in activation during emotion processing of negative stimuli, an analysis was conducted comparing areas of activation during the attended angry versus nonattended angry conditions. The results of the voxel-based random effects analyses showed significant genotype effects in the left amygdala, with significantly greater activation in "s/s" compared to "l/l" subjects. No main effect for group was evident in the maltreated versus control contrast, which may be due to the fact that the scans were completed 2 years after recruitment for the G × E studies, and 42% of the maltreated children included in this pilot study no longer met full criteria for PTSD or any other psychiatric diagnosis.

In terms of the interhemispheric transfer of information, during the dichotic listening task auditory information sent along ipsilateral pathways seems to be blocked or suppressed by information from the contralateral pathways (Plessen et al., 2007; Springer & Gazzaniga, 1975), such that auditory input received via the right ear in the forced right ear attend condition is initially processed in the left hemisphere. Processing of paralinguistic information (e.g., gender determination, prosody), however, is lateralized to the right hemisphere in the superior temporal gyrus (STG). Therefore, completion of this task in the right ear attend condition requires transfer of stimulus information from the left hemisphere to the right STG via the posterior region of the corpus callosum. Activation in the right STG in the right forced ear attend condition provides a test of interhemispheric transfer of information and corpus callosum integrity. During the right ear attend condition, when compared to maltreated children, control children showed significantly greater activation of the right STG. Group differences in this same region were also evident when comparing children with two "s" alleles to children with two "l" alleles of *5-HTTLPR*. As predicted, however, there were no differences in the activation of the right STG in the left ear attend condition when interhemispheric transfer of information is not necessary for processing the prosody stimuli. Imaging genomics research, especially when conducted in conjunction with translational research studies, holds significant promise in unraveling the mechanisms by which certain alleles and experiences confer vulnerability to psychopathology.

Translational Research Studies

Preclinical (e.g., animal) studies of the effects of stress provide a valuable heuristic in understanding the pathophysiology of depression and other stress-related psychiatric illnesses (Gorman, Mathew, & Coplan, 2002; Heim, Owens, Plotsky, & Nemeroff, 1997), with many of the biological alterations associated with early stress in preclinical studies reported in *adults* with these disorders. These studies also allow for an examination of molecular mechanisms that are simply not possible in living clinical populations. However, there appear to be developmental differences in some of the neurobiological correlates of stress across the life cycle, although little preclinical research has been conducted with prepubescent and early postpubescent animals. Thus, to address the gap we formed a collaboration with Coplan and colleagues. Coplan and colleagues developed an experimental model of early stress in nonhuman primates called variable foraging demand (VFD). VFD rearing is an early life–stress paradigm in which infant bonnet macaques are reared by mothers undergoing an experimentally induced "perception" of food unavailability (Rosenblum et al., 1994). Although adequate food is always available, the ease with which food is accessed is variable and unpredictable for 12–16 weeks within the first year of the infant's life. At times food is easily accessed, at other times mothers must forage for food in a bin of wood chips. There are no differences in weight between VFD and non-VFD mothers or infants, but VFD conditions are stressful for mothers. Stress is transmitted to the offspring via disruption of maternal attachment and affective reciprocity, with increased stress hormones observed in both mothers and infants (Coplan, Kaufman, et al., 2005). VFD rearing is associated with pervasive and sustained biobehavioral effects that closely resemble the biobehavioral abnormalities associated with human anxiety and depressive disorders throughout the developmental trajectory of the offspring and into adulthood (Coplan, Altemus, et al., 2005; Gorman et al., 2002).

Coplan and colleagues had data from 23 young adult male subjects who underwent MRI scans: 13 were reared under the VFD condition (eight "l/l" and five "s/l" or "s/s"), and nine age-matched male subjects were normally reared (seven "l/l" and two "s/l" subjects). Corpus callosum area measurements were obtained at the midsagittal slice using validated procedures (Witelson, 1976). Exploratory analyses revealed a significant effect for rearing condition and a gene × rearing effect in total corpus callosum area, with VFD-reared subjects with an "s" allele having the smallest corpus callosum area (Jackowski et al., in press).

Postmortem microarray studies are planned to look at changes in gene expression in key cortical areas. We are especially interested in examining the expression of myelin-related genes given the prominence of white matter changes reported in neuroimaging studies of maltreated children and adolescents (De Bellis et al., 1999, 2002; Jackowski et al., 2008, in press; Teicher et al., 2004), and results of postmortem studies of adults with depression documenting oligodendrocyte reduction in the amygdala (Hamidi, Drevets, & Price, 2004), and decreased expression of 17 genes related to oligodendrocyte function in the temporal cortex (Barley, Dracheva, & Byne, 2009). Oligodendrocytes are the myelinating cells of the central nervous system (CNS) which arise from progenitors in the subventricular zone and undergo a well-regulated process of proliferation, migration, and differentiation (Miller, 1996). One hypothesis emerging from our research is that genes involved in oligodendrocyte proliferation, migration, and differentiation may have a role in moderating the effects of stress.

More work is needed to unravel the mechanisms by which stress may confer vulnerability to depression and other stress-related psychiatric disorders. Multidisciplinary efforts that allow for cross-fertilization between basic and clinical investigators hold significant promise for delineating the mechanism of risk and identifying novel foci for future clinical research efforts. For example, recent data suggest that the epigenetic changes associated with variation in maternal care can be reversed in adult animals via infusion of the histone deacetylase inhibitor l-methionine or trichostatin A (Weaver, Meaney, & Szyf, 2006). Environmental enrichment in adolescent animals has also been found to reverse hypothalamus–pituitary–adrenal (HPA) axis hyperactivity, memory deficits, and other behavioral alterations associated with early nonoptimal rearing, with the reversal of many of these effects apparently mediated by enhancement of glutamate N-methyl-D-aspartate (NMDA) and α-amino-3hydroxy-5methyl-4isoxazolepropionic acid (AMPA) receptor subunit gene expression (Bredy et al., 2003, 2004). Improvement in stress and behavioral measures is not associated with reversal of glucocorticoid receptor changes, but with compensatory changes in the glutamate system. These findings highlight how better understanding of the mechanisms involved in stress-related psychopathology can lead to identification of novel targets for therapeutic interventions. It is becoming increasingly evident that there are multiple neurochemical systems that can be altered to modify the behavioral and biological sequelae associated with early stress.

IMPLICATIONS OF EMERGING G × E RESEARCH FINDINGS FOR DESIGNING INTERVENTIONS TO PROMOTE RESILIENCE IN MALTREATED CHILDREN

An important take-home message from the G × E studies is that neither high-risk genes nor high-risk environments guarantee deleterious outcomes. The availability of a positive caring adult support can moderate risk for deleterious outcomes in maltreated children—with the effect greatest for children with the highest genetic risk for psychopathology (Kaufman et al., 2004, 2006). Unfortunately, problems within the family of origin, extended lengths of stay in care, and multiple changes in foster care placements frequently compromise maltreated children's ability to have access to a positive stable adult support.

As noted briefly at the onset of this chapter, over 80% of the maltreated children in our study came from families struggling with substance use disorders. This is consistent with the findings of other investigators who have estimated that 60–70% of all substantiated child welfare cases, and 80% or more of parents whose children are placed in foster care, have substance use disorders (De Bellis et al., 2001; Osterling & Austin, 2008; Young et al., 2007). Among child welfare cases, parental substance abuse is associated with higher rates of child revictimization (Brook & McDonald, 2009; Ondersma, 2007), greater likelihood of out-of-home placement (U.S. Department of Health and Human Services, 1997), longer stays in care (Connell, Bergeron, Katz, Saunders, & Tebes, 2007; Vanderploeg et al., 2007), and higher rates of termination of parental rights and child adoption (Connell et al., 2007). Over time we observed similar trends in our sample.

This has led us to the hypothesis that learning how to optimally address substance abuse problems in the family of origin is the key to promoting resilience in maltreated children. As reviewed elsewhere (Oliveros & Kaufman, in press), over the past decade there has been growing interest in the problem of substance abuse within the child welfare system. Family treatment drug courts (FTDC) have emerged as the leading strategy in the United States for facilitating substance abuse treatment for parents involved in the child welfare system. While the services provided by FTDCs vary somewhat from one jurisdiction to next, these programs typically provide substance abuse evaluations within the court building, often completed immediately following the initial dependency hearing; regular, up to weekly, court hearings to monitor parents' treatment compliance; provision of office-based substance abuse treatment and adjunctive wraparound services; and frequent drug testing. In FTDC programs, rewards, sanctions, and intensity of judicial surveillance are linked to service compliance (Boles, Young, Moore, & DiPirro-Beard, 2007). FTDCs are associated with faster and greater rates of substance abuse treatment initiation (Green, Furrer, Worcel, Burrus, & Finigan, 2007; Worcel, Furrer, Green, Burrus, & Finigan, 2008), longer duration of treatment (Green, Furrer, et al., 2007; Worcel et al., 2008), and in two of the three studies conducted, greater likelihood of treatment completion (Boles et al., 2007; Green, Furrer, et al., 2007; Worcel et al., 2008). FTDCs have also consistently been associated with fewer days in out-of-home placement for children (Boles et al., 2007; Worcel et al., 2008), and higher rates of family reunification (Boles et al., 2007; Green, Furrer, et al., 2007; Worcel et al., 2008). Rates of treatment entry vary between 80 and 90% for FTDC cases, as compared to 55–60% for control cases that receive traditional child protective and substance abuse services. Also, while only about one-third of controls complete treatment, treatment completion rates are approximately two-thirds among FTDC cases. In one study, days in out-of-home care was significantly reduced from 495 to 403 (Worcel et al., 2008), and in the second that examined this outcome, days in out-of-home care was significantly reduced from 993 to 642 (Boles et al., 2007). Across studies, rates of reunification ranged from 42 to 69% for FTDC cases, and from 27 to 44% for controls, with reunification approximately twice as likely if parents completed at least one treatment cycle (Green, Rockhill, & Furrer, 2007). No consistent benefit of FTDC, however, has been demonstrated with regard to reentry into care or new substantiated reports of maltreatment. Boles and colleagues (2007) reported nonsignificant differences between FTDC cases and controls on rates of reentry into care, with 23% (83/362) of the children of parents who received FTDC services and 11% (5/47) of controls reentering care within 24 months of family reunification. Green and colleagues (2007) reported a similar pattern of findings, with rates for new substantiated reports of abuse (FTDC: 23% vs. control: 14%, ns), suggesting the need for further treatment refinement to better optimize the outcomes of families with substance use disorders who are involved with the child welfare system.

Recently Swenson, Henggler, and colleagues (2009) reported initial data on an alternative treatment model for providing substance abuse services to parents involved in the child welfare system: the Building Stronger Families (BSF) program. BSF integrates multisystemic therapy (MST) and reinforcement-based treatment (RBT) for adult substance abuse to provide home-based drug and alcohol treatment. MST is an empirically validated home- and community-based treatment for families with multiple complex treatment needs, and RBT is an incentive-based treatment for adults with addictive disorders. As many parents involved with child welfare meet criteria for PTSD, BSF clinicians are also trained in evidence-based PTSD treatments. BSF clinicians provide substance abuse, mental health, parenting skills, case management, and other services as needed, with 24/7 on-call services available to address crises that emerge afterhours. BSF is typically 6 months in duration. The goals of BSF are to eliminate parental substance misuse, address factors associated with child maltreatment, and keep children living with their families (parents or relatives), whenever possible. Family safety plans are developed with protective service workers and the BSF team, and ideally involve collaboration with members of the family's natural ecology. Breathalyzer and urine drug testing is conducted randomly in the home a minimum of three times per week for the duration of treatment. Within the BSF model, there is an understanding that relapse is a part of the recovery process. Decisions to remove children from their parents' homes are not based on the results on any particular drug test, but on parent adherence to safety plans and willingness to engage in substance abuse treatment. In a study of treatment feasibility with 54 families, 87% of the parents referred for BSF treatment initiated services, 93% of those who began treatment services completed the BSF program, and 75% of the parents retained custody of their children throughout the duration of treatment. Overall, 86% of the cases were discharged successfully with sustained sobriety, stable mental health, safe and secure housing, and placement permanency for children. These preliminary data are very promising and suggest an alternative model of care that warrants further evaluation.

We are in the initial planning phases to implement a randomized control study comparing the efficacy of FTDC and BSF for parents with substance abuse problems who are involved with the child welfare system and at risk of losing custody of their children. Treatment efficacy will be examined on (1) substance abuse treatment outcomes (e.g., treatment engagement, treatment completion, sobriety); (2) child welfare outcomes (e.g., need for out-of-home placement, number and duration of out-of-home placements, reabuse); (3) child and parent well-being measures (e.g., emotional well-being, social supports, concrete needs); and (4) cost-effectiveness.

Additional foci to optimize outcomes of maltreated children include eliminating use of congregate care settings for young children in care, assuring access to appropriate mental health care services for children, provision of enrichment opportunities, and continuity in care and sustained support. Significant advances have been made in treating trauma-related psychopathology (Cohen & Mannarino, 2002; Lieberman, Van Horn, & Ghosh Ippen, 2006); unfortunately evidenced-based treatments are not adequately available to children within the child welfare system (Landsverk et al., 2009). Enriched foster care programs that provide access to specialized mental health care services and a range of enrichment opportunities (e.g., camp, tutoring, music and dance lessons) have been found to decrease risk for depression, anxiety, and substance use disorders in young adult alumni from the foster care system (Kessler et al., 2008). To help promote resilience in children committed to care, a number of states have passed legislation to extend the age limit of foster care to 21, and added provisions for tuition assistance for foster care children seeking higher education (Child Welfare League of America, 2009). These initiatives hold significant promise for increasing the odds of youth aging out of the system succeeding in young adulthood, although the benefits of these programs have yet to be systematically examined.

RESEARCH UPDATE

Unfortunately, at the time of the writing of this chapter we were 4 years and 3 months into a moratorium on our G × E work in the State of Connecticut. With a change in leadership of the State Institutional Review Board, a moratorium was imposed on our work that letters of support from the Directors of the National Institute of Mental Health and National Institute on Alcohol Abuse and Alcoholism, the deans of the two medical schools in our state, the child advocate, and many others failed to affect. We have been forbidden to recruit new maltreated children, further characterize stored DNA specimens, or freely analyze data we had permission to collect. (This explains why we have never examined G × E predictors of PTSD in our sample.) Like other special needs populations, children in foster care deserve to benefit from advances in the biomedical sciences. Through organizations like Autism Speaks and the Child and Adolescent Bipolar Foundation, parents of these special needs children advocate for state-of-the-art biomedical research to improve the developmental outcomes of their children. Children receiving child protective services frequently do not have such support.

Table 9.1 outlines our responses to the major concerns raised regarding the incorporation of genetics research approaches in studies of children involved with the child protective services system. We are currently pursuing permission to resume our work in another jurisdiction. We remain committed to the perspective that incorporating genetics and utilizing a biopsychosocial approach is crucial to improving the life-course trajectory of the vulnerable population of children who enter foster care.

CLOSING REMARKS

The outcomes of maltreated children within the child protective services system are frequently compromised by failure to address substance abuse disorders in the family of origin, inadequate access to empirically validated child trauma treatments, multiple changes in out-of-home placements, excessive use of congregate care settings, and separation from siblings and other important supports (Kaufman, 2007). As noted above, an important take-home message from the G × E studies is that neither high-risk genes nor high-risk environments guarantee deleterious outcomes. Positive factors in the environment can reduce risk, but it does not alleviate risk as some children experience deleterious outcomes despite unyielding support from their caregivers. The more we understand about the relevant factors necessary to promote resilience, the more opportunity there will be to optimize child outcomes. It is our firm belief that the focus of clinical and research efforts for maltreated children must span from neurobiology to social policy. The cost of our ignorance is far too high.

TABLE 9.1. Promoting Positive Outcomes for Children in Care: The Role for Genetics Research

Risks/concerns	Discussion
1. Why study maltreated children?	• Maltreated children at high risk for a range of problems including depression, suicidality, posttraumatic stress disorder, aggression, and alcohol and substance use disorders. • Maltreated children overrepresented in psychiatric care settings. • Maltreated children comprise approximately one-third of all child psychiatric outpatients, and over 50% of child psychiatric inpatients.
2. Why not just study other traumatized groups of children?	• While all trauma is bad for children, child maltreatment and intrafamilial violence are associated with the highest risk for bad outcomes. • Among individuals with other types of trauma (e.g., community violence), it has repeatedly been demonstrated that those who also experience intrafamilial violence are at highest risk. • If excluding children involved with CPS, we'd be excluding the most vulnerable children.
3. Why genetics?	• In almost every area of medicine, genetics research has led to improved and earlier diagnosis, development of new and more effective treatments, and better patient–intervention matching. • The promise genetics holds for psychiatry as it does for other areas of medicine, even though most genes that are relevant for psychiatric disorders exert relatively minor effects compared to the genes involved in things like PKU or Huntington's disease. • Studies examining genetic *and* environmental factors are critical in this population given emerging understandings of epigenetic processes, the dynamic interplay of genes and environment, and the documented impact of environment on gene expression.
4. Why longitudinal research?	• Onset of several problems not evident until later in development (e.g., alcohol and substance abuse). • Ongoing follow-up will help to identify those at greatest risk, and help to identify positive factors that can decrease risk over time for bad outcomes. • Resilience changes over time. Understanding why some children bounce back and others experience chronic difficulties is essential for guiding prevention and intervention efforts.

(cont.)

TABLE 9.1. *(cont.)*

Risks/concerns	Discussion
5. Why not conduct research in adults to address the same questions?	• Children are not mini-adults. • Many of the medications that are extremely effective in the treatment of adult psychiatric disorders are totally *ineffective* in children. • Only studies with child populations can guide child clinical care and advance our understanding of psychiatric disorders in childhood.
6. Why recruit through CPS and not child guidance clinics or some other mechanism?	• Recruitment through CPS allows for the identification of the highest risk children, and children with *and* without problems. • If recruiting through child guidance clinics, by definition all children will be impaired.
7. Minorities overrepresented in CPS system Stigma concerns	• Minorities are typically *underrepresented* in research, leading to the identification of novel treatments with untested benefits in minorities. This has proven problematic in multiple areas of medicine. • The inclusion of comparison children who are demographically matched to the CPS sample (e.g., ethnicity, SES) minimizes the potential of stigmatization and misinterpretation of research findings.
8. Informed consent/assent	• Multiple consents and assents obtained • Birth parent/relative consent/assent • Assent from current guardian (e.g., foster parent) and CPS worker also obtained • Assent from child obtained in language that is comprehensible to child
9. Protection of DNA data	• Data protected with security codes and multiple protection methods standard in psychiatric and genetics research. • Certificate of Confidentiality obtained to prevent subpoenaing of research data. • In a recent survey of investigators conducting psychiatric genetics research who collectively recruited over 30,000 participants, there were no incidents of anyone getting access to the data who was not affiliated with the research.
10. Insurance company misuse of DNA data	• The Genetic Information Nondiscrimination Act (HR 493), passed in 2008, prohibits employers from using genetic information as a basis for hiring, firing, or promoting individuals. The act also forbids insurers from denying coverage or charging higher premiums to individuals based on genetic information.

(cont.)

TABLE 9.1. *(cont.)*

Risks/concerns	Discussion
11. Use of DNA specimens by law enforcement	• DNA data protected by Certificate of Confidentiality • Research DNA specimen of limited use to law enforcement • While individuals can be identified by testing a small number of markers in the research DNA sample, individual identification requires matching research sample with another DNA sample. If law enforcement had the reference DNA sample, there would be no reason to seek the research specimen.
12. Consent reaches into the future indefinitely unless affirmatively revoked	• Participants reconsented at each follow-up • Easy procedures for withdrawal—telephone or other communication • Train staff to ask all participants who wish to withdraw whether or not they would like their information eliminated from the databases, or if it would be okay for researchers to use information previously collected.
13. Consent is being provided on child's behalf, but is following child into adulthood	• This is true of all research studies involving children. • Children will be reassented as they grow older at each follow-up.
14. DNA specimens stored in perpetuity and used for multiple unspecified purposes	• With advances in science, new genetic markers will emerge that warrant testing in psychiatric research populations. • Using stored specimens of clinically characterized samples is cost effective. Societal investment in genetics research should be optimized (e.g., taxpayer dollars pay for federally funded research). • Given the pace at which science is advancing, it is impossible to know at the onset of a study all the relevant markers that may be informative in a given sample. For this reason the consent informs participants of plans to store DNA indefinitely and to conduct additional genetic tests.

Risk–Benefit Analysis: Spit DNA sample is benign. Major risks in genetics studies are loss of confidentiality or stigmatization of participants. Adequate protections against these risks are possible. In addition, short-term benefits for participation are possible (e.g., enrichment, comprehensive assessments, referral); great potential long-term gains in learning how to minimize the negative effects of abuse and neglect; and enormous need given the pervasiveness of problem of child maltreatment, limitations of current interventions, and tremendous cost to the individual and society for failed outcomes. Like other special needs populations, children in foster care deserve to benefit from advances in the biomedical sciences. Through organizations like Autism Speaks and the Child and Adolescent Bipolar Foundation, parents of these special needs children advocate for state-of-the-art biomedical research to improve the developmental outcomes of their children. Children receiving CPS likewise deserve to be the focus of state-of-the art biomedical research studies.

Note. CPS, child protective services.

REFERENCES

Barley, K., Dracheva, S., & Byne, W. (2009). Subcortical oligodendrocyte- and astrocyte-associated gene expression in subjects with schizophrenia, major depression and bipolar disorder. *Schizophrenia Research, 112*(1–3), 54–64.

Barr, C. S., Newman, T. K., Lindell, S., Shannon, C., Champoux, M., Lesch, K. P., et al. (2004). Interaction between serotonin transporter gene variation and rearing condition in alcohol preference and consumption in female primates. *Archives of General Psychiatry, 61*(11), 1146–1152.

Boles, S. M., Young, N. K., Moore, T., & DiPirro-Beard, S. (2007). The Sacramento Dependency Drug Court: Development and outcomes. *Child Maltreatment, 12*(2), 161–171.

Bredy, T. W., Humpartzoomian, R. A., Cain, D. P., Meaney, M. J., Morley-Fletcher, S., Rea, M., et al. (2003). Partial reversal of the effect of maternal care on cognitive function through environmental enrichment. *European Journal of Neuroscience, 18*(12), 571–576.

Bredy, T. W., Zhang, T. Y., Grant, R. J., Diorio, J., Meaney, M. J., Humpartzoomian, R. A., et al. (2004). Peripubertal environmental enrichment reverses the effects of maternal care on hippocampal development and glutamate receptor subunit expression. *European Journal of Neuroscience, 20*(5), 1355–1362.

Brook, J., & McDonald, T. (2009). The impact of parental substance abuse on the stability of family reunifications from foster care. *Children and Youth Services Review, 31*(2), 193–198.

Brunner, H. G., Nelen, M., Breakefield, X. O., Ropers, H. H., & van Oost, B. A. (1993). Abnormal behavior associated with a point mutation in the structural gene for monoamine oxidase A. *Science, 262*, 578–580.

Cases, O., Seif, I., Grimsby, J., Gaspar, P., Chen, K., Pournin, S., et al. (1995). Aggressive behavior and altered amounts of brain serotonin and norepinephrine in mice lacking MAOA. *Science, 268*, 1763–1766.

Caspi, A., McClay, J., Moffitt, T. E., Mill, J., Martin, J., Craig, I. W., et al. (2002). Role of genotype in the cycle of violence in maltreated children. *Science, 297*, 851–854.

Caspi, A., Sugden, K., Moffitt, T. E., Taylor, A., Craig, I. W., Harrington, H., et al. (2003). Influence of life stress on depression: Moderation by a polymorphism in the 5-HTT gene. *Science, 301*, 386–389.

Child Welfare League of America. (2009). Completed state foster youth 18–22 policies 4.1.09. Washington, DC: Author. Available at *www.cwla.org/advocacy/adoptionhr6893fostercarechart.pdf*.

Cohen, J. A., & Mannarino, A. P. (2002). Addressing attributions in treating abused children. *Child Maltreatment, 7*(1), 82–86.

Connell, C. M., Bergeron, N., Katz, K. H., Saunders, L., & Tebes, J. K. (2007). Re-referral to child protective services: The influence of child, family, and case characteristics on risk status. *Child Abuse and Neglect, 31*(5), 573–588.

Coplan, J. D., Altemus, M., Mathew, S. J., Smith, E. L., Sharf, B., Coplan, P. M., et al. (2005). Synchronized maternal–infant elevations of primate CSF CRF concentrations in response to variable foraging demand. *CNS Spectrums, 10*(7), 530–536.

Coplan, J. D., Kaufman, D., Shorman, I., Smith, E. L., Owens, M. J. Nemeroff, C. B., et al. (2005, December 13). *Variable foraging demand (VFD) exposure of primate maternal–infant dyads and impaired insulin action in juvenile offspring.* Paper presented at the American College of Neuropsychopharmacology annual meeting, Waikoloa, Hawaii.

Covault, J., Tennen, H., Armeli, S., Conner, T. S., Herman, A. I., Cillessen, A. H., et al. (2007). Interactive effects of the serotonin transporter 5-HTTLPR polymorphism and stressful life events on college student drinking and drug use. *Biological Psychiatry, 61*(5), 609–616.

De Bellis, M. D., Broussard, E. R., Herring, D. J., Wexler, S., Moritz, G., & Benitez, J. G. (2001). Psychiatric co-morbidity in caregivers and children involved in maltreatment: A pilot research study with policy implications. *Child Abuse and Neglect, 25*(7), 923–944.

De Bellis, M. D., Keshavan, M. S., Clark, D. B., Casey, B. J., Giedd, J. N., Boring, A. M., et al. (1999). Developmental traumatology: Part II. Brain development. *Biological Psychiatry, 45*(10), 1271–1284.

De Bellis, M. D., Keshavan, M. S., Shifflett, H., Iyengar, S., Beers, S. R., Hall, J., et al. (2002). Brain structures in pediatric maltreatment-related posttraumatic stress disorder: A sociodemographically matched study. *Biological Psychiatry, 52*(11), 1066–1078.

Deckert, J., Catalano, M., Syagailo, Y. V., Bosi, M., Okladnova, O., Di Bella, D., et al. (1999). Excess of high activity monoamine oxidase A gene promoter alleles in female patients with panic disorder. *Human Molecular Genetics, 8*(4), 621–624.

Drevets, W. C., Price, J. L., & Furey, M. L. (2008). Brain structural and functional abnormalities in mood disorders: Implications for neurocircuitry models of depression. *Brain Structure and Function, 213*(1–2), 93–118.

Duman, R. S., Heninger, G. R., & Nestler, E. J. (1997). A molecular and cellular theory of depression. *Archives of General Psychiatry, 54*(7), 597–606.

Famularo, R., Fenton, T., Kinscherff, R., & Augustyn, M. (1996). Psychiatric comorbidity in childhood post traumatic stress disorder. *Child Abuse and Neglect, 20*(10), 953–961.

Famularo, R., Kinscherff, R., & Fenton, T. (1992). Psychiatric diagnoses of maltreated children: Preliminary findings. *Journal of the American Academy of Child and Adolescent Psychiatry, 31*, 863–867.

Garland, A., Hough, R., McCabe, K., Yeh, M., Wood, P., & Aarons, G. (2001). Prevalence of psychiatric disorders in youths across five sectors of care. *Journal of the American Academy of Child and Adolescent Psychiatry, 40*(4), 409–418.

Glassman, L. H., Weierich, M. R., Hooley, J. M., Deliberto, T. L., & Nock, M. K. (2007). Child maltreatment, non-suicidal self-injury, and the mediating role of self-criticism. *Behaviour Research and Therapy, 45*, 2483–2490.

Gorman, J. M., Mathew, S., & Coplan, J. (2002). Neurobiology of early life stress: Nonhuman primate models. *Seminars in Clinical Neuropsychiatry, 7*(2), 96–103.

Grandjean, D., Sander, D., Pourtois, G., Schwartz, S., Seghier, M. L., Scherer, K.

R., et al. (2005). The voices of wrath: Brain responses to angry prosody in meaningless speech. *Nature Neuroscience, 8*(2), 145–146.

Grant, B. F., & Dawson, D. A. (1997). Age at onset of alcohol use and its association with DSM-IV alcohol abuse and dependence: Results from the National Longitudinal Alcohol Epidemiologic Survey. *Journal of Substance Abuse, 9*, 103–110.

Green, B. L., Furrer, C., Worcel, S., Burrus, S., & Finigan, M. W. (2007). How effective are family treatment drug courts?: Outcomes from a four-site national study. *Child Maltreatment, 12*(1), 43–59.

Green, B. L., Rockhill, A., & Furrer, C. (2007). Does substance abuse treatment make a difference for child welfare case outcomes?: A statewide longitudinal analysis. *Children and Youth Services Review, 29*, 460–463.

Hamidi, M., Drevets, W. C., & Price, J. L. (2004). Glial reduction in amygdala in major depressive disorder is due to oligodendrocytes. *Biological Psychiatry, 55*(6), 563–569.

Hariri, A. R., Mattay, V. S., Tessitore, A., Kolachana, B., Fera, F., Goldman, D., et al. (2002). Serotonin transporter genetic variation and the response of the human amygdala. *Science, 297*, 400–403.

Heim, C., Owens, M. J., Plotsky, P. M., & Nemeroff, C. B. (1997). The role of early adverse life events in the etiology of depression and posttraumatic stress disorder: Focus on corticotropin-releasing factor. *Annals of the New York Academy of Sciences, 821*, 194–207.

Herrington, J., Douglas-Palumberi, H., Meadows, A., Gelernter, J., Kaffman, A., Coplan, J., et al. (2007, May). *fMRI study of prosody processing in maltreated children*. Paper presented at the annual meeting of the Society of Biological Psychiatry, San Diego, CA.

Holmans, P., Zubenko, G. S., Crowe, R. R., DePaulo, J. R., Jr., Scheftner, W. A., Weissman, M. M., et al. (2004). Genomewide significant linkage to recurrent, early-onset major depressive disorder on chromosome 15q. *American Journal of Human Genetics, 74*(6), 1154–1167.

Jackowski, A., Douglas-Palumberi, H., Jackowski, M., Win, L., Schultz, R. T., Staib, L. H., et al. (2008). Corpus callosum in maltreated children with PTSD: A diffusion tensor imaging study. *Psychiatry Research: Neuroimaging, 162*(3), 256–261.

Jackowski, A., Perera, T., Garrido, G., Tang, C. Y., Martinez, J., Sanjay, M., et al. (in press). Early life stress, corpus callosum development, and anxious behavior in nonhuman primates. *Psychiatry Research: Neuroimaging*.

Karg, K., Shedden, K., Burmeister, M., & Sen, S. (in press). The serotonin transporter promoter variant (*5-HTTLPR*), stress, and depression meta-analysis revisited: Evidence of genetic moderation. *Archives of General Psychiatry*.

Kaufman, J. (1991). Depressive disorders in maltreated children. *Journal of the American Academy of Child and Adolescent Psychiatry, 30*(2), 257–265.

Kaufman, J. (2007). Child abuse. In *Lewis' child and adolescent psychiatry: A comprehensive textbook* (4th ed., pp. 629–700). Baltimore: Lippincott Williams & Wilkins.

Kaufman, J., Gelernter, J., Kaffman, A., Caspi, A., & Moffitt, T. E. (2010). Arguable assumptions, questionable conclusions. *Biological Psychiatry, 67*(4), 19–20.

Kaufman, J., & Henrich, C. (2000). Exposure to violence and early childhood trauma. In C. H. Zeanah, Jr. (Ed.), *Handbook of infant mental health* (pp. 195–207). New York: Guilford Press.

Kaufman, J., Plotsky, P., Nemeroff, C., & Charney, D. (2000). Effects of early adverse experience on brain structure and function: Clinical implications. *Biological Psychiatry, 48*(8), 778–790.

Kaufman, J., Yang, B. Z., Douglas-Palumberi, H., Crouse-Artus, M., Lipschitz, D., Krystal, J. H., et al. (2007). Genetic and environmental predictors of early alcohol use. *Biological Psychiatry, 61*(11), 1228–1234.

Kaufman, J., Yang, B. Z., Douglas-Palumberi, H., Grasso, D., Lipschitz, D., Houshyar, S., et al. (2006). Brain-derived neurotrophic factor-5-HTTLPR gene interactions and environmental modifiers of depression in children. *Biological Psychiatry, 59*, 673–680.

Kaufman, J., Yang, B. Z., Douglas-Palumberi, H., Houshyar, S., Lipschitz, D., Krystal, J., et al. (2004). Social supports and serotonin transporter gene moderate depression in maltreated children. *Proceedings of the National Academy of Sciences USA, 101*(49), 17316–17321.

Kendler, K. S., & Karkowski-Shuman, L. (1997). Stressful life events and genetic liability to major depression: Genetic control of exposure to the environment? *Psychological Medicine, 27*(3), 539–547.

Kessler, R. C., Pecora, P. J., Williams, J., Hiripi, E., O'Brien, K., English, D., et al. (2008). Effects of enhanced foster care on the long-term physical and mental health of foster care alumni. *Archives of General Psychiatry, 65*(6), 625–633.

Kilpatrick, D., Ruggiero, K., Acierno, R., Saunders, B., Resnick, H., & Best, C. (2003). Violence and risk of PTSD, major depression, substance abuse/dependence, and comorbidity: Results from the National Survey of Adolescents. *Journal of Consulting and Clinical Psychology, 71*(4), 692–700.

Kilpatrick, D. G., Koenen, K. C., Ruggiero, K. J., Acierno, R., Galea, S., Resnick, H. S., et al. (2007). The serotonin transporter genotype and social support and moderation of posttraumatic stress disorder and depression in hurricane-exposed adults. *American Journal of Psychiatry, 164*(11), 1693–1699.

Kim-Cohen, J., Caspi, A., Taylor, A., Williams, B., Newcombe, R., Craig, I. W., et al. (2006). MAOA, maltreatment, and gene–environment interaction predicting children's mental health: New evidence and a meta-analysis. *Molecular Psychiatry, 10*, 903–913.

Koenen, K. C., Aiello, A. E., Bakshis, E., Amstadter, A. B., Ruggiero, K. J., Acierno, R., et al. (2009). The serotonin transporter genotype and social support and moderation of posttraumatic stress disorder and depression in hurricane-exposed adults. *American Journal of Epidemiology, 169*(6), 704–711.

Kolko, D. (2002). Child physical abuse. In J. Myers, L. Berliner, J. Briere, C. T. Hendrix, C. Jenny, & T. A. Reid (Eds.), *The APSAC handbook on child maltreatment* (2nd ed., pp. 21–54). Thousand Oaks, CA: Sage.

Koob, G. F. (2003). Alcoholism: Allostasis and beyond. *Alcoholism: Clinical and Experimental Research, 27*(2), 232–243.

Koob, G. F., Le Moal, M., Barr, C. S., Newman, T. K., Lindell, S., Shannon, C., et al. (1997). Interaction between serotonin transporter gene variation and rearing condition in alcohol preference and consumption in female primates. *Science, 278,* 52–58.

Krishnan, V., & Nestler, E. J. (2008). The molecular neurobiology of depression. *Nature, 455,* 894–902.

Landsverk, J. A., Burns, B. J., Stambaugh, L. F., & Reutz, J. A. (2009). Psychosocial interventions for children and adolescents in foster care: Review of research literature. *Child Welfare, 88*(1), 49–69.

Lanktree, C., Briere, J., & Zaidi, L. (1991). Incidence and impact of sexual abuse in a child outpatient sample: The role of direct inquiry. *Child Abuse and Neglect, 15*(4), 447–453.

Lesch, K. P., Gross, J., Franzek, E., Wolozin, B. L., Riederer, P., & Murphy, D. L. (1995). Primary structure of the serotonin transporter in unipolar depression and bipolar disorder. *Biological Psychiatry, 37*(4), 215–223.

Lieberman, A. F., Van Horn, P., & Ghosh Ippen, C. (2006). Child–parent psychotherapy: Six-month follow-up of a randomized controlled trial. *Journal of the American Academy of Child and Adolescent Psychiatry, 45*(8), 913–918.

Malberg, J. E., Eisch, A. J., Nestler, E. J., & Duman, R. S. (2000). Chronic antidepressant treatment increases neurogenesis in adult rat hippocampus. *Journal of Neuroscience, 20*(24), 9104–9110.

McClellan, J., Adams, J., Douglas, D., McCurry, C., & Storck, M. (1995). Clinical characteristics related to severity of sexual abuse: A study of seriously mentally ill youth. *Child Abuse and Neglect, 19*(10), 1245–1254.

McGowan, P. O., Sasaki, A., D'Alessio, A. C., Dymov, S., Labonte, B., Szyf, M., et al. (2009). Epigenetic regulation of the glucocorticoid receptor in human brain associates with childhood abuse. *Nature Neuroscience, 12*(3), 342–348.

Miller, R. H. (1996). Oligodendrocyte origins. *Trends in Neuroscience, 19*(3), 92–96.

Molnar, B. E., Buka, S. L., & Kessler, R. C. (2001). Child sexual abuse and subsequent psychopathology: Results from the National Comorbidity Survey. *American Journal of Public Health, 91*(5), 753–760.

Munafò, M. R., Brown, S. M., & Hariri, A. R. (2008). Serotonin transporter (5-HTTLPR) genotype and amygdala activation: A meta-analysis. *Biological Psychiatry, 63*(9), 852–857.

Munafò, M. R., Durrant, C., Lewis, G., & Flint, J. (2009). Gene × environment interactions at the serotonin transporter locus. *Biological Psychiatry, 63*(3), 211–219.

Nilsson, K. W., Sjoberg, R. L., Damberg, M., Alm, P. O., Ohrvik, J., Leppert, J., et al. (2005). Role of the serotonin transporter gene and family function in adolescent alcohol consumption. *Alcoholism: Clinical and Experimental Research, 29*(4), 564–570.

Oliveros, A., & Kaufman, J. (in press). Addressing parents' substance abuse treatment needs in child welfare populations. *Child Welfare.*

Ondersma, S. J. (2007). Introduction to the first of two special sections on substance abuse and child maltreatment. *Child Maltreatment, 12*, 3–6.

Oroszi, G., & Goldman, D. (2004). Alcoholism: Genes and mechanisms. *Pharmacogenomics, 5*(8), 1037–1048.

Osterling, K. L., & Austin, M. J. (2008). Substance abuse interventions for parents involved in the child welfare system: Evidence and implications. *Journal of Evidence-Based Social Work, 5*(1–2), 157–189.

Pelcovitz, D., Kaplan, S. J., DeRosa, R. R., Mandel, F. S., & Salzinger, S. (2000). Psychiatric disorders in adolescents exposed to domestic violence and physical abuse. *American Journal of Orthopsychiatry, 70*(3), 360–369.

Plessen, K. J., Lundervold, A., Gruner, R., Hammar, A., Peterson, B. S., & Hugdahl, K. (2007). Functional brain asymmetry, attentional modulation, and interhemispheric transfer in boys with Tourette syndrome. *Neuropsychologia, 45*(4), 767–774.

Pritchard, J. K., Stephens, M., & Donnelly, P. (2000). Inference of population structure using multilocus genotype data. *Genetics, 155*(2), 945–959.

Risch, N., Herrell, R., Lehner, T., Liang, K. Y., Eaves, L., Hoh, J., et al. (2009). Interaction between the serotonin transporter gene (5-HTTLPR), stressful life events, and risk of depression: A meta-analysis. *Journal of the American Medical Association, 301*(23), 2462–2471.

Rosenblum, L. A., Coplan, J. D., Friedman, S., Bassoff, T., Gorman, J. M., & Andrews, M. W. (1994). Adverse early experiences affect noradrenergic and serotonergic functioning in adult primates. *Biological Psychiatry, 35*(4), 221–227.

Ruggiero, K., McLeer, S., & Dixon, J. (2000). Sexual abuse characteristics associated with survivor psychopathology. *Child Abuse and Neglect, 24*(7), 951–964.

Rutter, M., Giller, H., & Hagell, A. (1998). *Antisocial behavior by young people.* Cambridge, UK: Cambridge University Press.

Sabol, S. Z., Hu, S., & Hamer, D. (1998). A functional polymorphism in the monoamine oxidase A gene promoter. *Human Genetics, 103*(3), 273–279.

Sander, D., Grandjean, D., Pourtois, G., Schwartz, S., Seghier, M. L., Scherer, K. R., et al. (2005). Emotion and attention interactions in social cognition: Brain regions involved in processing anger prosody. *NeuroImage, 28*(4), 848–858.

Schaefer, M. (2007, November). *Public sector behavioral health for children and families: Aligning systems and incentives.* Paper presented at the Zigler Center in Child Development and Social Policy Colloquium Series, New Haven, CT.

Schuck, A. M., & Widom, C. S. (2003). Childhood victimization and alcohol symptoms in women: An examination of protective factors. *Journal of Studies on Alcohol, 64*(2), 247–256.

Springer, S. P., & Gazzaniga, M. S. (1975). Dichotic testing of partial and complete split brain subjects. *Neuropsychologia, 13*(3), 341–346.

Strauss, J., Barr, C. L., George, C. J., King, N., Shaikh, S., Devlin, B., et al. (2004). Association study of brain-derived neurotrophic factor in adults with a history of childhood onset mood disorder. *American Journal of Medical Genetics, Part B: Neuropsychiatric Genetics, 131*(1), 16–19.

Strauss, J., Barr, C. L., Vetro, A., King, N., Shaikh, S., Brathwaite, J., et al. (2004, June). *Brain derived neurotrophic factor gene and childhood-onset depressive disorder: Results from a Hungarian sample.* Paper presented at the Collegium International Neuro-Psychopharmacologicum (CINP) Congress, Paris.

Swenson, C. C., Schaeffer, C. M., Tuerk, E. H., Henggeler, S. W., Tuten, M., Panzarella, P., et al. (2009, Winter). Adapting multisystemic therapy for co-occurring child maltreatment and parental substance abuse: The Building Stronger Families Project. *Emotional and Behavioral Disorders in Youth,* pp. 3–8.

Teicher, M. H., Andersen, S. L., Polcari, A., Anderson, C. M., & Navalta, C. P. (2002). Developmental neurobiology of childhood stress and trauma. *Psychiatric Clinics of North America, 25*(2), 397–426, vii–viii.

Teicher, M. H., Dumont, N. L., Ito, Y., Vaituzis, C., Giedd, J. N., & Andersen, S. L. (2004). Childhood neglect is associated with reduced corpus callosum area. *Biological Psychiatry, 56*(2), 80–85.

U.S. Department of Health and Human Services. (1997). *National study of protective, preventive, and reunification services delivered to children and their families.* Washington, DC: Author.

Vanderploeg, J. J., Connell, C. M., Caron, C., Saunders, L., Katz, K. H., & Tebes, J. K. (2007). The impact of parental alcohol or drug removals on foster care placement experiences: A matched comparison group study. *Child Maltreatment, 12*(2), 125–136.

Weaver, I. C., Cervoni, N., Champagne, F. A., D'Alessio, A. C., Sharma, S., Seckl, J. R., et al. (2004). Epigenetic programming by maternal behavior. *Nature Neuroscience, 7*(8), 847–854.

Weaver, I. C., Meaney, M. J., & Szyf, M. (2006). Maternal care effects on the hippocampal transcriptome and anxiety-mediated behaviors in the offspring that are reversible in adulthood. *Proceedings of the National Academy of Sciences USA, 103*(9), 3480–3485.

Weder, N., Yang, B. Z., Douglas-Palumberi, H., Massey, J., Krystal, J. H., Gelernter, J., et al. (2009). MAOA genotype, maltreatment, and aggressive behavior: The changing impact of genotype at varying levels of trauma. *Biological Psychiatry, 65*(5), 417–424.

Westerhausen, R., Woerner, W., Kreuder, F., Schweiger, E., Hugdahl, K., & Wittling, W. (2006). The role of the corpus callosum in dichotic listening: A combined morphological and diffusion tensor imaging study. *Neuropsychology, 20*(3), 272–279.

Wichers, M., Kenis, G., Jacobs, N., Mengelers, R., Derom, C., Vlietinck, R., et al. (2008). The BDNF Val(66)Met × 5-HTTLPR × child adversity interaction and depressive symptoms: An attempt at replication. *American Journal of Medical Genetics, Part B: Neuropsychiatric Genetics, 147B*(1), 120–123.

Widom, C. (1989). The cycle of violence. *Science, 244,* 160–166.

Widom, C., & Ames, M. A. (1994). Criminal consequences of childhood sexual victimization. *Child Abuse and Neglect, 18*(4), 303–318.

Widom, C. S., Ireland, T., & Glynn, P. J. (1995). Alcohol abuse in abused and neglected children followed-up: Are they at increased risk? *Journal of Studies on Alcohol, 56*(2), 207–217.

Witelson, S. F. (1976). Sex and the single hemisphere: Specialization of the right hemisphere for spatial processing. *Science, 193*, 425–427.

Worcel, S., Furrer, C., Green, B. L., Burrus, S., & Finigan, M. (2008). Effects of family treatment drug courts on substance abuse and child welfare outcomes. *Child Abuse Review, 17*, 427–443.

Yoshimoto, K., McBride, W. J., Lumeng, L., & Li, T. K. (1992). Alcohol stimulates the release of dopamine and serotonin in the nucleus accumbens. *Alcohol, 9*(1), 17–22.

Young, N. K., Boles, S. M., & Otero, C. (2007). Parental substance use disorders and child maltreatment: Overlap, gaps, and opportunities. *Child Maltreatment, 12*(2), 137–149.

CHAPTER 10

Shaping Society through Social Policy

Will the Gene–Environment Revolution Make a Difference?

E. Jane Costello

This chapter on the gene–environment debate takes as its starting point what has been called the "Flynn effect." Flynn (1984; Lynn, 1990) noted that whereas the time frame of evolutionary change through random mutation and natural selection is a slow process, change on a range of human characteristics known to be highly heritable has been dramatically fast over the past century. Flynn and his colleagues have concentrated on intelligence, where measured scores, shown in twin studies to be highly heritable (Plomin & Spinath, 2004), have risen by about one standard deviation over 50 years. Height has also increased about the same extent in Europe and the United States (Lynn, 2009). In the realm of psychopathology, there have been several startling reports of rapid increases in some areas, particularly conduct problems (Collishaw, Maughan, Goodman, & Pickles, 2004) and anxiety (Twenge, 2000). The situation for childhood depression is less clear; some studies report a small secular increase (Collishaw, 2004), whereas others do not (Costello, Erkanli, & Angold, 2006; Twenge & Nolen-Hoeksema, 2002). Twenge, using data from high school and college students between 1938 and 2007, found increases of a standard deviation in scores on most of the subscales of the Minnesota Multiphasic Personality Inventory (MMPI; Hathaway & McKinley, 1940), including those measuring depression, anxiety, and antisocial tendencies (Twenge et al., 2010). All of these characteristics, whether classified as personality traits or clinical disorders, have also been shown to be at least moderately heritable (Benjamin, Ebstein, & Lesch, 1998; Blonigen, Hicks, Krieger, Patrick, & Iacono, 2005).

The Flynn paradox is relevant to the issue of gene–environment interplay because it deals with areas of human behavior which, while highly heritable, have changed so fast that the change must be driven by environmental factors in some way. The gene pool cannot have changed that rapidly, and so the genes have interacted with a rapidly changing environment to produce the observed secular trends. The question is: What are the environmental pressures, and how are they mediated through genes?

In this chapter I describe examples of the Flynn effect, set out a number of explanations for it that have been put forward, examine research that tests each of the explanations, and consider what the social policy implications of each explanation would be.

"DARWINIAN" EVOLUTION

One hundred and fifty years ago, Charles Darwin laid out the principles governing evolutionary change in living organisms: genetic variation in the population means that some organisms will be better adapted to the current environment, and will survive to reproduce more successfully than others in that environment. Natural selection acts on the phenotype of the organism, but the genetic basis of any phenotype that offers a reproductive advantage will become more common from one generation to the next. How fast the process works depends on the evolutionary disadvantage of the phenotype produced by alternative versions of the genes in question. The paradigmatic example of this process is the rise and fall of the dark-colored pepper moth (*Biston betularia*), a moth that exists in both a light-winged and a dark-winged form. In both the United States and the United Kingdom, "the rapid rise in the frequency of alleles producing melanic [dark-winged] phenotypes correlated with a general blackening of the environment following the nineteenth-century industrial revolution. . . . In recent years the frequency of melanics has been dropping steadily, apparently in . . . response to improved air quality" (Grant, 1996, p. 351).

The speed with which the dark and light pepper moths have changed their relative proportions in the population is exceptional in evolutionary history; they were clearly under extreme environmental pressure. Most changes driven by random mutation and natural selection (the basic principles of Darwinian evolution) occur much more slowly, as the fossil records show.

HERITABILITY OF HUMAN CHARACTERISTICS

One of the achievements of human genetics has been to document the extent to which many human characteristics are under genetic influence. For example, a recent study of over 30,000 twin pairs from eight predominantly Caucasian populations found that the heritability of height was 80–90% in all countries, despite considerable between-country differences in average height.

Evidence for the degree of heritability comes from genetically informative studies—that is, studies that permit a distinction to be made between the effects of heredity and the effects of the rearing environment. The most common of such designs compares monozygotic with dizygotic twins, but other researchers have studied twins reared apart; adopted children; complex families including twins, singletons, and stepchildren; and the children of twins, as well as migrant families. It is worth noting that, as Jensen (1969, p. 42) points out, "Heritability is a population statistic, describing the relative magnitude of the genetic component . . . in the population variance of the characteristic in question. It has no sensible meaning with reference to a measurement or characteristic in an individual. A single measurement, by definition, has no variance."

THE FLYNN EFFECT

Heritability, a process driven by random mutation and natural selection, is likely to produce change only quite slowly. Natural selection occurs when a particular random mutation increases the likelihood that its bearers will survive to reproduce successfully. Since different qualities increase the chance of survival to reproductive age in different environments, even characteristics that are "highly heritable" can become liabilities in a radically changed environment. The question is, how can we explain the extraordinary speed with which highly heritable characteristics have changed since we first began to measure them? For example, mean scores on an intelligence test administered to young males entering the military in Norway, a country that has universal conscription of males, rose by close to one standard deviation, an enormous increase, in less than 50 years. Similar increases on a test of general ability occurred in Danish conscripts over the same period. Figure 10.1 shows that the height of young adult males increased in a similar way over the same period (Sundet, Barlaug, & Torjussen, 2004).

There is evidence that this process has been going on for many decades. Schaie, Willis, and Pennak (2005) used data from a cohort-sequential study in Seattle to show a marked difference in a test of reasoning between the

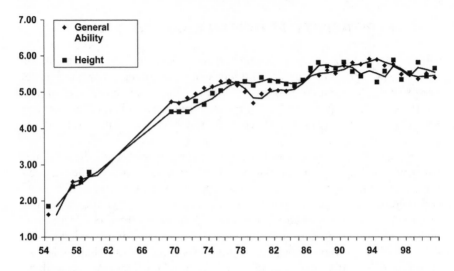

FIGURE 10.1. Mean standing height and mean general abilities test of Norwegian conscripts (both in z-score units + 5) by year of testing. Data from Sundet, Barlaug, and Torjussen (2004).

cohort born in the 1890s and those born in the 1940s and 1980s (Figure 10.2). The difference appears to persist into late life even when mean scores in general are starting to decline.

Rapid change of this sort has also been found in characteristics that are at first sight less advantageous than height and IQ, and more puzzling to explain within a gene–environment framework. For example, when Collishaw and colleagues (2004) used data from three birth cohort studies in the United Kingdom to construct a measure of antisocial behavior that was the same for each study, they found a steady and highly significant increase in the mean score between 1974 and 1999. Emotional problem scores (anxiety and depression) did not increase between the first two measurement points (1974 and 1986), but increased significantly between 1986 and 1999. As noted earlier, Twenge and colleagues found markedly higher scores on all the subscales of the MMPI (Twenge et al., 2010), as well as on narcissistic personality traits between 1982 and 2009 (Twenge & Foster, 2010). The list of "negative" human characteristics that appear to have changed much more rapidly than evolution would predict includes myopia, asthma, autism, and attention-deficit/hyperactivity disorder (ADHD) (Storfer, 1999).

In the face of this evidence that so many human characteristics are changing—for better or ill—at such speed, we need to pay attention to the social policy implications of such change. To give a single example, the

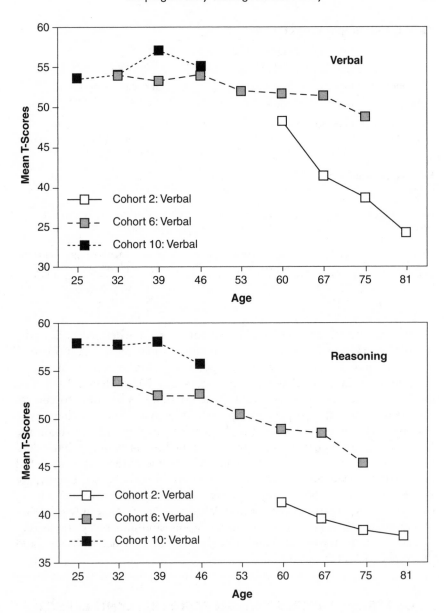

FIGURE 10.2. Within-cohort trajectories for the Abilities of Verbal Meaning and Reasoning from the Seattle Longitudinal Study (Schaie et al., 2005). Cohort 2: median birth year 1895; Cohort 6: median birth year 1924; Cohort 10: median birth year 1952

TABLE 10.1. Implications for Social Policy

Explanation	Evidence that would support the explanation	Policy implications
Methodological bias	Not clear	Increase support for monitoring studies
Increased environmental complexity	Gains across whole distribution; greater gains in past 20 years	Ensure equal access to environmental complexity, especially computers
Reduced environmental stressors	Greatest gains in the most stressed groups	Likely to reduce social inequality
Gene–environment correlation	Greatest gains in the most advantaged groups	Likely to increase social inequality
Heterosis	Greatest advantage to outbred societies	Encourage immigration from many places

percentage of children in U.S. public schools who were defined as mentally retarded (generally speaking, with a measured intelligence below 75) rose from less than 1% in the immediate postwar years to a peak of 2.16% in 1976, and since then has fallen back to around 1% (Nevin, 2009). We need to understand the reasons for these fluctuations not only to control their causes, but also to plan for appropriate services. In this chapter we consider five classes of reasons that have been put forward to explain the Flynn effect. For each class, we think about the kind of evidence that would be needed to test the explanation, and review some of that evidence (a full review of the evidence for all five classes would fill a book). Finally, we suggest some of the policy implications that would follow from accepting one type of explanation over another. We do not argue that only one class of explanation can be true—several may apply simultaneously. Table 10.1 presents a summary of the types of explanation, the evidence needed, and the implications for social policy.

CLASSES OF EXPLANATION FOR THE FLYNN EFFECT

There are roughly five groups of explanations put forward to explain changes in heritable human characteristics that exceed the expected speed of evolutionary change: (1) methodological bias, (2) increased environmental complexity, (3) reduced environmental stress, (4) heterosis, and (5) gene–environment correlation.

Methodological Bias

Nearly all the arguments presented for and against the various explanations of the Flynn effect take the form of correlations or, at best, regression models controlling for some alternative explanations. These are among the weakest forms of causal arguments (Shadish, Cook, & Campbell, 2002). There are untold possibilities for methodological error in assessing something as complex as change over long periods of time, and opponents of a particular explanation will be quick to see measurement error as bias. For example, the observed changes in intelligence test scores observed in Norwegian and Danish conscripts could be the result of changes in the tests, or in the criteria used to define the population tested (e.g., more boys of low intelligence could be excluded in later years). Older estimates of height based on records, or skeletal remains could be faulty, or the samples biased.

There is no question that methodological error is a constant danger; the question is to detect whether it introduces nonrandom bias in a certain direction rather than simply random noise. In each of the following sections we discuss what kinds of methodological error could result in bias.

Increased Environmental Complexity

This type of explanation is used mainly in relation to intelligence, and sometimes to psychopathology; it is not readily applicable to such changes as increased height. The argument is made that "increasing cognitive demands in developed countries promote an adaptive increase in cognitive ability" (Barber, 2005, p. 273). Barber (2005) used data from 81 countries to test the hypothesis that cross-national differences in IQ scores would be positively correlated with indices of cognitive demand, such as length of education and nonagricultural jobs. He found that after controlling for indices of environmental stress such as gross domestic product (GDP), low birth weight, and infant mortality, the hypothesis was supported. Barber concluded that

> children growing up in agricultural communities, where education is less important for social success, experience less cognitive challenge and have lower IQ scores consistent with the predictions of evolutionary social science. Modern populations are thus capable of responding to varying levels of intellectual stimulation with varied patterns of cognitive development. Education is one type of intellectual stimulation that increases in post-agricultural societies but further research will be necessary to determine whether other forms of modern intellectual stimulation (such as radio, television, and video games . . .) can modify national IQ scores in systematic ways. (p. 282)

Evidence That Would Support This Class of Explanation

The biggest sources of cognitive complexity in children's environment used, as Barber notes, to be provided by formal education. However, other types of stimuli are increasingly taking over from classrooms and books. Modern children in the developed world are expected to be able to use a computer to run Internet searches, to operate their own cell phone with a wide array of apps, to blog and twitter and contribute to Youtube and Facebook, and to live in parallel universes in interactive games—all developments of the very recent past. Therefore, if cognitive complexity were a major cause of increasing IQ, we would expect test scores to be increasing even in societies that have had universal education for many decades, or even to be showing an accelerating slope in recent years. In fact, the data are rather different. Figures 10.1–10.3 show that among Norwegian and Danish males beginning their military service, mean IQ scores peaked in the early 1990s and have not increased since then. A closer look at the Scandinavian data shows a significant drop since 1997, which is mirrored by a fall in the proportion of Danish youth attending advanced-level colleges (Sundet, Tambs, Harris, Magnus, & Torjusson, 2005; Teasdale & Owen, 2005, 2008). Height, which might not be expected to be driven by cognitive complexity one way or the other, has also leveled off in recent decades (Figure 10.2). It is possible to argue that increased cognitive complexity in the environment could have negative effects, and to adduce the still-continuing rise in conduct and emotional symptoms, asthma, and autism as evidence of this.

Reduced Environmental Stress

Societies frequently use as markers of progress factors that might well be linked to rapid increases in height, intelligence, and so on. These markers include smaller family size, better antenatal care and reduced infant and parent mortality, better nutrition, higher GDP, and lower disease load. The argument is that, like life expectancy, once released from the crippling effects of poverty and sickness these characteristics just naturally increase.

The "reduced stress" hypothesis has recruited many supporters, who sometimes endorse a general theory of stress reduction and sometimes espouse a particular theme, such as better nutrition (Lynn, 1990), smaller family size (Sundet, Borren, & Tambs, 2008), and prenatal care (Lynn, 2009).

The reduced stress hypothesis also has limitations. It is not clear how it would apply equally to "good" and "bad" characteristics—for example, why stress reduction should increase MMPI scores (Twenge et al., 2010) or conduct problems (Collishaw et al., 2004), as well as height and intelligence. It also begs the question of what controls the upper limits of human characteristics. Do they go on increasing forever unless constrained by lack of resources or an environmental catastrophe—are we destined to become as large as the dinosaurs?

Predictions from the reduced stress hypothesis differ from those of the environmental complexity hypothesis; increases should be proportional to the amount of stress reduction. It has proven remarkably difficult to find any clear tests of this, perhaps because of the necessity of measuring not only the outcome (IQ, height) but also the *relative* changes in different groups over time in exposure to stressors. For example, it is reasonable to make the assumption that increased availability of food benefits the poor more than the rich (Flynn, 2009) (at least until obesity becomes a problem), but it is hard to find studies that compare IQ or other changes in rich and poor groups. Instead, studies have compared slopes for those above and below the mean or median on the *outcome* measure (Flynn, 2009; Sundet et al., 2004; Teasdale & Owen, 2008) An indirect test of the hypothesis is to be found in a study of sibship size (Sundet et al., 2008), which shows that the increase in mean IQ between 1938 and 1985 birth cohorts of Norwegian conscripts was greater in those coming from large families. This implies that whatever caused the changes in IQ had a more marked effect in the presence of one stressor (large family) than in its absence (small family), or that being from a large family was progressively less stressful in each succeeding cohort. In short, the stress reduction hypothesis seems to be assumed rather than tested in the literature.

Heterosis

Heterosis is a genetic effect that will cause population-wide changes in a trait whenever three conditions are met. The first condition is that the population in question must initially have a mating pattern that is less than completely random prior to the occurrence of the trend. Such a deviation from pan-mixia, or random mating, creates an excess of homozygotes in the population and a deficit of heterozygotes. Second, the population must undergo a demographic change toward a closer approximation to random-mating conditions. This causes the frequency of homozygotes to decline and that of heterozygotes to increase. Of course, this second condition presupposes that the first condition is already met, as a trend toward more random mating cannot occur in a population already mating randomly. Third, the trait in question must display directional dominance, with more of the genes that influence the trait in one direction being dominant and more of those that influence the trait in the opposite direction being recessive. Given such nonadditive gene action, any increase in the ratio of heterozygotes to homozygotes will cause the distribution of the trait to shift over time in the dominant direction. Heterosis has been mentioned as a potential cause of the IQ trend by a number of researchers over the years (Anderson, 1982; Flynn, 1998; Jensen, 1998; Kane & Oakland, 2000; Mingroni, 2004; see also Dahlberg, 1942, chap. 10). "Few would dispute that heterosis could be responsible for at least some part of the trend; what is mainly at issue is whether it could be a major cause" (Mingroni, 2007, pp. 806–807).

Mingroni argues that whatever environmental factors account for the Flynn effect cannot occur after birth, because genetically informed studies (studies of twins reared together and apart, adoption studies, etc.) show that neither shared nor nonshared environments account for much of the difference in IQ. "One would need to posit prenatal environmental factors that vary among mothers over time but remain constant over the life of each individual mother" (2007, p. 809). For example, improved nutrition in one generation could result in a better prenatal environment for the next generation, through healthier mothers and/or improved sperm from the fathers (Storfer, 1999). These effects would have to apply across the whole population. Thus the heterosis explanation privileges genes over environment as an explanation of the Flynn paradox.

The corollary of heterosis as the explanation is that IQ (and other characteristics) will increase fastest where the population has moved from genetically undifferentiated to genetically mixed. So far there have been simulation studies (Mingroni, 2007), but little empirical evidence either to support or undermine heterosis as an explanation.

Gene–Environment Correlation

In the two decades since he propounded his paradox, Flynn has explored reasons why it exists. Working with W. T. Dickens of the Brookings Institution, Flynn has proposed an explanation based on the idea that there is a reciprocal causal relationship between phenotypic IQ and the environment that produces gene–environment correlation (rGE): the better the environment, the higher the IQ. "The process by which the ability of an individual and the environment of an individual are matched can increase the influence of any initial difference in ability—whether its source is genetic or environmental" (Dickens & Flynn, 2001, p. 350).

Dickens and Flynn (2001) use basketball skills as an analogy. A child who is naturally gifted is likely to enjoy basketball, to want to practice, and to be given more coaching and better facilities for play, as well as playing with better teammates, all of which will increase the child's level of skill. The authors present three models of increasing complexity to account for what they call "multiplier effects" by which an initial genetic predisposition interacts with environmental affordances.

Dickens and Flynn (2001) are clear that the explanation for the rapid rise in IQ scores lies in the cognitive demands of the modern world; theirs is a variant on the "cognitive complexity" hypothesis. However, as they explain:

We wish to stress that the way environment plays its role is very different from the traditional characterization. It appears that most environmental effects are relatively short-lived. At least for young children, experiences much more than a year old influence today's IQ only because of their effect on past IQ and the effect of past IQ on today's environment. Even then, the effects of environment decay, leaving only a narrow window in which transient environmental effects may influence IQ. If correct, our model suggests that improving IQs in childhood is not the way to raise the IQs of adults. Adult IQ is influenced mainly by adult environment. Enrichment programs may nonetheless be worthwhile because at least some seem to have long-term effects on achievement and life outcomes, and the temporary IQ boosts they provide may mediate those effects. However, our model suggests that such programs would be most likely to produce long-term IQ gains if they taught children how to replicate outside the program the kinds of cognitively demanding experiences that produce IQ gains while they are in the program and motivate them to

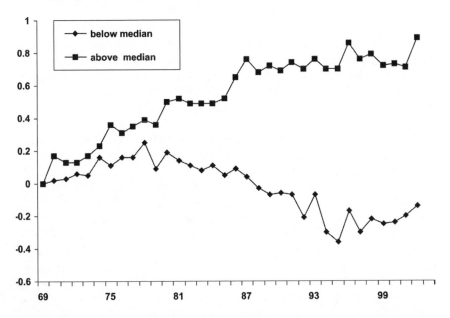

FIGURE 10.3. Mean height below and above the median height by year of testing: Data from a study of Danish conscripts, 1969–2004 (Sundet et al., 2004).

persist in that replication long after they have left the program. If the programs that were the subjects of longitudinal evaluations were trying to do this, those evaluations suggest that they were unsuccessful. Our model was motivated by a paradox in the study of IQ, but may be relevant for describing the development of a wider range of traits and behavior. Any trait that has a tendency to match itself to an environment that reinforces that trait will behave in the fashion our model describes. (p. 366)

The model could certainly be applied to neuroticism, self-esteem, and conduct problems, but it is hard to see how Dickens and Flynn's explanation could work for characteristics such as height, which tends to be fairly constant once adult height is reached. On the other hand, Sundet and colleagues (2004), using the data on Danish conscripts, showed that, relative to the 1969 draft cohort, the height of those above median increased, while the height of those below the median fell (Figure 10.3). This suggests the possibility of rGE even in height.

THE IMPLICATIONS OF THE FLYNN EFFECT AND RAPID CHANGES IN HUMAN CHARACTERISTICS FOR SOCIAL POLICY

What are the policy implications that different explanations would carry, were they partly or wholly correct? Overall, the implications are extraordinary; as Mingroni puts it, "in many countries today a person of average IQ would have been in approximately the top 15% of same-age scorers 50 years ago" (2007, p. 806). The average person today would also be much taller, more neurotic, delinquent, and vulnerable to asthma, autism, and ADHD (and also much fatter, but perhaps for different reasons). This suggests that social policy must at the very least expect succeeding generations not to be the same as past generations.

An interesting question is how long these changes can go on. As with life expectancy, there are questions about whether there is an upper limit to IQ, height, et cetera, or whether the Flynn effect is a temporary one.

Another way of looking at the picture is to wonder how and when the process began. The peoples who invented agriculture and writing, who built the pyramids and invented zero, certainly included some individuals of exceptional abilities by any standards. However, we may need to think more about the shape of the distribution than the mean. Several studies suggest that mean IQ, at least, has benefitted from a reduction in the numbers at the low end of the curve caused by, among other things, the removal of lead from paint and gas (Nevin, 2009). Clearly, it is good social policy to reduce the burden of very low IQ, whatever the dynamics of the distribution. Some social policies, such as the resources devoted to saving very low birthweight infants, may actually be adding to the numbers at risk for low IQ, as well as health and behavioral problems (Lynn, 2009). Poor-quality perinatal services, and lack of incentives for poor women to use them, also increase the risk of perinatal damage.

Social Policy Implications of the "Methodological Bias" Explanation

Methodological problems haunt this area of research: how should intelligence be measured? Are modern children being coached to take IQ tests? Is the selection process for conscripts the same now as 50 years ago? Many of the studies needed to solve these problems would be very expensive and take many decades (Schaie et al., 2005). The main implication is that, to the extent that it is important to understand what forces are driving these changes in population norms, resources will have to be devoted to monitoring them and testing competing theories. In particular, the overlapping cohorts design advocated by Schaie will be necessary.

Social Policy Implications of the "Increased Environmental Complexity" Explanation

The argument that our increasingly complex environment is force-feeding our intellectual development—and also, perhaps, our neuroticism, delinquency, and psychiatric disorders—has two types of social policy implications. First, unless the instruments of that complexity are equally distributed in the community, the IQ gap between the haves and have-nots will widen (cf. Ceci & Papierno, 2005). Second, it may be important to provide people, especially children, with some "quiet times" when they can rebalance themselves, if they are to avoid the risks to mental health.

Social Policy Implications of the "Reduced Environmental Stress" Explanation

All of the arguments for the role of reduced environment stress, whichever type of stressor they espouse, imply that the greatest social benefits will come from reducing pressures on the most stressed social groups. As noted above, there are few direct tests of this. However, such policies are in line with those of most developed and developing countries. Thus, improving access to health care for the poor could improve not only the health but also the intelligence of their children.

Social Policy Implications of the "Heterosis" Explanation

The argument for the "hybrid vigor" of greater genetic heterogeneity clearly implies policies that do not restrict immigration and mingling of gene pools, presumably at every level of social advantage. However, as noted above, there is little empirical evidence for or against this explanation. Does greater genetic heterogeneity also lead to an increase in neuroticism, delinquency, et cetera?

Social Policy Implications of the "rGE" Explanation

The real risk of this explanation to the social values of most democratic societies is that major disparities in the environmental affordances available to different social groups will increase inequalities (Ceci & Papierno, 2005). For example, evaluations of the effects of *Sesame Street* on disadvantaged and advantaged children suggest that the environmental enrichment provided to preschool children by the television program increased the skills of disadvantaged children—but also increased those of the advantaged children to the same extent, or possibly even more, thus increasing the gap between the groups (Cook & Shadish, 1994). Differences in mortality and morbidity associated with the size of the gap between the rich and poor have already been noted (Brunner, 1997; Kawachi & Kennedy, 1997; Subramanian & Kawachi, 2004; Wolfson, Kaplan, Lynch, Ross, & Backlund, 1999). If the rGE explanation is correct, it predicts (1) that conduct problems, anxiety, and possibly depression will increase at a faster rate among those with fewest advantages; (2) that height and IQ will increase at a faster rate among those with the most advantages. This suggests the need for policies to enrich the environment of those who need it most. In the language of prevention science, societies that want to shrink the disparities between haves and have-nots will need to use targeted interventions focused on those at greatest risk, rather than universal interventions that benefit everyone.

CONCLUSIONS

In this chapter we have discussed some surprising changes in population levels of characteristics that most people think of as "genetic": adult height, IQ, temperament, propensity to certain mental illnesses. We have compared some of the explanations offered, and discussed what the policy implications would be if a given explanation were true.

The biggest risk may be that rapid changes of the kind described here will increase inequalities within societies if, for whatever reason, benefits accrue to the already privileged, and disadvantages to the vulnerable. There are similarities between Dickens and Flynn's gene–environment explanation and the idea of "social selection" as a cause of mental illness (Dohrenwend et al., 1992; Fox, 1990; Jaffee, Caspi, Moffitt, Belsky, & Silva, 2001; Johnson, Cohen, Dohrenwend, Link, & Brook, 1999). According to Dohrenwend and colleagues, "social selection . . . posits that genetically predisposed people drift down or fail to rise out of [poverty]" (1992, p. 946). In his study of immigrants to Israel, he found that social selection seemed to explain the higher correlation between poverty and schizophrenia in the more settled European Israelis than in the more stressed Yemeni immigrants; over time, Europeans with mental illness drifted down the economic ladder, whereas among the recent Yemeni immigrants everyone was at a disadvantage, and the "sorting and sifting" process had not yet finished. As genes and environments become more highly correlated over time, the changes noted in this chapter may happen ever faster, unless societies make determined efforts to reverse them.

There is a growing literature arguing that, in developed countries, the size of the gap between the rich and the poor is a better predictor of many health outcomes, including violence and depression, than is actual income (Wilkinson, 1997). This means that processes leading to greater inequalities are likely to be increasingly harmful. There is much that societies can do, through income redistribution and provision of a social safety net, to limit at least the rate of increase of the difference between richest and poorest, and the gene–environment correlation explanation of the Flynn effect points to the importance of such interventions.

It is important for geneticists to help societies to understand what is going on so that they can create social policies that reduce inequities and increase social cohesion in future generations.

REFERENCES

Anderson, A. M. (1982). The great Japanese IQ increase. *Nature, 297,* 181–182.
Barber, N. (2005). Educational and ecological correlates of IQ: A cross-national investigation. *Intelligence, 33,* 273–284.
Benjamin, J., Ebstein, R. P., & Lesch, K.-P. (1998). Genes for personality traits: Implications for psychopathology. *International Journal of Neuropsychopharmacology, 1,* 153–168.
Blonigen, D. M., Hicks, B. M., Krieger, R. F., Patrick, C. J., & Iacono, W. G. (2005). Psychopathic personality traits: Heredity and genetic overlap with internalizing and externalizing psychopathology. *Psychological Medicine, 35,* 637–648.
Brunner, E. (1997). Stress and the biology of inequality. *British Medical Journal, 314,* 1472–1476.

Ceci, S. J., & Papierno, P. B. (2005). The rhetoric and reality of gap closing: When the "have-nots" gain but the "haves" gain even more. *American Psychologist, 60*, 149–60.

Collishaw, S., Maughan, B., Goodman, R., & Pickles, A. (2004). Time trends in adolescent mental health. *Journal of Child Psychology and Psychiatry, 45*, 1350–1362.

Cook, T. D., & Shadish, W. R. (1994). Social experiments: Some developments over the past fifteen years. *Annual Review of Psychology 45*, 545–580.

Costello, E. J., Erkanli, A., & Angold, A. (2006). Is there an epidemic of child or adolescent depression? *Journal of Child Psychology and Psychiatry, 47*, 1263–1271.

Dahlberg, C. (1942). *Race, reason and doubt.* London: Allen & Unwin.

Dickens, W. T., & Flynn, J. R. (2001). Heritability estimates versus large environmental effects: The IQ paradox resolved. *Psychological Review, 108*, 346–369.

Dohrenwend, B. P., Levav, I., Shrout, P. E., Schwartz, S., Naveh, G., Link, B. G., et al. (1992). Socioeconomic status and psychiatric disorders: The causation-selection issue. *Science, 255*, 946–952.

Flynn, J. R. (1984). The mean IQ of Americans: Massive gains 1932 to 1978. *Psychological Bulletin, 95*, 29–51.

Flynn, J. R. (1998). IQ gains over time: Toward finding the causes. In U. Neisser (Ed.), *The rising curve: Long-term gains in IQ and related measures* (pp. 25–66). Washington, DC: American Psychological Association.

Flynn, J. R. (2009). Requiem for nutrition as the cause of IQ gains: Raven's gains in Britain 1938–2008. *Economics and Human Biology, 7*, 18–27.

Fox, J. W. (1990). Social class, mental illness, and social mobility: The social selection-drift hypothesis for serious mental illness. *Journal of Health and Social Behavior, 31*, 344–353.

Grant, B. F. (1996). Prevalence and correlates of drug use and DSM-IV drug dependence in the United States: Results of the National Longitudinal Alcohol Epidemiologic Survey. *Journal of Substance Abuse, 8*, 195–210.

Hathaway, S. R., & McKinley, J. C. (1940). A multiphasic personality schedule (Minnesota): 1. Construction of a schedule. *Journal of Psychology, 10*, 249–254.

Jaffee, S., Caspi, A., Moffitt, T. E., Belsky, J., & Silva, P. (2001). Why are children born to teen mothers at risk for adverse outcomes in young adulthood?: Results from a 20-year longitudinal study. *Development and Psychopathology, 13*, 377–397.

Jensen, A. R. (1969). How much can we boost IQ and scholastic achievement? *Harvard Educational Review, 39*, 1–123.

Jensen, A. R. (1998). *The g factor: The science of ability.* Westport, CT: Praeger.

Johnson, J. G., Cohen, P., Dohrenwend, B. P., Link, B. G., & Brook, J. S. (1999). A longitudinal investigation of social causation and social selection processes involved in the association between socioeconomic status and psychiatric disorders. *Journal of Abnormal Psychology, 108*, 490–499.

Kane, H., & Oakland, T. D. (2000). Secular declines in Spearman's g: Some evidence from the United States. *Journal of Genetic Psychology, 161*, 337–345.

0

11

Kawachi, I., & Kennedy, B. (1997). Health and social cohesion: Why care about income inequality. *British Medical Journal, 314*, 1037–1040.

Lynn, R. (1990). Differential rates of secular increase of five major primary abilities. *Social Biology, 37*, 137–141.

Lynn, R. (2009). What has caused the Flynn effect?: Secular increases in the development quotients of infants. *Intelligence, 37*, 16–24.

Mingroni, M. A. (2004). The secular rise in IQ: Giving heterosis a closer look. *Intelligence, 32*, 65–83.

Mingroni, M. A. (2007). Resolving the IQ paradox: Heterosis as a cause of the Flynn effect and other trends. *Psychological Review, 114*, 806–829.

Nevin, R. (2009). Trends in preschool lead exposure, mental retardation, and scholastic achievement: Association or causation? *Environmental Research, 109*, 301–310.

Plomin, R., & Spinath, F. M. (2004). Intelligence: Genetics, genes, and genomics. *Journal of Personality and Social Psychology, 86*, 112–129.

Schaie, K. W., Willis, S. L., & Pennak, S. (2005). An historical framework for cohort differences in intelligence. *Research in Human Development, 2*, 43–67.

Shadish, W., Cook, T., & Campbell, D. (2002). *Experimental and quasi-experimental designs for generalized causal inference.* Boston: Houghton Mifflin.

Storfer, M. (1999). Myopia, intelligence, and the expanding human neocortex: Behavioral influences and evolutionary implications. *International Journal of Neuroscience, 98*, 153–276.

Subramanian, S. V., & Kawachi, I. (2004). Income inequality and health: What have we learned so far? *Epidemiologic Reviews, 26*, 78–91.

Sundet, J. M., Barlaug, D. G., & Torjussen, T. M. (2004). The end of the Flynn effect?: A study of secular trends in mean intelligence test scores of Norwegian conscripts during half a century. *Intelligence, 32*, 349–362.

Sundet, J. M., Borren, I., & Tambs, K. (2008). The Flynn effect is partly caused by changing fertility patterns. *Intelligence, 36*, 183–191.

Sundet, J. M., Tambs, K., Harris, J. R., Magnus, P., & Torjussen, T. M. (2005). Resolving the genetic and environmental sources of the correlation between height and intelligence: A study of nearly 2600 Norwegian male twin pairs. *Twin Research in Human Genetics, 8*, 307–311.

Teasdale, T. W., & Owen, D. R. (2005). A long-term rise and recent decline in intelligence test performance: The Flynn effect in reverse. *Personality and Individual Differences, 39*, 837–843.

Teasdale, T. W., & Owen, D. R. (2008). Secular declines in cognitive test scores: A reversal of the Flynn effect. *Intelligence, 36*, 121–126.

Twenge, J. (2000). The age of anxiety?: Birth cohort change in anxiety and neuroticism, 1952–1993. *Journal of Personality and Social Psychology, 79*, 1007–1021.

Twenge, J. M., & Foster, J. D. (2010). Birth cohort increases in narcissistic personality traits among American college students, 1982–2009. *Social Psychological and Personality Science, 1*, 99–106.

Twenge, J. M., Gentile, B., DeWall, C. N., Ma, D., Lacefield, K., & Schurtz, D. R. (2010). Birth cohort increases in psychopathology among young Americans,

1938–2007: A cross-temporal meta-analysis of the MMPI. *Clinical Psychology Review, 30,* 145–54.

Twenge, J. M., & Nolen-Hoeksema, S. K. (2002). Age, gender, race, SES, and birth cohort differences on the Children's Depression Inventory. *Journal of Abnormal Psychology, 111,* 578–588.

Wilkinson, R. G. (1997). Socioeconomic inequalities in morbidity and mortality in Western Europe. *Lancet, 350,* 516–517.

Wolfson, M., Kaplan, G., Lynch, J., Ross, N., & Backlund, E. (1999). Relation between income inequality and mortality: Empirical demonstration. *British Medical Journal, 319,* 953–955.

CHAPTER 11

Gene–Environment Interactions, Criminal Responsibility, and Sentencing

Stephen J. Morse

Imagine a defendant who has been charged with murder, the intentional homicide of a victim he was robbing with a weapon. He has a history of three previous convictions and imprisonments for armed robbery. Prior to being released from the third term, he publicly threatened to kill any future armed robbery victims who might be able to identify him. When the current victim looked our armed robber in the eye, the robber said to the victim, "You looked the wrong way at the wrong guy," pulled the trigger, and killed the victim. (We know this because his accomplice has turned state's evidence and, unbeknownst to the robber, there was a witness who will corroborate the accomplice's evidence.)

This is a desperate case. Assume that a lawyer has been assigned to defend the killer and she needs to discover evidence that will help her make an argument to defeat the charges against the defendant or that will help her seek mitigation at sentencing if the defendant is convicted. The lawyer is aware of the Caspi and colleagues (2002) study and its later replications that found a vastly increased risk for criminal behavior among males who had been subject to severe abuse as children *and* who had a genetic defect that caused an monoamine oxidase A (*MAOA*) deficiency. The lawyer is easily able to confirm from family members, teachers, and neighbors that the robber was severely abused as a child, and a genetic analysis confirms that the robber also has the specific defect associated with increased risk for crime.

207

The question is whether the presence of this well-studied and mostly well-confirmed gene–environment interaction (G × E) is relevant to support claims on behalf of the armed robber or the prosecution at trial or sentencing.

The case just described is not simply hypothetical. An Italian judge recently reduced a convicted murderer's sentence on the ground that the killer was predisposed to be particularly aggressive in stressful situations because he had the same *MAOA* deficiency studied by Caspi and colleagues (Feresin, 2009). There have also been a small number of U.S. cases in which such evidence has been introduced (Bernet, Venecak-Jones, Farahany, & Montgomery, 2007; Denno, 2009). It is seldom explained why a genetically driven predisposition justifies a sentence reduction. Various experts criticized the Italian's judge's decision. Nevertheless, the use of G × E for making decisions about criminal responsibility and sentencing will surely increase. The question for the law is what the relevance of such explanations of behavior might be. For example, does a G × E suggest that the hypothetical murder defendant has diminished culpability or enhanced dangerousness? Was the Italian judge justified in reducing the murderer's sentence based on genetic predisposition?

My task in this chapter is to consider the relevance of G × E to criminal responsibility and sentencing. I begin with a number of preliminary assumptions that will inform the analysis. I then turn to the law's view of the person, including the law's implicit psychology, and the criteria for criminal responsibility. False starts and distractions about responsibility are addressed next. This section explains in detail why arguments based on free will and causation that are rooted in scientific explanations of crime, including G × E, do not have the implications for criminal responsibility that proponents often claim.

The extended discussion of the foregoing topics is necessary before one can even begin to consider the relation between G × E (or any other causal variable) to criminal responsibility and sentencing. With this necessary background in place, I then turn specifically to the relation between G × E and criminal responsibility. I next address sentencing and consider whether G × E is relevant to mitigation and aggravation. I conclude by considering briefly how knowledge of G × E might otherwise influence criminal justice policy and practice.

I claim that G × E causes of criminal behavior have no relation to current conceptions of responsibility per se, but they may be relevant to culpability if valid research discloses an association between G × E and a genuine excusing or mitigating condition. Thus, although G × E is unlikely to have a major transformative effect on responsibility doctrines and practices unless it transforms basic conceptions of human agency, it may well play an important role in the adjudication of individual cases. I also propose that G

× E is likely to play its largest role in criminal justice at sentencing. I suggest that the same considerations governing responsibility ascriptions apply to sentencing mitigation and that the prediction of future dangerousness will be a common sentencing application for aggravation and mitigation.

PRELIMINARY ASSUMPTIONS

Genes, environments, and their interactions do not commit crimes; acting people commit crimes. We do not praise and reward or blame and punish G × E; these are attitudes and actions we direct at people. Bedazzled by the newest scientific findings in behavioral genetics, neuroscience, and other rapidly advancing disciplines, we often forget this simple truth about our actual social and legal practices of praising and blaming, rewarding and punishing. Unless we cease to treat each other as acting agents, as persons, no major alteration of these practices is likely to result.

G × E raises no new issues about criminal responsibility or the prediction of future dangerousness that have not been raised previously by other alleged causal explanations for crime, such as social structural explanations, psychodynamic and behavioral psychological explanations, genetic explanations, and neuroscientific explanations. Such explanations allegedly prove the truth of determinism, but as the chapter later shows, determinism is not inconsistent with criminal responsibility. Similarly, many people think that discovery of a causal explanation, such as G × E, is per se excusing or mitigating, but this is not the case, as the chapter also explains. Again, unless a causal explanation threatens human agency, which G × E does not purport to do, the basic structure of criminal responsibility and punishment is not likely to change substantially. G × E may affect the adjudication of individual cases and sentencing decisions, but it is unlikely to lead to major changes.

The basic questions for the law are always the same. What is the relevance of this causal information to legal doctrine and practice? Does the evidence seem to suggest the need for radical, fundamental restructuring or reform of law or for more limited, discrete reforms, if any, of particular doctrine or practices. Advocates often tend to make overclaims based on science (Morse, 2006), but experience indicates that most of what we learn suggests no major overhaul of law.

Human behavior is generally the product of immensely complex factors that include biological, psychological, and sociological variables. Human beings are fundamentally biological machines that always interact with their environments (Noe, 2009). In particular, G × E is surely part of the explanation of many and perhaps most behaviors. Although this is true, human beings are a special type of causal end product of the interaction between biology and environment. Our unique capacities, such as our ability to use fully developed propositional language and our ability to deliberate about what we have reason to do, have enormous moral and legal implications.

It is important to stress that responsibility is a distinguishable issue from prophylactic or rehabilitative concerns. Even if particular scientific knowledge has no bearing on responsibility, it may well have implications for the ex ante (i.e., before the fact) prevention of undesirable behavior, the ex post (i.e., after the fact) prevention of recidivism, the control of predictably dangerous people, and the promotion of desirable behavior.

Criminal responsibility and its consequences, such as whether and how much to punish a wrongdoer, are normative moral, political, and ultimately legal questions. They address how we should live together. Empirical discoveries about behavior can make profound contributions to debates about what we have reason to do, but they do not by themselves dictate any normative conclusion. On the ultimate issue of how we should live, science must fall silent because how we should live is a matter of practical and not theoretical reason (but see Harris, 2010, for a contrary argument). The issue is normative and not factual.

Finally, and with few exceptions, retribution—giving people their just deserts—is a necessary precondition for blame and punishment in the U.S. criminal justice system and it plays a role in all developed Western legal systems. Most criminal justice theorists justify punishment on mixed retributive and consequential grounds. Consequential concerns do matter to the definition of crimes and to the appropriate sentence to be imposed, but U.S. and Western criminal justice systems agree that no one should be punished unless he or she deserves it and no more than he or she deserves. Retribution is a well-recognized justification for the state infliction of pain on its citizens and it must be distinguished from revenge, with which it is often confused. Revenge is the primitive desire to hurt those who have hurt you. It usually involves anger and often includes psychological catharsis. Retribution, in contrast, is a theory of justice. There are many different accounts of retribution, but all agree that it is a good in itself to give people what they morally and legally deserve. It is not a primitive and prescientific form of human response, but a considered theory of justice. Blaming and punishing people for wronging others because they deserve such a response is the mirror image of praising and rewarding people for helping others because they deserve such a response. Accepting a retributive theory of punishment does not entail whether or how much criminals should be punished. One could be permissive or obligatory about whether retribution demands punishment, and a retributivist can be harsh or tender about how much punishment is deserved. The only basic commitment is that people should not be punished unless they deserve it and then no more than they deserve.

THE LAW'S PSYCHOLOGY
AND CRIMINAL RESPONSIBILITY

The law—anyway a reification—has not explicitly adopted any psychology or concept of the person. What follows is a rational reconstruction of the criminal law's implicit psychology and concept of the person and why these are necessary if law is to make coherent sense and to serve a useful function in society.

Lawyers take the criminal law's implicit psychology for granted because there is seldom any need to identify or question it. G × E and other scientific findings may appear to call the law's psychology into question, however, so it is crucial consciously to recognize it and to understand what would be entailed if it were undermined.

Criminal law presupposes the "folk psychological" view of the person and behavior. This psychological theory causally explains behavior in part by mental states such as desires, beliefs, intentions, willings, and plans. Biological, other psychological, and sociological variables also play a role, but folk psychology considers mental states fundamental to a full explanation of human action. Human behavior cannot be adequately understood if mental state causation is completely excluded or eliminated. Lawyers, philosophers, and scientists do of course argue about the definitions of mental states and about theories of mind and action, but that does not undermine the general claim that mental states are fundamental to law. Indeed, the arguments and evidence disputants use to convince others itself presupposes the folk psychological view of the person. Brains don't convince each other; people do.

For example, the folk psychological explanation for why you are reading this chapter is, roughly, that you desire to understand the relation of G × E to criminal responsibility and sentencing, you believe that reading the chapter will help fulfill that desire, and thus you formed the intention to read it. This is a "practical" explanation rather than a deductive syllogism.

Folk psychology does not presuppose the truth of free will (which will be discussed further below), it is not dualist (although it, and ordinary speech, sound that way), it is perfectly consistent with the truth of determinism, and it presupposes no particular moral or political view. It does not presuppose that all mental states are necessarily conscious or that people go through a conscious decision-making process each time that they act. It allows for "thoughtless," automatic, and habitual actions, and for nonconscious intentions. For example, consider the behavior of putting on your undershorts in the morning. You probably have not considered which leg to put through first since you learned to dress yourself. There is no decision; the behavior is utterly automatic and habitual. This makes sense because there is no reason to give any thought to which leg goes first. Absolutely nothing turns on this. Suppose, however, that you had good reason to put the other leg first, say, a threat to kill you if you put the usual leg through first. You would then bring this automatic behavior under the control of reason. This example is an illustration of folk psychology's presupposition that human action will at least be rationalizable by mental state explanations or that it will be responsive to reasons, including incentives, under the right conditions.

The definition of folk psychology this chapter uses does not depend on the truth of any particular bit of folk wisdom about how people are motivated, feel, or act. Any of these bits, such as that experiencing disrespect often produces anger, might turn out to be wrong after further empirical investigation. The definition insists only that human action is in part causally explained by mental states.

Consider the criteria for criminal responsibility. The prosecution must first prove the "elements" of the crime, which is simply the legal term for the criteria for criminal conduct. These elements are composed primarily of acts and mental states. All are infused with mental states. All crimes include a "voluntary" act requirement, which is defined, roughly, as an *intentional* bodily movement (or an omission in cases in which the person has a duty to act) done while the agent is in a reasonably integrated state of consciousness. Although the meaning of an intentional bodily movement is seldom specified, the best definition is a bodily movement that in principle can be understood according to the person's mental state. One can almost always ask of any act, "Why did you do that?," and expect some explicit or implicit mental explanation. If there is none even implicitly possible, it is probable that the agent's bodily movement was not an act at all. For example, reflexes and neuromuscular spasms involve bodily movements, but they are not actions because they were not intentional bodily movements and cannot respond to reasons or incentives.

With few exceptions that are themselves controversial, all crimes also require a culpable further mental state, such as purpose, knowledge, or conscious awareness that one is risking a prohibited harm (a mental state lawyers call "recklessness"). Some crimes are also defined with the mental state of negligence, which is defined as an unreasonable failure to be aware of the risk of a prohibited harm. Negligence appears to be the absence of a mental state. This is a controversial issue among legal scholars, but the best explanation for criminalizing negligence is that the failure to pay attention when the agent was creating a substantial and unjustifiable level of risk is itself a type of culpable omission. On the other hand, some scholars believe that negligence is an insufficiently culpable mental state to support criminal liability.

To make this discussion more concrete, consider the following standard definition of murder mentioned in the opening hypothetical about the homicidal armed robber: killing another human being with the intent to cause death. Any intentional killing conduct—for example, shooting, stabbing, strangling, poisoning, or bludgeoning—is sufficient to meet the act requirement as long as the agent was in a state of reasonably integrated consciousness when engaging in the killing conduct. Furthermore, the agent must engage in the conduct with the intent to cause death. If the agent lacked that intent and, say, just risked killing the victim, then the agent will not be guilty of intentional murder, but may be guilty of some other homicide crime that requires a different mental state.

Even if the prosecution is able to prove all the elements of crime, the defendant may still avoid criminal liability by successfully establishing what is called an affirmative defense of justification or excuse. In cases of justification, conduct that would otherwise be criminal is right or at least permissible under the circumstances. Self-defense is a classic example. Intentionally killing another human being is ordinarily murder, but an agent may be justified in killing if the other person is threatening the agent with wrongful, deadly force. In such cases, intentional killing is considered right or at least permissible. Note that in cases of justification, the agent is a fully responsible person.

In contrast, cases of excuse involve wrongful action performed by an agent who is not responsible. Roughly speaking, lack of rational capacity, external compulsion (e.g., acting in response to a "do-it-or-else" threat of death or grievous bodily injury), and, more controversially, lack of the capacity to control oneself (sometimes referred to as "internal compulsion") are the basic grounds for criminal law's doctrinal excuses. Note that in the cases of lack of rational capacity or lack of the capacity to control oneself, responsibility requires only the possession of the general capacity at the time in question, even if the agent did not exercise the capacity on that occasion. For example, acting irrationally, arationally, and foolishly are common even among people with the greatest capacity for rational conduct. Failure to exercise a capacity does not necessarily mean that one lacks that capacity. For the law, if the person is capable of exercising the capacity for rationality or self-control if there is good reason to do so—as there always is when important interests of potential victims are at stake—then the person may be held responsible even if he or she failed to exercise that capacity.

If the person lacks the relevant capacity, an excuse is warranted. Legal insanity is a classic example. Suppose a person delusionally believes that he or she is about to be killed by a secret agent and kills the suspected secret agent in what the person believes is self-defense. The person has wrongfully killed intentionally, but he or she would be excused because he or she was not a rational agent when he or she killed. In a very real sense, the killer did not know what he or she was doing.

All affirmative defenses involve an inquiry into the person's mental state, such as the person's belief that self-defensive force was necessary or his or her lack of knowledge of what he or she was doing or that what he or she was doing was wrong.

In short, criminal responsibility is established if the prosecution can prove all the elements of the crime charged and the defendant cannot establish an affirmative defense. Criminal responsibility is defeated if the prosecution cannot prove all the elements of the crime charged or if the defendant can establish an affirmative defense. The elements and affirmative defenses all involve mental states. Of course the person's mental state is influenced by biological, psychological, and sociological variables, including $G \times E$, and knowledge of these variables may help determine what the person's mental state was. Nevertheless, the law is ultimately concerned with the person as an acting agent who has acted for reasons. The final explanatory pathway for criminal law is always folk psychological (directly or indirectly). Any relevant data from $G \times E$ or other sciences must be translated into the law's folk psychological criteria.

We will turn to the relation of $G \times E$ to criminal law's responsibility criteria below. Before doing so, however, I describe why the law's psychology must be folk psychology and will briefly discuss some false starts and distractions about responsibility.

THE INEVITABILITY OF FOLK PSYCHOLOGY IN LAW

Brief reflection should indicate that the law's psychology must be a folk psychological theory, a view of the person as a conscious (and potentially self-conscious) creature who forms and acts on intentions that are the product of the person's other mental states, such as desires, beliefs, willings, and plans. Law is primarily action guiding (Sher, 2006) and could not guide people ex ante and ex post unless people could use rules as premises in their reasoning about how they should behave. Otherwise, law as an action-guiding, normative system of rules would be useless, and perhaps incoherent. Law is a system of rules that, at the least, is meant to guide or influence behavior and thus to operate as a potential cause of behavior. As philosopher John Searle (2002) wrote:

> Once we have the possibility of explaining particular forms of human behavior as following rules, we have a very rich explanatory apparatus that differs dramatically from the explanatory apparatus of the natural sciences. When we say we are following rules, we are accepting the

notion of mental causation and the attendant notions of rationality and existence of norms. . . . The content of the rule does not just describe what is happening, but plays a part in making it happen. (p. 35)

Legal rules are not simply mechanistic causes that produce "reflex" compliance, although they can certainly help to inculcate law-abiding "habits." They operate within the domain of folk psychology. Agents are meant to and can only use these rules as potential reasons for action as they decide about what they should do. Legal rules are thus action guiding primarily because they provide an agent with good moral or prudential reasons for forbearance or action.

Unless people are capable of understanding and then using legal rules to guide their conduct, law would be powerless to affect human behavior (Shapiro, 2000). Law can directly and indirectly affect the world we inhabit only by its influence on human beings who can potentially use legal rules to guide conduct. For example, no "instinct" governs how fast a person drives on the open highway. Among the variables that explain the speed at which a person drives, the posted speed limit and the belief in the probability of suffering the consequences for exceeding it surely play a large role in the driver's choice of speed. The law thus guides action.

Human behavior can be modified by means other than influencing deliberation, and human beings do not always deliberate before they act. Nonetheless, the law presupposes folk psychology, even when we most habitually follow the legal rules. All citizens constantly act in the "shadow of the law," especially when criminal conduct is at stake.

The legal view of the person does not hold that people must always reason or consistently behave rationally according to some preordained, normative notion of rationality. Rather the law's view is that people are capable of acting for reasons and are capable of minimal rationality according to predominantly conventional, socially constructed standards. The type of rationality the law requires is the ordinary person's commonsense view of rationality, not the technical notion that might be acceptable within the disciplines of economics, philosophy, psychology, computer science, and the like.

Virtually everything for which agents deserve to be praised, blamed, rewarded, or punished is the product of mental causation, and, in principle, responsive to reason. I do not mean to imply dualism here. I am simply accepting the folk psychological view that mental states—which are fully produced by and realizable in the brain—play a genuinely causal role in explaining human behavior. Machines may cause harm, but they cannot do wrong and they cannot violate expectations about how people ought to live together. Machines do not deserve praise, blame, reward, punishment, concern, or respect because they exist or because of the results they cause.

Only people, intentional agents with the potential to act, can violate expectations of what they owe each other and only people can do wrong.

Many scientists and some philosophers of mind and action consider folk psychology to be a primitive or prescientific view of human behavior. No one, however, has even remotely suggested a replacement psychology for the law that would conceivably be practical—and law is an intensely practical enterprise. For the foreseeable future, then, the law will be based on the folk psychological model of the person and behavior, and this chapter will proceed on that premise. Until and unless scientific discoveries convince us that our view of ourselves is radically wrong—and nothing science has discovered begins to support this claim (Morse, 2008)—the basic explanatory apparatus of folk psychology will remain central. The folk psychological theory of personhood that the law implicitly adopts seems secure. As eminent philosopher of mind Jerry Fodor (1987) has written:

> If commonsense intentional psychology were really to collapse, that would be, beyond comparison, the greatest intellectual catastrophe in the history of our species; if we're that wrong about the mind, then that's the wrongest we've ever been about anything. The collapse of the supernatural, for example, doesn't compare. . . . Nothing except, perhaps, our commonsense physics . . . comes as near our cognitive core as intentional explanation does. We'll be in deep, deep trouble if we have to give it up. . . . But be of good cheer; everything is going to be all right. (p. xii)

It is vital that we not lose sight of the folk psychological model lest we fall into confusion when various claims based on G × E or other causal variables are made. Once again, any G × E data or evidence must always be relevant to the law's folk psychological criteria. If G × E is to have any influence on legal decisions about criminal responsibility and sentencing, it must be almost entirely through this framework.

DISTRACTIONS AND FALSE STARTS IN CRIMINAL RESPONSIBILITY ANALYSIS

In this section of the chapter I consider the following distractions that have bedeviled attempts to understand the relation between scientific explanations for criminal behavior and criminal responsibility: the free will debate, the belief that causation is per se an excusing condition, the belief that causation by abnormal variables is per se an excusing condition, and the belief that causation is the equivalent of compulsion. Many of the arguments in this section probably will be unfamiliar to many scientists, but they are crucial to proper understanding and therefore deserve careful consideration.

The Non-Problem of Free Will in Criminal Law

There is a problem about free will, but not in criminal law (Morse, 2007). Free will, as the term is used in the philosophical debate about free will and responsibility, is not a criterion for any legal doctrine. Criminal law criteria involve questions genuinely related to responsibility, including issues concerning consciousness, the formation of mental states such as intention and knowledge, the capacity for rationality, and compulsion, but they never address the presence or absence of free will. People sometimes use "free will" loosely to refer to genuine responsibility doctrines, but this simply distracts attention from the real issues and perpetuates confusion.

The philosophical problem of free will is metaphysical and often clouds clear thinking about the foundation for criminal responsibility. Specialists in the philosophy of free will and responsibility often distinguish between freedom of action, the freedom to do as one chooses, and freedom of the will, the freedom to choose what one would prefer to choose (Kane, 2006). This chapter will subsume both under the locution "freedom of the will" or "free will."

Roughly, the notion of free will used in the debate refers to whether an agent has the ability to cause his or her own behavior uncaused by anything else. In a phrase, the buck stops entirely with the agent. This ability is sometimes called contra-causal freedom, agent origination, metaphysical libertarianism, and other like phrases. Only a small number of philosophers adhere to this view, which has been termed a "panicky" metaphysics (P. F. Strawson, 1980, p. 80) because it is so implausible (Bok, 1998).

Even if this type of free will is not a criterion for any criminal law doctrine, many people nonetheless believe that this type of power or ability is a foundational assumption for legal responsibility and for justifying the fair imposition of blame and punishment. Thus, if people do not possess this god-like power, then doctrines and practices relating to responsibility may be entirely incoherent. But, as we shall see, contra-causal freedom is not a necessary support for current responsibility doctrines and practices.

Most philosophers and, I speculate, virtually all scientists, believe that the universe is deterministic or universally caused, or nearly so, especially above the subatomic level. There is no uncontroversial definition of determinism and we will never be able to confirm that it is true or not. As a working definition, however, let us assume, roughly, that all events have causes that operate according to the physical laws of the universe and that were themselves caused by those same laws operating on prior states of the universe in a continuous thread of causation going back to the first state. Even if this is too strong, the universe seems so sufficiently regular and lawful that rationality demands that we assume that universal causation is approximately correct. Philosopher G. Strawson (1989) terms this assumption the "reality constraint."

It is important to understand that, for the determinist, biological causes, including interactions of biology with the environment, pose no more or less challenge to responsibility than nonbiological or social causes. As a conceptual and empirical matter, we do not necessarily have more control over psychological or social causal variables than over biological causal variables. More important, in a world of universal causation or determinism, causal mechanisms are indistinguishable in this respect and biological causation creates no greater threat to our life hopes than psychological or social causation (Richards, 2000). For purposes of the metaphysical free will debate, a cause is just a cause, whether it is biological, psychological, sociological, or astrological.

If determinism is true, the people we are and the actions we perform have been caused by a chain of causation over which we mostly had no rational control and for which we could not possibly be responsible. We do not have contra-causal freedom. How can responsibility be possible for action or for anything else in such a universe? How can it be rational and fair for criminal law to hold anyone accountable for anything, including blaming and punishing people because they allegedly deserve it?

Those who believe that responsibility is not compatible with determinism are called "incompatibilists" and adopt different conclusions depending on their view of determinism. "Libertarian" incompatibilists believe that determinism is not true for most action because we have metaphysical libertarian freedom, and therefore we are responsible. "Hard determinist" incompatibilists believe that determinism is true, deny that we have contra-causal freedom, and conclude that responsibility is impossible. "Compatibilists" believe that determinism is true, deny that contra-causal freedom is necessary for responsibility, and hold that responsibility is possible under the right conditions.

No analysis of this problem could conceivably persuade everyone. There are no decisive, analytically incontrovertible arguments to resolve the metaphysical question of the relation between determinism, libertarian free will, and responsibility. And the question is metaphysical, not scientific. Indeed, the debate is so fraught that even theorists who adopt the same general approach to the metaphysical challenge substantially disagree. Nevertheless, the view one adopts has profound consequences for legal (and moral) theory and practice.

Let us begin with hard determinist incompatibilism. (I have already rejected libertarianism as empirically implausible. The rest of the discussion will therefore focus only on hard determinist incompatibilism, which is a coherent position held by many.) Incompatibilism does not try either to explain or to justify our responsibility concepts and practices. It simply assumes that genuine responsibility is metaphysically unjustified. For example, a central incompatibilist argument is that people can be responsible only if they could have acted otherwise than they did, but if determinism is true, they could not have acted other than they did. This is sometimes called the "principle of alternate possibilities." It has generated endless disputes between incompatibilists, who believe it is flatly inconsistent with responsibility, and compatibilists, who believe that it is not inconsistent with responsibility (Wallace, 1994). Based on this principle and similar arguments, the incompatibilist claims that even if an internally coherent account of responsibility and related practices can be given, it will be a superficial basis for responsibility, which is only an illusion (Smilansky, 2000).

Incompatibilism based on any level of scientific cause, including G × E, thus provides an external critique of responsibility. To see why, remember that causal determinism "goes all the way down." It applies to all people, to all events. Thus, if determinism is true and is inconsistent with responsibility, then no one can ever be really responsible for anything and responsibility attributions cannot properly justify further action. But Western theories of morality and the law do hold some people responsible and excuse others, and the law responds accordingly. And when we do excuse, it is not because there has been a little local determinism at work. For example, young children are not considered fully responsible because they are incapable of recognizing and of properly weighing the right reasons for action and forebearance, not because they are determined creatures but adults are not. Determinism does not loosen its grip on us as we age.

The question, then, is whether as rational agents we must swallow our pride, accept incompatibilism because it is so self-evidently true, and somehow transform the legal system accordingly into a system that abandons desert and relies on a prediction and prevention model of social control that is untethered from considerations of genuine responsibility. Such systems have been proposed (e.g., Wootton, 1963), but they have been criticized for their harsh and potentially inhumane implications that profoundly threaten liberty and dignity (Hart, 1968; Lewis, 1953). Once again, until scientific explanations, whether from G × E or others, convinces us that we are not acting agents, such a system is exceptionally unlikely to gain assent.

Compatibilists, who agree with hard determinist incompatibilists that determinism is true, have three basic answers to the incompatibilist challenge. First, they claim that responsibility attribution and related practices are human activities constructed by us for good reason and that they need not conform to any ultimate metaphysical facts about genuine or "ultimate" responsibility. Indeed, some compatibilists deny that conforming to ultimate metaphysical facts is even a coherent goal in this context. Second, compatibilism holds that our positive doctrines of responsibility are fully consistent with determinism. Third, compatibilists believe that our responsibility doctrines and practices are normatively desirable and consistent with moral, legal, and political theories that we firmly embrace. The first claim is theoretical; the third is primarily normative. There are very powerful arguments for the first and third claims (Lenman, 2006; Morse, 2004). For our current purpose of determining whether criminal law has a free will problem, the second claim is the most important.

Let us begin with the most general responsibility and excusing conditions. Recall that the capacity for rationality is the primary responsibility criterion and its lack is the primary excusing condition. Now, it is simply a fact about human beings that they have different capacities for rationality in general and in specific contexts. Once again, for example, young children in general have less rational capacity than adults. It is also true that rationality differences differentially affect agents' capacity to grasp and to be guided by good reason. Differences in rational capacity and its effects are real even if determinism is true. Compulsion is also an excusing condition, but it is simply another fact about human beings that some people act in response to external or internal hard choice threats to which persons of reasonable firmness might yield and most people most of the time are not in such situations when they act. This is true even if determinism is true and even if people could not have acted otherwise.

For a specific example, consider again the specific doctrines of criminal responsibility. Assume that the defendant has caused a prohibited harm. Recall that responsibility requires that the defendant's behavior was an action and performed with a requisite mental state. Now it is simply true that some bodily movements are intentional and performed in a state of reasonably integrated consciousness and some are not. It is also true that some defendants possess the requisite mental state and some do not. The truth of determinism does not mean that actions are indistinguishable from nonactions or that people do not have different mental states when they act. These facts are true and make a perfectly rational legal difference, even if determinism is true. Determinism is fully consistent with making distinctions among defendants about whether the elements of the crime charged can be proven.

Now consider the defense of legal insanity, which was briefly addressed above. Some people with mental disorder do not know right from wrong; others do. Once again, legally differentiating these cases makes perfect sense according to dominant retributive and consequential theories of punishment. A causal account, including from G × E in an appropriate case, can explain how these variations were caused to occur, but it does not mean that they do not exist. Determinism is fully consistent with both the presence and the absence of affirmative defenses. In sum, the legal criteria used to identify which defendants are criminally responsible map onto real behavioral differences that justify differential legal responses.

A causal determinist account would become inconsistent with our responsibility practices only if our scientific investigations convinced us that we are not the types of creatures the law takes us to be—conscious and intentional creatures who act for reasons. If it is true, for example, that we are all automatons, then no one is acting and no one can be responsible for action. I have termed this the "No Action Thesis" (Morse, 2003b, 2008). Unlike the claimed inconsistency between determinism and responsibility, which is a metaphysical question, this critique is empirical and in principle capable of resolution. The conclusion that we are essentially automatons would once again provide an external critique of responsibility and leave no rational room for legal decision making about genuine responsibility. Although some scientists are gesturing in this direction (Wegner, 2002), there is little in current science that suggests that most people most of the time are not conscious and intentional creatures who act for reasons or whose behavior can be guided by reason and incentives (Morse, 2008).

Compatibilism is consistent with our criminal responsibility doctrines and practices, and there is no convincing theoretical reason to reject it. All participants in the criminal justice system, including scientists who contribute to legal policymaking and decisions in individual cases, have good reason to embrace compatibilism. Scientists can comfortably continue to play a crucial role in assisting the promotion of more rational criminal justice without being distracted by the irrelevant issue of free will.

Causation Per Se Does Not Excuse: The "Fundamental Psycholegal Error"

The most persistent confusion about our actual doctrines and practices concerning responsibility, which I have termed the "fundamental psycholegal error" (Morse, 1994), is the mistaken belief that causation, especially by an abnormal cause, is per se an excusing condition. In brief, this error relies on the same argument the incompatibilist makes, but without recognizing that it provides an external critique that must deny the possibility of any responsibility. If the truth of determinism or universal causation is an excusing condition, it applies not just in any particular legal context, such as guilt or sentencing proceedings. It applies everywhere and always.

In a causally deterministic universe, all phenomena, including human actions, are fully caused. If causation were per se an excusing condition, no one could ever be responsible for anything. Thus, causation cannot be an excusing condition in law and morals, both of which hold some people responsible and excuse others. Although this is a simple and straightforward analytic point, the error persists (e.g., Kaye, 2005). If the causal chain were different, the ensuing action would be different. The question for law is not whether behavior was caused. It is whether the legal criteria have been satisfied. For purposes of assessing responsibility, it does not matter whether the cause of the behavior in question is biological, psychological, sociological, or some combination of the three. Adducing a genetic or neurophysiological cause does no more work than adducing an environmental or interactive cause. The question is always whether the legal criteria for nonresponsibility are met, however the behavior in question may have been caused. A person who is mentally disordered and does not know right from wrong will be excused from criminal responsibility whether his or her rationality impairment was primarily a product of faulty genetics, a neurotransmitter defect, bad parenting, social stress, the alignment of the planets, or some combination of the above, including $G \times E$. The most important question for criminal law is whether the legal excusing condition was present, not how it was caused. Causal knowledge, if sufficiently precise, may help establish whether or the likelihood that the legal criterion in question was satisfied, but the person will be excused if the excusing condition is present, even if we have no idea how the condition was caused.

For example, in *Roper v. Simmons* (2005) the Supreme Court addressed the question of whether adolescents who committed capital murder when they were 16 or 17 years old should be categorically excluded from being sentenced to death. Advocates for abolition for this group of murderers argued that the demonstrated lack of complete myelination of the cortical neurons of the adolescent brain was reason to believe that 16- and 17-year-old murderers were insufficiently responsible to deserve capital punishment. Rigorous behavioral studies had already confirmed the average differences in rational capacity between adolescents and adults. The moral and constitutional implications of the data may be controversial, but the data are not. At most, the neuroscientific evidence provided a partial causal explanation of why the observed behavioral differences exist and thus some further evidence of the validity of the behavioral differences. The neuroscience was thus of only limited and indirect relevance to responsibility assessment, which is based on behavioral criteria concerning rationality. Diminished responsibility follows from diminished rationality, however the latter is caused.

Finally, it follows logically that if full causation is not per se an excusing condition, then "partial causation" also does not partially or fully excuse the agent. Most of the time, we possess only imperfect, partial understanding of the causes of behavior. It is important to remember, however, that not possessing knowledge of the complete causal account of a person's behavior does not mean that a complete causal account does not exist. Indeed, the notion that only some phenomena are caused or determined, but others are not, is incoherent. If this is a universally caused or deterministic universe, all phenomena are caused, whether or not we have knowledge of those causes.

In any case, discovering a partial normal or abnormal cause for behavior does not partially or completely excuse the agent unless that cause produces a genuine mitigating or excusing condition. For example, various causes we discover may in part explain why an agent's rationality is fully or partially impaired, but then it is the impairment of rationality, not causation, that is doing the excusing work.

Abnormal Causation Does Not Excuse Per Se

Abnormal causation, say, by mental disorder, also does not excuse per se, but excuses only if it produces a genuine excusing condition, such as lack of capacity to appreciate the criminality of one's actions. For example, a person suffering from mental disorder that plays a causal role in the sufferer's behavior may nonetheless retain sufficient capacity for rationality to be held fully responsible. A clinically hypomanic robber, for example, may be especially energetic, mentally acute, and confident when the agent mugs. Indeed, but for the clinical condition, the robber may not have mugged, but there is no question about the agent's criminal responsibility in this case. The robber is sufficiently rational to be held fully responsible.

Causation Is Not Compulsion

Causation is also not the equivalent of compulsion, even if some type of normal or abnormal causal variable played a role in explaining the criminal behavior in question. All behaviors are lawfully caused, but as philosopher David Hume observed, the laws of nature are not coercive (Hume, 1978; Scanlon, 2008). Not all behavior is the product of the external or internal coercive conditions that meet moral and legal criteria for compulsion. If causation were the equivalent of compulsion, everyone would always be compelled and excused. For example, just because a person is predisposed to antisocial activity by a G × E interaction, it does not mean that the person was compelled to act. For another example, a delusional belief or a hallucination may produce irrational reasons for action, but irrational reasons are not per se more compelling than rational reasons. A person who delusionally believes in the need to use deadly self-defense is no more compelled to act than a nondelusional agent with the same honest belief. The former may be excused because he or she is irrational, but compulsion plays no role in such cases. By the same logic, discovering part of the causation of behavior does not mean that the behavior was compelled to that degree. Causation is not per se compulsion and "partial causation" is not per se partial or complete compulsion.

In conclusion, G × E will not affect responsibility analysis simply because it is a cause of criminal behavior, even if it produces an immensely predisposing cause. G × E will be relevant only if it helps prove or disprove the existence of actual criminal law criteria. Let us therefore next examine the specific relevance of G × E to those criteria.

G × E AND CRIMINAL RESPONSIBILITY

The question of the relation of G × E to criminal responsibility reduces to whether G × E evidence or data cast doubt on the elements of crimes, such as action and mental states, or helps to establish (or cast doubt about) the existence of a complete or partial affirmative defense. G × E causation, no matter how powerful its explanatory role may be, will only negate responsibility if it prevents a defendant from meeting the responsibility criteria of the criminal law.

Using the example of the armed robber and the G × E interaction of childhood abuse and a genetic *MAOA* deficiency with which this chapter began, let us consider how this G × E affects responsibility. Although I will concentrate on this specific example, the argument is fully generalizable to any G × E that might causally contribute to criminal behavior.

The first criterion for responsibility is the "act" requirement. The defendant's bodily movements that appear to have violated the law must have been intentional and performed in a state of reasonably integrated consciousness. In other words, the agent must have acted. There is no evidence in the G × E literature under consideration to suggest that the agents thereby predisposed to criminal behavior are not acting when they commit crimes. Their bodily movements are not the equivalent of reflexes or spasms and they are not performed in a dissociative state, such as sleepwalking. Unless some other explanation for lack of action is forthcoming, our armed robber's behavior is clearly action even if G × E played a causal role.

A similar analysis applies to whether the defendant possessed the mental state, the "mens rea," such as intention, knowledge, recklessness, or negligence, when the crime was committed. Again, nothing in the literature of the G × E interaction in question suggests that this causal variable prevents people from forming culpable mental states. Our armed robber, for example, surely had both the intent to steal using a weapon as a threat, and, ultimately, the intent to kill.

It is possible, however, that the effect of the interaction on a defendant's mental capacities may interfere with the formation of some culpable mental states. For example, in some states, intentional killings that are performed after relatively cool, rational deliberation (so-called premeditated murder) are considered especially heinous and punished accordingly.

Although I know of no such data, suppose it could be demonstrated that G × E made it extremely difficult to plan coolly and rationally for those subject to it. In that case, the G × E evidence would help the law decide if an intentional killer in fact premeditated. Notice, however, that it is lack of premeditation, not G × E itself, which might explain why the killer is not guilty of the aggravated degree of intentional homicide. If there were clear behavioral evidence that the defendant did premeditate or was capable of doing so despite the G × E—and, of course, there will be variation among people with this G × E—then the defendant would be guilty of aggravated homicide despite the evidence that G × E tends generally to make it difficult to premeditate.

Another example would be recklessness. Recall that the criminal law's definition of recklessness is conscious awareness that one's conduct is creating a high risk of a prohibited harm. It is a subjective mental state. Suppose good evidence suggested that people with G × E are extremely poor estimators of the consequences of their conduct. If so, the G × E evidence would be relevant and probative of whether a defendant actually was aware of the risk created. And again, if the behavioral evidence suggested that the defendant was actually aware of the risk despite the G × E, say by adverting to it in comments to accomplices, then G × E data would be trumped.

Consider negligence as a final example. Negligence is the failure to be aware that one's conduct is creating a high risk of a prohibited harm in situations in which a reasonable person should have been aware of the risk. It is considered an "objective" mental state because we are comparing the defendant to a hypothetical reasonable person. Suppose good evidence suggests that G × E makes it very difficult for those subject to it to behave as reasonable people should. Although there is a good argument for negating the presence of negligence in that case (Hart, 1968), the law is unforgiving about negligence. Everyone is held to the standard of the reasonable person, including those people who may find it supremely difficult to meet that standard through no fault of their own. Any mitigation based on the defendant's deficiencies would only be considered at sentencing, which I address in the next section.

In short, G × E is not likely to have much if any effect on the formation of the act and mental state elements of the crime charged.

G × E is most likely to be relevant to the generic excusing conditions: lack of rational capacity and lack of the capacity to control oneself. G × E is not likely to be relevant to compulsion, criminal action compelled by "do-it-or-else" threats using death or grievous bodily harm as the "or-else" because these threats must be external. Lack of rational and of control capacity have technical legal doctrinal criteria, but for our purposes it is sufficient to use the generic justifications for the doctrinal excuses, such as infancy, legal insanity, and duress.

Before we can answer whether G × E is relevant to rational and control capacity, it is necessary to explore what we mean by these capacities in a bit more detail. There is no consensual definition of rationality in any of the relevant disciplines, such as psychology, psychiatry, economics, and philosophy, that study this issue. Likewise, there is no uncontroversial legal definition of rationality or of what kind and how much is required for responsibility in various legal contexts. Rationality for the law must be understood according to some contingent, normative notion both of rationality and of how much capability is required. For example, legal responsibility might require the capability of understanding the reason for an applicable rule, as well as understanding the rule's narrow behavior command and the consequence for failure to comply. These are matters of moral, political and, ultimately, legal judgment about which reasonable people can and do differ. These are normative issues about intentional behavior guided by reasons.

If one examines the various legal responsibility and competence doctrines that implicitly address rationality defects, however, one can infer that the law's general definition is a congeries of abilities that closely track an ordinary person's commonsense definition. For example, the agent must be able to get the facts right, to know what he or she is doing, to be able to respond reasonably to reasons and incentives in the context in question, and the like. For example, one criterion for legal insanity is that the agent does not know what he or she is doing. For another example, one criterion for incompetence to stand criminal trial is that the defendant is unable to understand the nature of the charges against him or her and the nature of the trial proceedings that are about to occur. Deciding whether such criteria are met requires an implicit, commonsensical folk psychological definition of rationality of the sort we all use everyday to evaluate our own conduct and the conduct of others.

It is much harder to provide a folk psychological account for the lack of capacity to control oneself that is independent of a rationality defect. People commonly use locutions like "I can't help myself," "I lost control of myself," and like expressions, but what do they mean? When people "lose control" and act badly, they are surely acting, but what is the folk psychological process that suggests loss of control? Various models have been used to try to inject content into the process, including a collapse of control problems into rationality defects (Morse, 2002), but none has seemed conclusive. Moreover, at present we have no way of distinguishing action that a person cannot control from action he or she simply did not control. Such practical difficulties in part accounted for why both the American Bar Association and the American Psychiatric Association recommended abolishing "control" criteria for legal insanity in the mid-1980s.

The definitional problems persist. A recent, influential legal example is the Supreme Court's decision in *Kansas v. Crane* (2002), in which a criterion of "serious difficulty" controlling oneself was constitutionally required to be proven before a state could civilly commit a so-called mentally abnormal sexually violent predator. There was a withering dissent about the difficulty of making this conclusory judgment and the courts that have since tried to interpret this requirement have been unable to do more than simply repeat the "serious difficulty" formula without further operationalization.

A current example from psychiatry is the conclusion that the drug seeking and using of addicts is "compulsive." It is question begging to say the addict cannot control seeking and using because those behaviors are signs of a disease. Actions are different from the purely mechanistic signs and symptoms of most diseases, such as fevers or metastases. The lack of ability to control action must be demonstrated independently (Fingarette & Hasse, 1978). The psychiatric conclusion about compulsion is not based on such an independent, operationalized measure. It is based on the commonsense conclusion that people who persist in behavior that often creates ruinous medical, psychological, fiscal, personal, and legal problems and who report feelings such as craving must not have good control over their drug-related behavior. Although there is reason to question this conclusion, especially in its strongest form (Heyman, 2009), no folk psychological process has been specified even if we do accept it.

In short, adequately defining control capacity is a problem for criminal law that science has not yet solved. Nonetheless, the ensuing discussion will assume for the sake of argument that we can make sense of control problems. Like the rationality criterion for responsibility, the degree of control the law will require is a normative matter that can vary from one legal context to another.

To be relevant to legal excuses, G × E data will have to be translated into the law's folk psychological definitions of rational capacity and control capacity. The G × E studies in question were not clinical or thick phenomenological descriptions of the high-risk subjects. For the sake of general argument, however, let us assume a number of folk psychological variables that might in part account for the high rates of offending among these subjects. Nothing turns on whether these are the correct variables because the argument that will be made is general and would apply to whatever variables are doing the explanatory work. Consequently, let us simply assume that the subjects may have been highly sensation seeking, impulsive, or suffering from poor judgment.

These types of folk psychological variables are relevant to commonsense notions of rational and control capacity. Moreover, science can help operationalize and measure such variables. For example, the amicus ("friend of the court") briefs of the American Psychological Association in the *Roper v. Simmons* (2005) case and in the recently decided Supreme Court case concerning the constitutionality of sentencing juvenile offenders to life in prison without the possibility of parole (JLWOP) for nonhomicide crimes, *Graham v. Florida* (2010), are replete with studies of the decision-making abilities and other psychological variables that are relevant to whether adolescents as a class are on average less responsible than adults because they have less rational capacity. Whether the differences between adolescents and adults are sufficiently large in quantity and quality to warrant differential treatment is, of course, a normative moral and legal question that science cannot answer, but the data are surely relevant to the legal decision that must be made.

The same type of analysis applies to G × E offenders, including our armed robber. Assuming that the folk psychological process G × E produces adversely affects rational and control capacities, the question will be whether the adverse effects are sufficiently large to warrant excuse or mitigation for criminal conduct. Treated as a general matter of legal policy, a question would be whether the effects are so marked that we should mitigate the culpability of G × E offenders as a class and forego individualized evaluation on a case-by-case basis. The law generally disfavors such general as opposed to individualized decision making, although it has been willing to prohibit the capital punishment of murderers from the reasonably well-delineated classes of people with retardation (*Atkins v. Virginia*, 2003) and of killers who were 16 or 17 years old at the time of the capital crime (*Roper v. Simmons*, 2005).

Assuming that G × E does have psychological effects that bear on responsibility, it is virtually certain that G × E offenders would have their culpability assessed individually through doctrinal excuses or at sentencing. Recall that the offender's actual behavior will be more probative than the group data. If the offender's history and conduct at the time of the crime indicate no substantial defects, the group data will be of little avail. Actions speak louder than G × E. If the offender's capacities are unclear, however, the group data might help.

Unfortunately for G × E offenders, no general excusing condition seems to apply. The insanity defense may seem like the strongest opportunity, but G × E offenders will not qualify for the insanity defense unless they also suffer from a major mental disorder that causes them to lose touch with reality. This is required by many jurisdictions and in practice suffering from gross loss of contact with reality is necessary to succeed with an insanity defense even if the legal rule does not specify that the disorder must have psychotic features. No other general excusing condition is even remotely applicable. Criminal law has few mitigating doctrines that are considered at trial to which the folk psychological processes G × E produces would apply. I have proposed that criminal law should adopt a generic "partial responsibility" doctrine based on diminished rationality that would be considered at trial and that would mitigate the offender's degree of conviction and punishment if the claim were successful (Morse, 2003a). Alas, no jurisdiction has adopted or is even considering this proposal. Again, such factors may be considered at sentencing, which I consider in the next section.

The arguments that I have been making about the G × E that Caspi and colleagues (2002) discovered are fully generalizable to any future G × E discoveries. The evidence would have to be relevant to the criminal law's folk psychological criteria for whether the defendant acted, whether he or she possessed the mental state required by the definition of the crime, and whether an excusing condition, such as lack of rational or control capacity, is established. Whether G × E played a causal role in explaining the criminal behavior is legally irrelevant unless one falls prey to the "fundamental psycholegal error" of thinking that causation is an excuse. This conclusion applies even in the unlikely event that *every* person subject to the G × E in question commits a crime. A genuine excusing or mitigating condition would still have to be established to defeat the allegation of criminal responsibility. After all, in a lawful causal world, all human behavior is fully explained by the causal background that produced it. If causes were excuses, no one would be responsible. That is not the legal and moral world we inhabit and it is not likely to be.

In short, G × E will seldom play much role in guilt determinations, but it may play a more extensive role in sentencing and parole decisions, to which I now turn.

G × E AND SENTENCING

Questions concerning mitigation and potential future dangerousness are primarily the province of sentencing decisions. The question at sentencing is how G × E evidence would be relevant to sentencing criteria. This section begins by considering sentencing practices generally, and then turns to how G × E might be relevant.

In most U.S. jurisdictions, there is a range of permissible sentence for each crime and the sentencing judge has virtually complete discretion to impose any sentence within that range or to place the defendant on probation. A minority of jurisdictions, including the federal system, have guidelines that constrain judicial discretion, but even in such constrained systems judges have some discretion about the sentence to be imposed. Thus, sentencing judges can consider mitigating and aggravating factors not considered at trial to adjust the offender's sentence up or down within the statutorily permitted range of sentence for the crime. Sentencing criteria in noncapital cases are undertheorized and often not specified, thus leaving judges unguided discretion. Capital punishment must be decided by a jury (*Ring v. Arizona*, 2002), and there are typically statutory aggravating and mitigating factors the jury must consider. In addition, beginning with *Lockett v. Ohio* (1978), the Supreme Court made clear in many decisions that the defendant facing capital punishment may present virtually any evidence that could conceivably be mitigating even if the statutory mitigating factors do not include the factor the evidence supports.

Consider mitigation first. Sentencing practices are often considerably less clear than the criteria for guilt. For example, the erroneous "causal theory of excuse" appears to be taken into account for mitigation. The rationale seems to be that understanding the causes of the defendant's behavior somehow reduces responsibility per se. The Italian judge's reduction of the defendant's sentence on the ground that the defendant was predisposed to violence when stressed suggests that the judge was implicitly adopting this rationale. On the other hand, the evidence introduced at sentencing may suggest that mitigation is warranted because the defendant suffered from substantial rationality or control deficits, even if they were not sufficiently substantial to rise to the level of a full legal excuse. Such a claim would be entirely supported by retributive and perhaps consequential justifications for punishment that we firmly embrace. Even if the defendant was criminally responsible, he or she may deserve a lesser sentence if he or she was not fully rational at the time of the crime.

A central aggravating factor is the predicted future dangerous conduct of the defendant, which is considered not only at sentencing itself, but also for parole decisions. In capital sentencing statutes, future dangerousness is often expressed by criteria based on past behavior, such as prior convictions, and sometimes it is expressed directly. This ground for aggravation or for denial of parole is purely consequential—the protection of the public. Of course, by the same logic, defendants who are less predictably dangerous should receive lesser sentences on consequential grounds. The major practical issue is determining how accurately we can predict future dangerous conduct and how much contribution to such accuracy evidence such as G × E might contribute. Current law is accepting of predictions based on weak evidence (e.g., *Barefoot v. Estelle*, 1983), but well-validated prediction factors have the potential to make prediction decisions more rational and just. Other aggravating factors include the defendant's failure to show remorse, and committing the crime in a particularly dangerous or cruel manner (which is a culpability factor as well as an indication of dangerousness).

Note one final feature of using prediction of future dangerousness as an aggravating factor. It appears to deny the offender's agency and dignity by suggesting that the offender cannot be guided adequately by reason (Duff, 2007). This may be justified by consequential justifications and there is no problem concerning retribution as long as the sentence remains within the statutorily authorized range, but it is nonetheless an undesirable aspect of prediction practices concerning responsible agents.

Now let us consider the relation of G × E to this brief account of sentencing, returning to our armed robber for final consideration. There is little dispute that people with his G × E are highly predisposed to committing criminal or otherwise antisocial acts. To the extent that the judge or jury in a capital case accepts the "causal theory of mitigation," the sentence may be reduced despite any clear rationale for doing so. Another theory might also be lurking to support mitigation, although it depends on only the abuse part of the interaction. The rationale is that the hard life suffered by the defendant has been "payment in advance" (Klein, 1990) or sufficient previous suffering that should reduce the amount of suffering that should be imposed now. This theory has no legal basis, but it may play a role psychologically. In any case, note that this theory has little to do with the G × E specifically. It is possible, however, that the same psychological characteristics G × E produces that predispose the armed robber to crime are rationality or control defects. If so, there will be good theoretical reason to mitigate the armed robber's sentence.

Now let us turn to how G × E might be relevant to sentencing aggravation, parole, or commitment decisions. The very same evidence of G × E predisposing the armed robber to future criminal behavior would certainly be considered a risk factor for future criminality, and thus would support a longer sentence and denial of parole. The issue would be the practical one of accurately assessing how much G × E predisposes to future criminal behavior. Also, if this G × E were linked not only to future dangerousness, but also to lack of remorse, then it might be further confirmation of behavioral indications that this defendant lacked remorse.

In brief, G × E evidence can be a knife that cuts both ways, supporting both mitigation and aggravation.

G × E FOR CRIMINAL LAW ISSUES OTHER THAN RESPONSIBILITY AND SENTENCING

Understanding the causes of criminal behavior may be vitally useful within and without the criminal justice system to questions concerning rehabilitation and prevention. For example, outside the criminal justice system, it may be useful for establishing policies and programs that will reduce the risk of antisocial behavior. Fully discussing these uses raises complex issues and would require a chapter in itself, but I will gesture at them in this section.

For many reasons, including issues of retributive and distributive justice and civil liberties, rehabilitation is no longer considered a prime goal of the criminal justice system and it is of diminished importance within the delinquency jurisdiction of juvenile justice and especially when juveniles who commit crimes are tried as adults. Nonetheless, if causal knowledge could help create effective, cost–benefit justified rehabilitation methods for some prisoners, there would be impetus to use them because recidivism imposes major costs on our society. Whether a particular G × E that predisposes people to criminal offending is amenable to specific rehabilitation methods derived from that causal knowledge is of course an open empirical question that good research can help answer. Whether an apparently effective intervention is cost–benefit justified is of course a normative moral, political, and legal question that science cannot decide.

Causal G × E knowledge may also be the key to prophylactic policies and programs that would be established outside the criminal justice system. Yet again, whether specific policies and programs would be effective and cost–benefit justified are open empirical and normative questions. There are risks associated with identifying classes of people and individuals as "at risk" for criminal behavior. Labeling effects, interventions that are unnecessary and often counterproductive for many recipients, and privacy issues are examples of the potential negative effects of such policies and programs. Let us hope, however, that advancing causal knowledge, whether from G × E or other fields, does point the way to successful preventive intervention and that the potential negative effects could be minimized.

REFERENCES

Atkins v. Virginia, 536 U.S. 304 (2002).

Barefoot v. Estelle, 463 U.S. 880 (1983).

Bernet, W., Venecak-Jones, C., Farahany, N., & Montgomery, S. (2007). Bad nature, bad nurture, and testimony regarding MAOA and SLC6A4 genotyping at murder trials. *Journal of Forensic Science, 52*, 1–10.

Bok, H. (1998). *Freedom and responsibility*. Princeton, NJ: Princeton University Press

Caspi, A., McClay, J., Moffit, T., Mill, J., Martin, J., Craig, I., et al. (2002). Role of genotype in the cycle of violence in maltreated children. *Science, 297*, 851–854.

Denno, D. (2009). Behavioral genetics evidence in criminal cases: 1994–2007. In N. Farahany (Ed.), *The impact of behavioral sciences on criminal law* (pp. 317–354). New York: Oxford University Press.

Duff, A. (2007). *Answering for crime: Responsibility and liability in the criminal law*. Oxford, UK: Hart.

Feresin, E. (2009). Lighter sentence for murderer with "bad genes." Retrieved November 21, 2009, from *www.nature.com/news/2009/091030/full/news.2009.1050.html*.

Fingarette, H., & Hasse, A. (1978). *Mental disabilities and criminal responsibility*. Berkeley and Los Angeles: University of California Press.

Fodor, J. (1987). *Psychosemantics: The problem of meaning in the philosophy of mind.* Cambridge, MA: MIT Press.

Graham v. Florida, 130 S.Ct. 2011, 560 U.S. __ (2010).

Harris, S. (2010). *The moral landscape: How science can determine human values.* New York: Free Press.

Hart, H. L. A. (1968). *Punishment and responsibility: Essays in the philosophy of law.* New York: Oxford University Press.

Heyman, G. (2009). *Addiction: A disorder of choice.* Cambridge, MA: Harvard University Press.

Hume, D. (1978). *A treatise on human nature* (P. Nidditch, Ed.). Oxford, UK: Oxford University Press.

Kane, R. (2006). *A contemporary introduction to free will.* New York: Oxford University Press.

Kansas v. Crane, 534 U.S. 407 (2002).

Kaye, A. (2005). Resurrecting the causal theory of the excuses. *Nebraska Law Review, 83*, 1116–1177.

Klein, M. (1990). *Determinism, blameworthiness and deprivation.* Oxford, UK: Oxford University Press.

Lenman, J. (2006). Compatibilism and contractualism: The possibility of moral responsibility. *Ethics, 117*, 7–31.

Lewis, C. S. (1953). The humanitarian theory of punishment. *Res Judicatae, 6*, 224–230.

Lockett v. Ohio, 438 U.S. 586 (1978).

Morse, S. (1994). Culpability and control. *University of Pennsylvania Law Review, 142*, 1587–1660.

Morse, S. (2002). Uncontrollable urges and irrational people. *Virginia Law Review, 88*, 1025–1078.

Morse, S. (2003a). Diminished rationality, diminished responsibility. *Ohio State Journal of Criminal Law, 1*, 289–308.

Morse, S. (2003b). Inevitable mens rea. *Harvard Journal of Law and Public Policy, 27*, 51–64.

Morse, S. (2004). Reason, results and criminal responsibility. *Illinois Law Review, 2004*, 363–444.

Morse, S. (2006). Brain overclaim syndrome and criminal responsibility: A diagnostic note. *Ohio State Journal of Criminal Law, 3*, 397–412.

Morse, S. (2007). The non-problem of free will in forensic psychiatry and psychology. *Behavioral Sciences and the Law, 25*, 203–220.

Morse, S. (2008). Determinism and the death of folk psychology: Two challenges to responsibility from neuroscience. *Minnesota Journal of Law, Science, and Technology, 9*, 1–35.

Noe, A. (2009). *Out of our heads: Why you are not your brain, and other lessons from the biology of consciousness.* New York: Hill & Wang.

Richards, J. R. (2000). *Human nature after Darwin: A philosophical introduction.* London: Routledge.

Ring v. Arizona, 536 U.S. 584 (2002).

Roper v. Simmons, 543 U.S. 551 (2005).

Scanlon, T. (2008). *Moral dimensions: Permissibility, meaning, blame.* Cambridge, MA: Belknap Press.

Searle, J. (2002). End of the revolution. *New York Review of Books, 49,* 33–35.

Shapiro, S. (2000). Law, morality, and the guidance of conduct. *Legal Theory, 6,* 127–170.

Sher, G. (2006). *In praise of blame.* Oxford, UK: Oxford University Press.

Smilansky, S. (2000). *Free will and illusion.* Oxford, UK: Oxford University Press.

Strawson, G. (1989). Consciousness, free will and the unimportance of determinism. *Inquiry, 32,* 3–27.

Strawson, P. F. (1982). *Freedom and resentment.* In G. Watson (Ed.), *Free will* (pp. 59–80). Oxford, UK: Oxford University Press.

Wallace, R. J. (1994). *Responsibility and the moral sentiments.* Cambridge, MA: Harvard University Press.

Wegner, D. (2002). *The illusion of conscious will.* Cambridge, MA: MIT Press.

Wootton, B. (1963). *Crime and the criminal law: Reflection of a magistrate and social scientist.* London: Stevens & Sons.

CHAPTER 12

Gene–Environment Studies in the Era of Full-Genome Sequencing

Some Lessons from Eugenics and the Race–IQ Debates

Robert Cook-Deegan

The study of gene–environment interactions (G × E) lies at the confluence of two powerful streams of 20th-century science. On one branch we have the systematic study of behavior, cognition, and perception. As the 20th century progressed, psychology, neurology, psychiatry, and the biology of brain function separated into different fields, but these fields strongly interacted through their common focus on brain and behavior. Genetics is the other scientific stream that meets psychology in gene interaction studies. The rediscovery of Mendel's 1865 particulate theory of inheritance in 1900, and its integration into evolutionary theory and human population genetics in the grand synthesis so ably summarized by Provine (1971), gave rise to one of the 20th century's most powerful scientific torrents. Genetics began as the study of inheritance, but by century's end it was primarily the study of DNA structure and how DNA sequence encoded instructions for RNAs and proteins that mediate the molecular biology of cell function. Genetics became integrated into a broader molecular biology of the cell. Genetics is now going organismal, and even social, through population genetics and statistical analysis of large data sets. One point of convergence in these dual streams is the individual human organism, the object of natural selection and the focus of many studies of behavior.

Both behavioral psychology and human population genetics became embroiled in social controversy. There was unequivocal scientific progress in both fields, yet both psychology and genetics gave rise to social movements based in part on inferences drawn from the science but pushing well beyond the bounds of experiment and evidence. Some controversy is normal in science, indeed controversy is part of its process of organized skepticism. Controversy associated with drawing social and policy implications from science, however, is often about facts and values outside the consensual base of evidence. It may be instructive to inspect the claims made for each field in thinking about how to avoid needless and destructive controversy in contemporary science as we try to bring these two fields together, particularly as research findings are translated into policy options.

Other chapters in this volume address the interpretation of G × E in longitudinal population studies, or in cross-sectional studies that follow behavioral outcomes while also studying social and environmental differences associated with those outcomes. The main argument of Herrnstein and Murray's The Bell Curve in 1994 was that population differences in IQ and educational achievement were highly heritable and not amenable to social interventions, for example, a hotly contested interpretation. In this volume, by way of contrast, one of the findings reported by Costello (Chapter 10) is that a simple social intervention—distribution of earnings from the casino operated by the Eastern Band of Cherokee Indians—had a salutary effect on outcomes of children in families getting income supplements compared to controls in the same age and region who did not. Caspi, Hariri, Holmes, Uher, and Moffitt report more complex interactions between genotype and phenotype (see Chapter 2). Some behavioral outcomes appear to be contingent on extent and timing of stressors during individual development.

THE ARROGANCE OF STRONG BEHAVIORISM

J. B. Watson famously observed, in his 1930 book Behaviorism:

> Give me a dozen healthy infants, well formed, and my own specified world to bring them up in and I'll guarantee to take anyone at random and train him to become any type of specialist I might select—doctor, lawyer, artist, merchant, chief, and yes, even beggarman and thief—regardless of his talents, pensions, tendencies, abilities, vocations, and race of his ancestors. I am going beyond my facts and I admit it, but so have the advocates of the contrary, and they have been doing it for many thousands of years. (p. 82)

On first blush, this appears to be a grandiloquent and overweening claim of behavioral determinism, and indeed it is. But perhaps we should forgive Watson for a bit of puffery that presaged his conversion to the advertising industry, of which he became a famous cofounder. On closer inspection, however, the claim is less powerful than it initially appears. It is, after all, a claim about influence on *occupational* choice. If he had made claims about sexual behavior, alcohol use, or family dynamics, his claims might have met with considerable skepticism even at the time (although just such strong determinist claims about being able to control those behaviors are part of the history of behaviorism too). His insight was that reward and punishment affect behavior, and behaviorism certainly ratcheted up the methodological sophistication of psychology as a discipline. But Watson edged into unsupportable ideology in excluding social and biological factors, factors that are not entirely mediated by reward and punishment as studied in his psychology. He was indeed going beyond his facts—well beyond them. If we took Watson's claims seriously, he had it all figured out; but he didn't. The emphasis here is on "all." The rigorous experimental testing of behavioral hypotheses in psychology was a major 20th-century advance, and behaviorism contributed to it (as did other schools of psychology). Psychologists today would not, or at least should not, indulge in Watson's arrogance. To the extent that psychology as a field has learned some humility, it is the better for it.

Let us look at the nature of the choice Watson claimed to be able to control: career. As a premajor advisor in a freshman dormitory, it seems to me that occupational choices are often almost arbitrary, and relatively easy to influence at the margin. So being able to influence that kind of choice is not all that spectacular an accomplishment even if it were possible. If Duke University gave faculty complete control over access to food and sex, could we turn every aspiring undergraduate into a premedicine major? No, but we could probably increase the odds. (Throw in Skinner boxes and electrodes and perhaps we could increase them even more, and call ourselves Harvard Yard.) The point is, however, that even Watson's claims about choices in the limited domain of occupation are not sustainable. Roughly half my first-year undergraduate advisees say they are interested in becoming doctors. Half of those half stop being premeds, and it is generally not for want of motivation, lack of punishment, or insufficient reward for good grades. One big force for change in career choice is the course requirements for all those who plan to attend medical school. Watson may have been persuasive and talented, but even he could not make more than half the undergraduates in organic chemistry get above-average grades in a tough course. Achievement in physics, chemistry, organic chemistry, and college mathematics seem to do a lot of work in changing career choice, so it suggests that Watson was just flat wrong. It does not seem plausible that rewarding performance with good food or ample sex (even more than we already do—remember I live in a dorm) would get him where he promised to go. Watson's dismissal of biological factors is simply not credible in the end. Yet a strain of behavioral determinism persists in our culture, and those of us who are educators do think we make a difference, at least at the margin. The lesson to take from Watson is to be wary of overpromising on what education, social factors, and behavioral interventions can deliver. That does not seem to be a terribly controversial stance to take in 2011.

EUGENICS, RACIAL HYGIENE, AND THE LIMITS OF GENETIC DETERMINISM

Even as Watson was building his case for the power of the new psychology in 1930, another, quite different strain of determinism was gathering force. Genetic determinism attributed human differences primarily to inherited genetic variations. Human genetics as a scientific field was associated with the social movements of eugenics and racial hygiene. Cowan (2008) rightly points out that not all of human genetics was enamored of eugenics, and it is easy to oversimplify the overlap between the science and the social movement. The development of medical genetics, for example, can be seen to be largely independent of eugenics (Cowan, 2008). Many who were prominent in basic genetics and in understanding how specific Mendelian disorders were inherited, and how they could be prevented and treated, were generally not among the cheerleaders for eugenic social policies.

Yet the history of the eugenics and racial hygiene movements did rest in part on the human genetics of its day. Scholarship about the social history of eugenics emerged in the 1980s with the publication of Kevles's four-part series in *The New Yorker* and his book *In the Name of Eugenics* (Kevles, 1984, 1985). This became a hot topic in the history of genetics even as the Human Genome Project was taking flight, and the generation of scientists that populated the new field of genomics took the backlash against the overreach of eugenics and racial hygiene as a given. Knowing at least a bit about the social history of eugenics was seen as important in doing human genetic research, in part as a negative model for how one's future reputation could be harmed by claiming more for science than the evidence could support.

It would be nice to think that the world changed during the 20th century, so that the controversy and skepticism that greeted *The Bell Curve* when it was published in 1994 (Allen et al., 1996) contrasts with the generally enthusiastic reception for Francis Galton's *Hereditary Genius* in 1869 or *Essays in Eugenics* in 1909, Davenport's *Heredity in Relation to Eugenics* in 1911 (1911/2008), or Harry Laughlin's *Eugenical Sterilization in the United States* in 1922. Herrnstein and Murray's prescriptions for education policy were met mainly by scholarly challenge and resistance rather than adopted into national immigration policy and state sterilization statutes.

The use of eugenics as a cautionary tale for scientists continues to this day. Jan Witkowski and John Inglis call eugenics "pathological science" in the preface to their 2008 book *Davenport's Dream*. Charles Davenport was one of the deans of the eugenics movement, and became director of the Cold Spring Harbor Laboratory, now mainly known as the Mecca of molecular biology. Historian Elof Carlson says, "In the verdict of history, Davenport is seen . . . not as an idealist but as an opinionated mischief maker whose eugenic movement . . . fed the prejudices of the middle class and led to a dubious compulsory sterilization movement and blatant discriminatory immigration policy in the 1920s" (2008, p. 61). According to Carlson, Davenport's lieutenant, Harry Laughlin, is "universally perceived as the Iago of the American Eugenics Movement" (p. 61). There is disagreement among historians about the relative importance of class, the relative role of individuals, and the relative importance of science in how the eugenics movement played out, but there is historical consensus that human genetics, particularly human population genetics, got tangled up in eugenics as a social movement. For aspiring scientists, the main lesson is to avoid being a modern Charles Davenport or Harry Laughlin. But how?

Davenport's Dream starts with an essay by another Watson (2008), James Dewey Watson of double helix fame, who for several decades had the same job Davenport did as director of the Cold Spring Harbor Laboratory. Watson's theme is the relationship between science and public policy. His main argument is that the science was bad, the psychiatry of the day was also poorly founded on unreliable scientific knowledge, and the social policies were driven by powerful ideological agendas that illegitimately drew on the credibility of science and scientists, some of whom themselves contributed to the fiasco. He ends by arguing that a much more robust genetics emerged from the molecular biology of the last third of the 20th century. Its scientific insights and practical fruits will be greeted warmly by a public that will learn to distinguish the dark early history of eugenics and racial hygiene from the tangible benefits of better science and rapidly advancing technology. There is surely great truth here, but the argument is not entirely persuasive because it is hard to be confident that if the science was so bad, why wasn't that obvious at the time? Why didn't scientists of the day condemn it more strenuously, and work as hard to block its premature and destructive application as its proponents promoted eugenics and racial hygiene? Cowan (2008) points out that some did. The leaders of genetics, such as Thomas Hunt Morgan, did distance themselves from Davenport, and Davenport gained a reputation as a somewhat prickly and insecure director with an imperious style who surrounded himself with yes-people who dared not criticize him (Carlson, 2008). And perhaps more scientists would have stepped forward publicly if they had fully foreseen the wreck down the track this train was on.

HUMAN POPULATION GENETICS AND THE GRAND SYNTHESIS

Darwin's cousin, Francis Galton, was fascinated by the role of heredity in explaining human differences (Galton, 1869, 1907, 1909). To get at these questions, he helped develop many of the statistical tools that we still use to study population distributions and variations of many kinds. This includes the famous bell-shaped curve that arises from the accumulated effects of many small differences that affect a given measured attribute. He forged the tools to carry out studies of variations in height and other human attributes including intelligence. It was obvious that inheritance influenced many human traits. And here inheritance did not mean money or housing stock, but something biologically transmitted from ancestors through parents. The nature of the substance that was transmitted was unknown, but that biological inheritance mattered was apparent, and Galton and others crafted the tools to study the associations between inheritance (what we would now call *genotype*) and characters or measurable traits (which we would now call *phenotype*). Galton coined the term *eugenics*, referring to deliberate efforts to promote improvement of the human race by breeding to produce desirable traits (1909; see "Definitions" chapter).

One of the great achievements of early 20th-century science was harmonizing findings about inheritance of human variation with Mendel's particulate theory of inheritance as well as with evolutionary theory. Sewall Wright, Ronald Fisher, and others pioneered the study of population genetics and showed how the inheritance of genetic differences could assemble into observable variations in populations. They gave us the normal distribution, regression methods, and other tools of statistical inference that are still in use to this day, not only in human genetics, but in many other fields.

One example is Fisher's classic 1918 paper, which introduced the formal statistical "analysis of variation" (ANOVA) method. In it, Fisher said he was "using the term environment formally for *arbitrary* external causes independent of heredity" (Fisher, 1918, p. 420; emphasis added). Analysis of variation was a methodological innovation. The paper addressed variation in height, but the same methods were later applied to human attributes such as intelligence, cognition, and other factors that have less precise and less universally accepted outcome measures. Fisher's focus was on isolating the effects of heredity through mathematical analysis of population differences, and specifically by identifying what fraction of variation in a population sample was attributable to inheritance. It was great statistical method, but it set the stage for social mischief, in part because factors other than inheritance took a back seat under this statistical method, and the almost careless use of the term "environment," which really meant any factor not consistently aligned with genetic inheritance.

The statistically dichotomous methods set the stage for persistent confusion of the meaning of "heritability," for example, by forcing a choice between "genetic" and "environmental" sources of variation, when in fact the methods were applied to variations in phenotype in a sample derived from a given environment, and thus inherently confined the environmental variation. Thus was born a virulent and persistent conceptual virus to which I will return below: the belief that heritability implies lack of environmental malleability, when in fact heritability can change with environment (and population sample) and *the effects of* inherited factors can be highly malleable.

Fisher's agenda was to identify the amount of variation that genetically inherited factors accounted for, but this came at a cost of uninspected assumptions about both the other sources of variation, and overdeterministic interpretation of inherited factors. This carried on Galton's tradition, most flamboyantly displayed in his multiple editions of *Hereditary Genius*, that attributed intelligence, personality, and character to genetic inheritance (1869). Galton went still further to make claims about race differences that at the time surely seemed quantitative and objective, but are offensive and obviously poorly founded to modern eyes.

First, the negro race has occasionally, but very rarely, produced such men as Toussaint l'Ouverture. . . . Secondly, the negro race is by no means wholly deficient in men capable of becoming good factors, thriving merchants, and otherwise considerably raised above the average of whites . . . the average intellectual standard of the negro race is some two grades below our own. . . . A native chief has as good an education in the art of ruling men, as can be desired; he is continually exercised in personal government, and usually maintains his place by the ascendency of his character, shown every day over his subjects and rivals. . . . It is seldom that we hear of a white traveler meeting with a black chief whom he feels to be the better man. I have often discussed this subject with competent persons, and can only recall a few cases of the inferiority of the white man,—certainly not more than might be ascribed to an average actual difference of three grades, of which one may be due to the relative demerits of native education, and the remaining two to a difference in natural gifts. Fourthly, the number among the negroes of those whom we should call half-witted men, is very large. Every book alluding to negro servants in America is full of instances. I was myself much impressed by this fact during my travels in Africa. The mistakes the negroes made in their own matters, were so childish, stupid, and simpleton-like, as frequently to make me ashamed of my own species. . . . (1892, second edition of *Hereditary Genius*, appendix on ".The Comparative Worth of Different Races," pp. 338–339)

Galton's method was to study families and their members' accomplishments, much the same approach that Davenport and Laughlin carried into the America Eugenics Movement, through the Eugenics Record Office at Cold Spring Harbor Laboratory on Long Island, New York. It is almost as if in studying genetically inherited factors, Galton, Fisher, and others forgot about other forms of inheritance that also affect human phenotypes: education, family privilege, wealth, and culture—indeed the terms originally most associated with the idea of "inheritance."

Fisher was one of many in his field who contributed to the science but also joined the eugenics movement. One argument often raised against eugenics is that eugenicists did not appreciate how long it would take to change human populations through genetic means, by changing who bred with whom. This problem might be true of some, but Paul (1998, pp. 117–132) clearly shows that Fisher and others were well aware that eugenics would take a long time and would exert its effects only over long periods and at the margin, and they supported it anyway. Fischer was not alone in his enthusiasm for eugenics, but not all human population geneticists were associated with eugenics. In the wake of the Holocaust, and with the rise of human medical genetics in the 1950s and 1960s, there was a strong anti-eugenic backlash.

The centerpiece of human *medical* genetics during that period was Mendelian inheritance in man. The scientific strategy was to understand the actions of particular genes that were inherited in Mendelian fashion and could explain unusual diseases attributable to individual genes with major effects. A distinguished lineage of medical geneticists ran from Archibald Garrod—who catalogued *Inborn Errors of Metabolism* in his 1909 book and described alcaptonuria as the first human disease attributable to single-gene inheritance in 1902 (Garrod, 1902)—to the modern dean of human genetics, the late Victor McKusick, who lovingly curated 12 editions (1966–1998) as a book and then the online database *Mendelian Inheritance in Man* until his death in 2008. Most human Mendelian conditions were rare. Classic examples were phenylketonuria, alkaptonuria, cystic fibrosis, and sickle cell disease.

Sickle cell disease became a particularly interesting scientific story as it was the first molecular disease of humans, described by Linus Pauling in 1949 (Pauling, Itano, Singer, & Wells, 1949). Pauling used the novel technique of isoelectric focusing to separate two protein components of hemoglobin, one associated with sickle cell disease and the other not. The DNA sequence variation that encoded an amino acid substitution in the beta chain of hemoglobin was described in the mid-1950s (Ingram, 1956). It was a beautiful, clean story of a DNA sequence change giving rise to a protein change that affected hemoglobin solubility, in turn associated with the sickling of red blood cells and the symptoms of sickle cell disease. The hypothesis that heterozygosity (inheriting one wild type or normal allele and one sickle cell allele from one's parents) was associated with resistance to malaria became an intriguing story of natural selection for hemoglobin variants among human populations in the "Malaria Belt": northern Africa, Southeast Asia, and the Mediterranean Rim.

The story is also relevant to G × E as a classic instance. It is one of the few cases in which natural selection on human populations has become widely accepted as an explanation of population genetic differences. That story, by definition, entails strong G × E. It is worth noting, however, that the beginning of this scientific story was not so much newly observed population variations as the characterization of the beta chain of hemoglobin and the reconstruction of a plausible biological mechanism. The story of selection was constructed to explain the high population frequency of a deleterious mutation. That mutation was discovered first by noticing a difference at the protein level, then by explaining it at the level of DNA. Moreover, even this elegant and classic "genetic" disease is highly variable in its severity, and the sickling of red cells depends on low oxygen levels.

Those who have hereditary persistence of fetal hemoglobin, which fails to shut down the production of hemoglobin F that usually occurs in newborns, have much milder disease. The hemoglobin F mitigates the effects of the mutated sickle cell globin chain. Sickle cell disease can be treated by antibiotics to combat the associated infections, and even with drugs to induce expression of fetal hemoglobin. So even sickle cell disease—the prototype of an inherited Mendelian disorder attributable to a single basepair change—has an environmental trigger (oxygen saturation), shows highly variable severity depending on which other genes are expressed in a given individual, and can be treated to change outcomes dramatically. Most Mendelian disorders described since have been even more variable in expression and many are at least as amenable to treatment. Inheriting a genetic mutation is thus only a partial predictor of outcome even with this gene of major effort and whose mechanism is far better understood than most genetic factors associated with disease. The genetic influences on pathways influencing cognitive and behavioral characters are generally going to be even more variable and complicated, and we can base hopes that they can be changed by social and behavioral interventions on solid precedent from other genetic diseases.

THE RISE OF HUMAN GENETICS
STARTING FROM DNA VARIATIONS

Starting in the 1980s, with the advent of human genetic linkage maps, the strategy for finding genes associated with human traits took a U-turn. The molecular characterization of most initial Mendelian diseases started by looking for genes associated with known protein function (or malfunction). Good "guesses" about protein function led to finding the associated genes and the mutations associated with altered (usually diminished or absent) protein function. The new approach was to study human families in search of DNA differences strongly associated with phenotype differences, without having to make guesses about which protein might be affected. The study of Huntington's disease, cystic fibrosis, neurofibromatosis, hemochromatosis, breast cancer, and Alzheimer's disease exemplified the new approach. The idea was to construct pedigrees and look for strong phenotype–genotype associations. The phenotype in medical genetics was typically a disease inherited in Mendelian fashion. The genotype differences were inherited variations, usually of unknown functional significance, presumably located as specifiable positions on the human chromosomes.

What was needed was a map of human variations to guide searches for the genotype–phenotype associations (Botstein, White, Skolnick, & Davis, 1980). Variations in DNA sequence among human individuals were systematically collected and catalogued starting in the early 1980s, and once the locations were mapped to the human chromosomes, they could be used as "markers" to locate regions of DNA associated with a given phenotype. The resulting genetic linkage map was a tool to study families that showed Mendelian inheritance of a disease or interesting trait. Once a trait was linked to a marker, DNA from that part of the human chromosomes could be studied in those same families to look for specific mutations associated with the disease. Genetic linkage was a way to narrow the amount of DNA that had to be analyzed looking for specific mutations directly associated with disease. This strategy culminated in the discovery of mutations associated with many human diseases. It was a powerful strategy that carried well into the 1990s.

THE SHIFT TO SCANNING COMMON VARIATIONS
THROUGHOUT THE HUMAN GENOME

With the construction of a human reference genomic sequence in 2000 (Lander et al., 2001; Venter et al., 2001), genetics took another new turn. The old strategy did not disappear, but it was augmented by the ability to scan quickly the entire genome for common variations. The human reference genome was a major scientific landmark and a powerful scientific tool. Understanding human disease, and human biology, however, required tools to study human *variation*, not just a reference sequence. Finding disease associations meant finding genetic differences that correlated with observable individual differences. The bridge was the so-called HapMap, a systematic survey of common DNA sequence variations in human populations. Those DNA sequence differences were put onto chips and became tools for rapidly studying thousands and even millions of common DNA variations in large numbers of people, and gave rise to the current wave of genomewide association studies (GWAS).

STUDYING FULL GENOME SEQUENCES IN MANY INDIVIDUALS

Genomics is now on the verge of yet another shift. GWAS studies can only be used to look for known common human variations, because only those sequence variations have been put on the microarray chips. But now the technologies for individual full genome sequencing are becoming cheap enough and fast enough to envision population-based full-sequence genomic studies. This will not only get at common variations, but also structural rearrangements, rare variations, and other differences detectable at the level of DNA sequence. The main driver is the technology itself, which for the past half decade has been getting cheaper by roughly an order of magnitude per year (G. Church, lecture, June 9, 2009). The human reference genome produced from 1995 until 2003 cost a billion dollars, to one significant figure. By 2007, when Jim Watson's genomic sequence was given to him on a hard disk, the cost was two orders of magnitude lower (G. Church, lecture, June 9, 2009; Drmanac et al., 2009; Singer, 2009). In June 2009, Illumina announced a commercial service for full genome sequencing of an individual costing $48,000, another two orders of magnitude drop in 2 years. The company Complete Genomics published full-genome sequences in November 2009, reporting reagent costs per genomic sequence from over $8,000 to less than $1,800 (Drmanac et al., 2009). The cost of DNA sequencing is expected to continue to drop for the next few years at least. Already the costs of data gathering, tracking, and characterizing samples at the front end, and computational analysis of the resulting sequence data at the back end, exceed the cost of generating the DNA sequence data itself. DNA sequencing will soon stop being a limiting constraint on how much and how fast genomic analysis is done.

This remarkable technological change has implications for the science. It suggests that the study of DNA sequence will progress faster at lower cost, and therefore more scientists will pick up these tools and use them. It does not mean that what can be studied through analysis of DNA is more important or a more powerful explanation. It merely means that progress in studies that require studying DNA variations will move faster than other kinds of studies, and the genetic study of many phenomena will become much more pervasive. But note that the meaning of "genetic" has changed here, from studying inheritance to studying DNA sequence variation, which can be either inherited or can arise from changes within cells or over time in the body.

Studying DNA is thus not always the same as studying inherited genetic factors. Many of the explanations we can expect to flow out of full-genome sequence analysis and the new tools of single-molecule DNA detection will be about how the expression of DNA is turned off and on, how proteins alter DNA structure, and real-time changes at the level of molecules in cells. This is not the traditional realm of genetics, which was about what you inherited from your parents. Many of the stories will be about differences that occur in a person over time, or in particular physiological states (e.g., how brain cells adapt or gene expression patterns change in response to environmental change), or about how one set of cells differs from others (e.g., the differences between cancer cells and other cells of the same tissue type).

Results of complex G × E experiments are already beginning to emerge. Yamamoto and colleagues (2009) have intriguing results comparing caloric restriction to fasting–refeeding protocols in mice, for example, showing different expression of hundreds of genes in the amygdala and other brain regions, most affecting expression of genes in the alpha-adrenergic and dopamine pathways. This study used microarray technology. The next wave of functional studies may well move up to the highest level of resolution at the DNA level, full-genome sequencing.

DNA sequencing technology—and its close cousin DNA synthesis technology for making stretches of DNA *de novo*, another technology that is improving with remarkable speed—have set the stage, then, for a period of highly productive genetic studies of many phenomena, including G × E.

G × E STUDIES OF DEVELOPMENTAL PSYCHOPATHOLOGY ARE OF INTENSE INTEREST, BOTH SCIENTIFICALLY AND BECAUSE OF THEIR IMPLICATIONS FOR POLICY

The social stakes are high. It is reasonable to assume that science, including genomics, can contribute some answers to questions that really do matter in people's lives. What are the causes of addiction, and what can we do about addictive disorders? What are the long-term sequelae of physical and psychic trauma, and what can we do about them? These questions touch on education policy, child protection services and foster care, criminal justice, reproductive choice, substance use treatment and prevention, and of course prevention and treatment of medical conditions. This is important stuff.

It is important to get the science right, and to be careful in translating it into policy options because of that importance. It is all too easy to look at high heritability estimates and assume that genetic studies will capture most of what needs to be discovered. The dangers lurking in this line of reasoning are all too apparent. The race–IQ debate teaches us that it is easy to move from findings of population differences to assumptions that those differences are inherited genetically to arguments for social policies that presume immutability of genetic risk. The stepping-stones across the turbulent stream of research on the pathophysiology of behavioral and cognitive development are all slippery, and quite a few researchers have fallen in.

Science in general has become a central pillar of our culture. Within science tools of genetics have gotten more powerful very fast and have enabled the study of DNA structure. Individual differences and cellular and molecular biological phenomena can be studied at a pace even faster than other domains of science.

CONFLATION OF HERITABILITY AND IMMUTABILITY: AN INERADICABLE CONCEPTUAL VIRUS?

The conceptual virus noted earlier—the conflation of heritability with a simplistic genetic determinism—is particularly important to avoid in studies of G × E. Indeed, the field is centered on studying the interactions, which clearly implies rejecting inheritance and responsiveness to environment as dichotomous variables. The study of G × E, particularly as it refers to human behavior, confronts one particular problem with greater intensity than many other areas of human biology. How can the field avoid the persistent confusion between the statistical notion of heritability and the inference that *the effects of* what is inherited cannot be changed?

At one level, this seems obvious, even tautological. If the variations in a trait can be attributed to inheritance, doesn't this imply that there's nothing we can do about it since we don't choose our parents and don't control which genes we inherit from them? The insight that we can't control what we inherit does not, however, imply that we cannot influence the outcome. The reason is that almost all genetic effects, even very strong ones, are contingent on a particular environment, and if that environment changes, the outcome can change. This is the importance of the G × E effect for policy. We are complex organisms and not simple machines programmed by our genes. Indeed, the most complex genetic systems are cybernetic circuses, with components specifically adapted to respond to environmental change, with elaborate systems of functional redundancy, error tolerance, and capacity to learn. Organisms have evolved to respond to their environment, which means that only rarely will knowing the status of one gene or one chromosomal change give strong predictions about the fate of the entire organism, unless we also fully know the organism's environment across time.

A few examples illustrate how main-effect thinking in genetics can go awry, even in a relatively simple case of a single-gene disorder. One of the classic diseases first described to explain human Mendelian inheritance was phenylketonuria (PKU). Until the 1960s, it accounted for about 1% of those classified in the quaint term of the day as "mentally retarded." PKU was a classic Mendelian condition in which the DNA sequence inherited from both the mother and the father encoded a phenylalanine hydroxylase enzyme protein that did not process phenylalanine, which led to accumulating toxic levels that killed nerve cells. Asbjorn Folling first hypothesized in 1934 that this might be a genetic disease and suggested dietary management (Folling, 1934). Robert Guthrie developed a quick and inexpensive test in the early 1960s (Guthrie & Susi, 1963; Paul, 1997) and by the late 1960s it was incorporated into population-wide newborn screening. By the 1970s, this was a prototypical success story for newborn screening of other treatable childhood conditions (Simopoulos et al., 1975; for a history and review, see Simopoulos, 2008). The justification for newborn screening for PKU was precisely because dietary intervention blocked most of the deleterious effects on brain development, but had to be started soon after birth— that is, a G × E. There was a good reason to do genetic testing because the dietary intervention, avoiding foods with phenylalanine, could alter the outcome if started before brain damage occurred.

Here is another case where we can explain genetic inheritance down to the level of nucleotides and proteins, and the explanation of cause is obviously genetic inheritance; yet it does not follow that the people who inherit PKU mutations inevitably suffer the brain deterioration that befell those who were born before we understood the causal pathway. The causal story depends on a particular environment. Once the G × E was discovered, an obvious environmental change could be engineered to lead to dramatic changes in outcomes. Inherited factors and response to environmental factors can be orthogonal and interactive, rather than dichotomous. Ridley (2003) gives many other examples of this phenomenon in *Nature Via Nurture*.

Most of the phenomena being studied in G × E studies today are far more complex than PKU. Many of the genes involved encode proteins that function in brain cells that are parts of networks in an organ defined by its ability to learn from, and in turn project, changes onto the external environment. Some relevant DNA sequences will not even encode proteins, but rather control the transcription and translation of genes, or alter proteins that affect cellular structures in extraordinarily complicated cybernetic networks. We can predict from the get-go that these networks are highly redundant, fault-tolerant, and yet, paradoxically, fragile because of their complexity. Schizophrenia, bipolar disorder, alcohol dependence, and physiological responses to physical and emotional trauma have proven remarkably refractory to simple Mendelian genetic dissection despite being highly heritable. GWAS studies looking for common sequence variations found few statistical associations in a large study of 1,460 patents and almost 13,000 controls, but there was an intriguing association between large genomic deletions of DNA in those with symptomatic schizophrenia (Need et al., 2009). Such genomic rearrangements will not be detected by chips with common sequence variations, the state of the art until recently, but instead will depend on the more elaborate full-genome analysis possible with emerging technologies.

Most of the genetic factors that we know must be there to be found because of high heritability estimates remain undiscovered. That is probably because they do not trace their origins to a break in a single pathway, like the "broken genes" detected in Mendelian single-gene disorders, but rather involve perturbations of networks that involve interactions of molecules, and interactions with systems that change with social and environmental history and stress. There is no reason to believe, a priori, that they are not amenable to treatment just because they are heritable. Indeed, we know that treatments for many such conditions are better than they were in the 1950s, and we can hope they have a long future of significant improvement ahead. Teasing out the causal pathways at the molecular, subcellular organelle, cellular, organ, organismal, and social levels will be a tough slog. The genetic tools are getting better, and so they may be an important part of the science that unfolds, and part of the story is likely to be how genes influence and are influenced by experience and behavior. We have early examples of that in the other chapters in this volume (e.g., Meyer-Lindenberg, Chapter 4; Uher, Chapter 8), and surely many more to come.

Estimates of heritability derive primarily from studies of twins, and particularly from studying variations among identical (monozygotic) twins compared to fraternal (dizygotic) twins or siblings, or from "snapshot" statistical studies of human populations. At the highest level, these studies can help us answer the question, Do genes play a role? The deep and pervasive confusion that has plagued both psychology and genetics is the assumption that if the answer is yes, it follows that other factors do not also affect the outcomes. The PKU example illustrates the fallacy of this assumption that genetic factors and environmental factors are dichotomous. In fact, genetic and "environmental" factors are often independent and interactive. That is, a genetic character can be highly heritable and highly malleable, and contingent on environmental conditions.

High heritability thus does not imply low malleability. In studies of heritability estimates, the total variance in an outcome such as psychopathology is always one, and the proportions are allocated to genes or environments as a forced choice. Because the estimates must sum to one, it appears that if the heritability quotient is high, then the environmental quotient is necessarily low. The problem with this conclusion is that the estimates are contingent on the context in which the measurements are drawn (i.e., the range of genes and environments that exist in that context) and fail to take into account the possibility that the environment might, at least theoretically, be very different. In a new population in which the range of environments is suddenly great, heritability estimates might change radically. Changing the environment (perhaps through intervention) could change heritability estimates. Malleability is generally best studied in intervention studies and longitudinal population studies such as those reviewed by Costello (Chapter 10, this volume).

This confusion between heritability and immutability has obvious implications for social policy. The race and IQ debate of the 1970s, and the resurgence of that debate with publication of *The Bell Curve* in 1994 (Herrnstein & Murray, 1994) exposed the noxious persistence of the "heritability implies inevitability" conceptual virus. Of course genes matter a great deal in the construction of various forms of intelligence; and of course so do education, nutrition, experience, and avoidance of toxic exposures (e.g., lead). Those working in this field should beware of how the science of genetics and human behavior can easily be imported into prognostications for public policy that rest on assuming that high heritability justifies environmental nihilism, an assumption that is demonstrably false in case after case, once we have pieced together a story. Sometimes genetic factors will indeed limit the power of interventions such as education. We can do much to help those with Down syndrome or fragile X, but those with those genetic conditions cannot be raised to the species-normal mean for cognitive performance. A child with a brain damaged by lead exposure is also constrained in how much education can change his or her cognitive performance. Here biology is not destiny, but it is a serious constraint on cognition (even if it is arguably *not* a major impediment to living a life that is meaningful for that person and those around him or her). Genetic inheritance and environmental exposures are among the crucial contingencies to study. Cases such as PKU show how assuming that genetics is destiny can be an unsafe assumption at the individual level, and even more suspect at the population (and thus policy) level. Assessing malleability requires understanding a full causal pathway. Stopping at the genetics does not get us there, and pointing to heritability tells us little about whether outcomes are fated or malleable.

The best forms of inoculation against the conceptual virus is understanding the technical meaning of heritability and its limits, with a booster shot of another form of understanding: awareness of the cyclical history of the race–IQ debate and knowledge of the history of eugenics and genetic determinism. At the other extreme, some attenuated strains of behavioral determinism are probably still persistent in our culture as well. Learning psychology should entail learning that history.

DO SCIENTISTS HAVE SPECIAL RESPONSIBILITIES?

Given the predictable rapid advances on the genetic front, and sustained fascination with and real-world implications of the study of behavior, cognition, and personality, what can we say about the responsibility of science and of scientists? Do scientists have a special responsibility?

The overbearing behavioral determinism of Watson and the disastrous consequences of eugenics and racial hygiene should give us pause. But the message cannot be to retreat from public engagement. This science is likely to be relevant to policy whether we like it or not.

Optimism that science can improve the world does rest on real achievements. To illustrate how science can improve health through public policy, consider how the field of public health chalked up remarkable achievements during the last century. In 1900, life expectancy at birth in even the wealthiest nations was in the 50s, but by century's end it had increased to the low 80s. Three decades of life extension over the course of 10 decades is staggering in its implications. This change utterly transformed how we expect to live our lives. Rising life expectancy, and particularly the reduction of childhood and infant mortality, led to fewer births, greater investment in those born, and expectations of long and healthy life unfathomable before the generations now living.

Most of the story is explained by improved sanitation, nutrition, transportation, and general affluence during the first half of the last century. But starting midcentury, new scientific knowledge began to contribute to preventing, detecting, and treating the conditions that shorten and degrade human lives. The epidemiology of tobacco use in the 1950s gave rise to preventive strategies for public education, banning public smoking, raising tobacco taxes, and other interventions including strong incentives to quit smoking. Smoking rates are less than half what they once were, despite nicotine being one of the most addictive substances ever discovered. The fact that most of this research was primarily epidemiological, social, and behavioral rather than chemical or biological did not make it anytheless scientific. The story of how mortality from heart disease, stroke, and high blood pressure dropped steadily for five decades also rested heavily on epidemiology and longitudinal studies such as the Framingham Heart Study and the National High Blood Pressure Education Program (Jones & Hall, 2002; Levy & Brink, 2005). It also depended on many new drug treatments, diagnostic techniques, and systematic study of medical management strategies incorporated into health care. And biological risks and medical care go only so far. As Deans and colleagues (2009) note in a recent epidemiological study in Glasgow, Scotland, "Classic cardiovascular risk factors did not fully explain the difference in plaque presence between participants from the most deprived areas and those from the least deprived areas, suggesting that current public health messages directed at classic risk factors (diet, blood pressure, smoking) may not adequately address the continuing socioeconomic gradient in cardiovascular disease" (p. 11). The gains in life expectancy attributable to lower cardiovascular mortality are spectacular nonetheless, even if we do not yet fully understand all the reasons for them.

Can we promise similar achievements for G × E studies focused on behavior, cognition, and personality? Here we have to be cautious. If these interactions were not complex, we would already understand them. It is not lack of caring about human behavior, both individual and collective, that has constrained the field. Rather, it is the immense difficulty of doing good science—controlling for variables in experiments, designing careful intervention studies, and the expense of longitudinal population studies—that imposes stringent limits on expectations. Genetics cannot speed up studies like Framingham or accelerate the accumulation of data in decade-long observation trials. Genetics will be layered onto such studies, and we surely hope there will be major findings. But we should not promise quick results because the underlying process is still about following many people over long periods of time. The acceleration of progress in experimental genomic molecular laboratory systems and model organisms that comes from the prodigious advance of sequencing and synthesis technologies will come from studying more people and other organisms in greater genetic detail at lower cost, but interpretation will also still depend on studies of people in their environment over time.

There is also an obvious difference between studying heart disease, diet, and exercise, or studying tobacco use and lung cancer, and the kind of gene–environment studies of human behavior addressed in this volume. The heart and lung are complex organs that respond to the environment, but they are orders of magnitude less complex, and the nervous system is inherently about responding to the environment. That is, the most distinctive features of the nervous system are perception, cognition, learning, adaption, and intervention, in contrast to respiration or circulation. This means there are many more intervening variables between cause and effect. The functional difference between brain cells in different neuroanatomical locations vastly exceeds the difference between cells at the apex and base of the lung, or the different ventricles of the heart. Synapses and action potentials may be common among neurons, but connection, location, and history matter immensely to neural function. Neuroscience faces three-dimensional, electrical, and gene-regulatory complexity far, far beyond the study of other organ systems, and the degree of genetic diversity is also greater in the brain. Our grandchildren will still be busy studying $G \times E$ in human behavior. We should set public expectations accordingly, not to put a damper on enthusiasm but to narrow the gap between what we can study with the tools in hand now and public expectations about how quickly we will achieve full understanding and apply it to practical ends.

Scientists do not have any particular expertise in ethics, nor do they have a distinctive claim on moral authority. They do, however, have a distinctive responsibility in the public debate. J. B. Watson, Fisher, Davenport, and Laughlin were guilty of making scientific claims with public policy implications that went well beyond their evidence. Eugenics and racial hygiene point to dangers of commingling the science of human genetics with simplistic and unchallenged social policy prognostication. Let's admit there were disasters and those disasters had something to do with science, and scientists. But there is no need to stay hunkered down in scientific bunkers or retreat to ivory towers.

Scientists should indeed be cautious when they engage with social policy, but it does not mean they should not do it. Quite the contrary, public policy depends on the best science of the day. Those making policy decisions depend on a scientific community that is debating not only what is true, but also why it matters in the real world and how to apply what it knows. Scientists do have a responsibility to ensure that they conduct their science responsibly and ethically, for example, by respecting the rights and interests of people who participate in research. They also have a role to play in ensuring that the translation of that science and public policy is done in full view. The Mertonian norms of organized skepticism, open sharing, objectivity, and vigorous debate (Merton, 1973) are just as relevant for translating science into public policy as they are in conducting the science itself.

It is quite clear that gene–environment studies of human behavior will be difficult, complicated, and hotly contested. Some studies will take years or decades to bear fruit. The science will be hard, and its interpretation messy and contentious. The ongoing process of interpreting that science for those making policy decisions will likewise be difficult, complicated, and sometimes controversial, and rightly so.

Several practical implications flow from the history of psychology, genetics, and public health. One is that a field that pays conscious attention to its social implications is less likely to make catastrophic mistakes than one oblivious to how its work will be translated into social policy. The danger is not engagement with policy, but rather that only one faction of the scientific community will engage—with credible scientists leaving policy translation to the charlatans—or that scientific disagreement will not be acknowledged in the policy debate. One can hope that modern scientists will not let shoddy science stand unchallenged to the degree that geneticists let eugenicists hold sway 80 and 90 years ago. Indeed, there may be a ray of hope in the story of *The Bell Curve*. While it sold well and caused a major ruckus, unlike the eugenics movement of the 1920s and 1930s, *The Bell Curve* elicited a firestorm of criticism in academe, and some of that debate spilled over into policy circles. The books produced by Laughlin and Davenport fed a national movement that passed legislation restricting immigration and enabled forced sterilization, encroaching on the freedoms of whole groups (Davenport, 1911/2008; Laughlin, 1922). The U.S. sterilization laws were lauded in Germany, which took several disastrous further steps in its march to the Holocaust (Proctor, 1988). But as noted above, *The Bell Curve* did not have anything like the major national policy impact of Davenport and Laughlin, although some of the nihilistic prescriptions for Head Start and education policy would have had disparate effects on African American and indigent populations if implemented. One lesson here is that an academic community was able to thwart the policy translation of science by debating its implications and by engaging with those making policy decisions.

A corollary lesson is that those practicing in the field can learn from history, and indeed knowing some of the history of eugenics, racial hygiene, and the race–IQ debate may be an essential ingredient of training for those studying G × E. Translating that learning into the conduct of research and into debates about public policy will entail political processes—and here I mean "politics" in the sense of collective action to solve real-world problems in its positive, functional meaning and not as a pejorative term. Politics necessarily mediates the professional and scientific debate about both the science and its application for public policy. The prescription for those in the field is clear: learn some history, and accept the idea that politics is part of both doing good research and translating its implications for those making policy decisions. Devoting some attention to ensuring that the political processes for doing science and translating it into policy is constructively critical, open, and civil should pay off.

REFERENCES

Allen, A., Anderson, B., Andrews, L., Beckwith, J., Bowman, J., Cook-Deegan, R., et al. (1996). *The bell curve*: Statement by the NIH-DOE Joint Working Group on the Ethical, Legal, and Social Implications of Human Genome Research. *American Journal of Human Genetics, 52*, 487–488.

Botstein, D., White, R. L., Skolnick, M., & Davis, R. W. (1980). Construction of a genetic linkage map in man using restriction fragment length polymorphisms. *American Journal of Human Genetics, 32*, 314–331.

Carlson, E. A. (2008). The eugenic world of Charles Benedict Davenport. In J. A. Witkowski & J. R. Inglis (Eds.), *Davenport's dream: 21st century reflections on heredity and eugenics* (pp. 59–76). Cold Spring Harbor, NY: Cold Spring Harbor Laboratory Press.

Cowan, R. S. (2008). *Heredity and hope: The case for genetic screening.* Cambridge, MA: Harvard University Press.

Davenport, C. B. (2008). *Heredity in relation to eugenics.* New York: Henry Holt and Company. In J. A. Witkowski & J. R. Inglis (Eds.), *Davenport's dream: 21st century reflections on heredity and eugenics* (pp. 192–298). Cold Spring Harbor, NY: Cold Spring Harbor Laboratory Press. (Original published 1911)

Deans, K. A., Bezlyak, V., Ford, I., Batty, G. D., Burns, H., Cavanagh, J., et al. (2009). Differences in atherosclerosis according to area level socioeconomic deprivation: Cross sectional, population based study. *British Medical Journal, 339,* b4170.

Drmanac, R., Sparks, A. B., Callow, M. J., Halpern, A. L., Burns, N. L., Kermani, B. G., et al. (2009). Human genome sequencing using unchained base reads on self-assembling DNA nanoarrays. *Science, 327*, 78–81.

Fisher, R. A. (1918). The correlation between relatives on the supposition of Mendelian inheritance. *Transactions of the Royal Society of Edinburgh, 52*, 399–433. Retrieved from *digital.library.adelaide.edu.au/coll/special//fisher/9.pdf.*

Folling, A. (1934). Excretion of phenylpyruvic acid in urine as a metabolic anomaly in connection with imbecility. *Nordisk Medicinsk Tidskrift, 8*, 1054–1059.

Galton, F. (1869). *Hereditary genius: An inquiry into its laws and consequences.* New York: Appleton.

Galton, F. (1907). *Probability: The foundation of eugenics.* Oxford, UK: Clarendon Press.

Galton, F. (1909). *Essays in eugenics.* London: Eugenics Education Society.

Garrod, A. E. (1902). The incidence of alkaptonuria: A study in chemical individuality. *Lancet, 2*, 1616–1620.

Garrod, A. E. (1909). *Inborn errors of metabolism.* London: Frowde.

Guthrie, R., & Susi, A. (1963). A simple phenylalanine method for detecting phenylketonuria in large populations of newborn infants. *Pediatrics, 32*, 338–343.

Herrnstein, R. J., & Murray, C. (1994). *The bell curve: Intelligence and class structure in American life.* New York: Free Press.

Illumina. (2009, June 10). Illumina announces personal genome sequencing service, offering to provide comprehensive image of individual whole genome.

Retrieved from *investor.illumina.com/phoenix.zhtml?c=121127&p=irol-newsArticle&ID=1298128&highlight=%20.*

Ingram, V. M. (1956). A specific chemical difference between the globins of normal human and sickle-cell anaemia haemoglobin. *Nature, 178,* 792–794.

Jones, D. W., & Hall, J. E. (2002). The National High Blood Pressure Education Program: Thirty years and counting. *Hypertension, 39,* 941–942.

Kevles, D. J. (1984, October 8, October 15, October 22, October 29). Annals of eugenics: A secular faith. *New Yorker,* pp. 51–115 (part 1), pp. 52–125 (part 2), pp. 92–151 (part 3), pp. 51–117 (part 4).

Kevles, D. J. (1985). *In the name of eugenics.* New York: Knopf.

Lander, E. S., Linton, L. M., Birren, B., Nusbaum, C., Zody, M. C., Baldwin, J., et al. (2001). Initial sequencing and analysis of the human genome. *Nature, 409,* 860–921.

Laughlin, H. (1922). Eugenical sterilization in the United States. Psychopathic Laboratory of the Municipal Court of Chicago. Retrieved from *dnapatents.georgetown.edu/resources/EugenicalSterilizationInTheUS.pdf.*

Levy, D., & Brink, S. (2005). *A change of heart: How the people of Framingham, Massachusetts, helped unravel the mysteries of cardiovascular disease.* New York: Knopf.

Merton, R. K. (1973). *The sociology of science: Theoretical and empirical investigations.* Chicago: University of Chicago Press.

McKusick, V. A. (1966–1998). *Mendelian inheritance in man: A catalog of human genes and genetic disorders.* Baltimore: Johns Hopkins University Press.

Need, A. C., Ge, D., Weale, M. E., Maia, J., Feng, S., Heinzen, E. L., et al. (2009). A genome-wide investigation of SNPs and CNVs in schizophrenia. *PLoS Genetics, 5,* e1000373.

Paul, D. (1997). Appendix 5: The history of newborn phenylketonuria screening in the U.S. In N. A. Holtzman & M. S. Watson (Eds.), *Promoting safe and effective genetic testing in the United States: Final report of the task force on genetic testing.* Baltimore: Johns Hopkins University Press. Retrieved from *biotech.law.lsu.edu/research/fed/tfgt/index.htm.*

Paul, D. (1998). *The politics of heredity: Essays on eugenics, biomedicine, and the nature–nurture debate.* Albany: State University of New York Press.

Pauling, L., Itano, H. A., Singer, S. J., & Wells, I. C. (1949). Sickle cell anemia, a molecular disease. *Science, 110,* 543–548.

Proctor, R. (1988). *Racial hygiene: Medicine under the Nazis.* Cambridge, MA: Harvard University Press.

Provine, W. B. (1971). *The origins of theoretical population genetics.* Chicago: University of Chicago Press.

Ridley, M. (2003). *Nature via nurture: Genes, experience and what makes us human.* London: Fourth Estate.

Simopoulos, A. P. (2008). Genetic screening: Programs, principles, and research—thirty years later. *Public Health Genomics, 12,* 105–111.

Simopoulos, A. P., Childs, B., Committee for the Study of Inborn Errors of Metabolism, Division of Medical Sciences, Assembly of Life Sciences, National Research Council. (1975). *Genetic screening: Programs, principles, and research.* Washington, DC: National Academy of Sciences.

Singer, E. (2009). Interpreting the genome. *Technology Review, 112*(1), 48–53.

Venter, J. C., Adams, M. D., Myers, E. W., Li, P. W., Mural, R. J., Sutton, G. G., et al. (2001). The sequence of the human genome. *Science, 291,* 1304–1351.

Watson, J. (1930). *Behaviorism.* Chicago: University of Chicago Press.

Watson, J. (2008). Genes and politics. In J. A. Witkowski & J. R. Inglis (Eds.), *Davenport's dream: 21st century reflections on heredity and eugenics* (pp. 1–34). Cold Spring Harbor, NY: Cold Spring Harbor Laboratory Press.

Witkowski, J. A., & Inglis, J. R. (2008). Preface. In J. A. Witkowski & J. R. Inglis (Eds.), *Davenport's dream: 21st century reflections on heredity and eugenics* (pp. xii–xiii). Cold Spring Harbor, NY: Cold Spring Harbor Laboratory Press.

Yamamoto, Y., Tanahashi, T., Kawai, T., Chikahisa, S., Katsuura, S., Nishida, K., et al. (2009). Changes in behavior and gene expression induced by caloric restriction in C57BL/6 mice. *Physiological Genomics, 39,* 227–235.

CHAPTER 13

Genes, Environments, and Public Policy

Kenneth A. Dodge *and* Michael Rutter

In Chapter 1 of this volume, Rutter described the multiple types of gene–environment interplay that can affect behavioral outcomes, particularly gene–environment interaction (G × E), and he highlighted the challenges facing scholars in trying to understand how G × E operates on behavior through intermediate phenotypes. Rutter and Dodge (Chapter 5) then summarized the significant leaps forward being made by the work of Caspi, Hariri, Holmes, Uher, and Moffitt (Chapter 2), Hariri (Chapter 3), and Meyer-Lindenberg (Chapter 4) in providing a biological basis for G × E effects. Rutter and Dodge concluded that the G × E effects are real, they have been replicated, and their implications are not yet fully realized. Virtually every paradigm shift and major advance in science is followed quickly by claims of applications and calls for radical reform in clinical practice or public policy. Some of these calls represent true advances in the translation of science to practice, but many "implications" overreach and are proven to be misguided over time. The G × E discoveries in developmental psychopathology will be no exception. In this chapter, we address several issues in the state of science-to-policy translation of G × E in three domains: science policy, health services policy, and judicial policy.

SCIENCE POLICY

Without a doubt, the discovery of G × E and gene–environment interplay in developmental psychopathology changes the way that science must proceed over the next decades. In fact, the most immediate implications of G × E discoveries are for scientific theory itself. Main effects of genetic variation tell us little about the process of how psychopathology develops, and main effects of environments are usually confounded with genetic or environmental variables such that any causal interpretation is guarded. However, the intersection of gene and environment not only describes behavior, it guides us toward understanding processes of development when we understand how gene and environment are related. Even though statistical analyses de-confound the separate effects of gene and environment, it is the interaction that brings theoretical advances by helping us understand the nature of a disorder. For example, by knowing that conduct disorder can be predicted from early experiences of maltreatment, particularly among children who have a polymorphism in monoamine oxidase A (*MAOA*, which codes for a protein that may interfere with one's ability to regulate or temper a behavioral response to provocation), we have a clue that conduct disorder may be a disorder of behavioral regulation in response to threats or constraints. Likewise, by knowing that depressive disorder can be predicted from a life of stressful experiences primarily among those individuals who have a polymorphism in *5-HTTLPR* (which has been associated with a dysregulated stress response), we learn that depression may be a disorder of regulation of response to stressors.

Of course, findings must be replicated, and caution must be taken with regard to generalization across populations. Beyond these usual points, though, we suggest that supporting inquiry into G × E should be a highest priority for science policy. The scientific field will benefit from attention to matters of (1) how environment data are collected in studies of individuals over time; (2) how public policies can enhance the collection of environment data and gene data in large populations; and (3) how theory must guide the analysis of data through the search for pivotal phenotypes.

Collect Good Environment Data

The finding that the impact of genes varies across environments may prove to be the most important event in the study of environments, because now this field of inquiry must be taken more seriously and must be conducted more rigorously than in the past. Without deprecating past environment research, we acknowledge that the goal of some past work had been merely to establish that the environment is important, rather than to understand *how* the environment influences behavior. For example, past studies have sometimes confounded the measure of the environment with the self's interpretation about the environment. Although interesting theoretically, because one mechanism of action of the environment might well operate through the individual's appraisal of it, the environment still must be measured independently and objectively. This task is complicated by the fact that culturewide appraisals of events (which are independent of an individual's appraisal) also shape the impact of an event, as in the case of medical-surgical procedures on children that are not interpreted as torture (although they might well be stressful experiences).

The cultural normativeness of an experience also influences its impact on a child. Lansford and colleagues (2005) found that corporal punishment has relatively little impact on child anxiety and aggressive behavior when experienced in a cultural context of high normativeness of this practice (such as Kenya or India); in contrast, in cultures in which this practice is less common (such as Thailand), individual differences in experience have a larger impact on child outcomes.

A major potential contribution of G × E science is to identify novel and important domains of environment that could provide leverage for clinical interventions. Reiss and Neiderhiser (Chapter 6), for example, found that some genetic processes influence clinical outcomes by operating on the environment. They point toward parents' marriage as an environmental event that mediates some genetic impacts and that could be targeted for policy interventions.

Sometimes environment measures have been so broad that they confound multiple environment variables. Furthermore, because the time of measurement is often retrospective, the enivronment variable confounds current symptoms with recollections of past events. And, of course, research designs that fail to control genetic influences risk confounding a parent's genes with that parent's socializing behaviors. These problems, and some potential solutions, are illustrated in the study of two of the most important environment constructs in G × E research to date: stress and early maltreatment.

The study of life stressors has a rigorous precedent in the work of Brown and Harris (1978), which has been summarized by Monroe and Reid (2008), who noted, "Groundbreaking studies on life stress and depression have advanced both research designs for testing etiological hypotheses and methods for specifying types of life stress that most commonly precede depression's onset. Yet almost none of this knowledge has informed recent research on gene–environment interactions in depression" (p. 947). They go on to note that stress has been variously conceptualized, measured, and scored across studies, with wide-ranging operationalizations that include parental marital breakup, the experience of chronic illness, and natural disasters. Some stressful events are recent and acute (e.g., failure on an exam, death of a parent), whereas others started long ago and are chronic (e.g., growing up with an alcoholic father). Such variation in the morphology of environment is justified on the ground that these diverse events have a common impact on the individual through a stress process (Rutter, 1985). Indeed, Caspi and colleagues (2003) found similar impact on depression for two very different kind of stressors, one that is in line with the original Brown and Harris concept of a provoking factor that precipitates the onset of a new episode and a second kind that is an index of long-standing adversities.

Stress indexes tally the number of stressful events that are experienced, with underlying assumptions that these events have similar valence and strength of impact and need not have psychometric coherence or high inter-item internal consistency. Muddying the science, however, is the fact that items that "count" as stress vary across studies. This current state of the science of environmental stress reflects both the wisdom of a theory of stress but also the long way that still must be traversed in future studies to sort out how different stressful environments exert different impacts.

Monroe and Reid (2008) follow from Brown and Harris (1978) to propose that stress is best measured as: "(a) acute (i.e., distinct onset), (b) very recent (within approximately 3 to 6 months), (c) major (i.e., very threatening or unpleasant), and (d) primarily focused on the participant" (p. 951). Although this advice is grounded in empirical literature, we contend that the book should remain open on the topic because future studies may well reveal that different genetic variables interact with different forms of stressors to produce different forms of psychopathology. The stressor that ignites an initial depressive episode might be different from the stressor that increases the probability of relapse or interferes with successful treatment. More work needs to be completed on a taxonomy of stressful environments, and this work takes a new turn when considered in the context of G × E.

The measurement of child maltreatment is similarly fraught with inconsistency across studies (Dodge, Bates, & Pettit, 1990). Some studies have identified maltreated children from an official registry of "proven" perpetrators, which has the advantage of a high degree of certainty that a maltreating event occurred. However, such studies overweight single, acute maltreating traumatic events over chronic experiences, and they confound the traumatic event with the public-agency treatment of the child received postevent (e.g., the child might be removed from the home and placed into foster care). Other studies rely on retrospective recollections that an individual had been maltreated as a child (thoroughly confounding the measurement of environment with current symptoms and appraisals). Still other studies rely on interviews with community samples of key observers (e.g., parents). Although these studies partially disentangle the maltreatment experience from its consequences, they suffer from uncertainty about the veracity of the observer's perspective.

Taxonomies of maltreatment need to move beyond simple categories of physical abuse, environmental neglect, and sexual abuse. The perpetrator (e.g., parent, other family member, nonrelative), the victim's context of relationships with other adults (e.g., a supportive nonabusive parent), and the chronicity of the experience all may affect the strength and quality of impact on the victim. Furthermore, these factors may interact with genetic variables in diverse ways.

These challenges in the measurement of environment are formidable. They point toward the need for nuanced, in-depth studies of how environment variables operate, but those studies are complicated by the emerging findings that environment operates differently in different genetic contexts. Objective characteristics of an environment event must be distinguished from its filtered experience by the individual. Furthermore, the errors that can ensue are great when distinctions among environment variables are not appropriately considered. In this volume, Caspi and colleagues (Chapter 2) point out the erroneous interpretations that have been made of 5HT-by-stress studies of depression when environment variables are misinterpreted (Risch et al., 2009). Nonetheless, G × E studies clearly point toward the importance of expanded, accurate measurement of environment in future studies. Prospects for doing so can come by adding the measurement of environment to genomewide association studies (GWAS) or by adding the collection of DNA to ongoing longitudinal studies that had previously highlighted only the measurement of environment. The former is a controversial topic because the new collection of high-quality environment data in existing large GWAS samples that had previously assembled only genetic data may be difficult to achieve. The need for environment data has been questioned by advocates of GWAS studies (Risch et al., 2009), as has the importance and robustness of G × E findings, perhaps precisely because the collection of such data in those studies is not feasible.

The addition of gene data to an existing prospective study of the environment has been attempted by Caspi in the Dunedin study (Chapter 2), by Guo in the Add-Health study (Chapter 7), and by Reiss and Neiderhiser in the NEAD study (Chapter 6). The payoff for these attempts depends on the scientific contributions that get made.

Public Policies Should Support the Collection of Environment and Gene Data

Consistent with the historically grounded mandate to improve public health, governments can nurture the routine collection of environment data at both the individual and community levels. Recent G × E findings increase the importance of these data for current studies, and the wisdom of such data collection by governments will be revealed in future studies.

At the individual level, an obvious beginning is the expansion of relevant environment data that can be recorded in birth records and made available to scholars. Prenatal care and illness history, prenatal substance use, smoking, alcohol use, stressors, family demography, and context of material affordances and income all can be added to birth records stored by local governments. Similar records can be recorded and stored across the lifespan. School records have a long history of important use in developmental research (e.g., Rutter, Maughan, Mortimore, & Ouston, 1979) and can be enhanced to include family context, demographics, and residential addresses that can be geocoded for neighborhood context. Health records can be similarly enhanced to include broader individual information and relevant environmental context information.

Governments can also collect and share information at the school, neighborhood, and community levels. For example, school information can be collected and shared about size, demographic constitution, teacher–student ratio, teacher qualifications, expenditures-per-pupil, schoolwide achievement, and schoolwide behaviors that are summarized from anonymous surveys. Neighborhood census information is increasingly available about socioeconomic distribution, crime, and population density. Community information is available in many districts about average quality of day care, availability and quality of health care, and normativeness of experiences of crime, parenting, and family life. The scope of government-supported environment data collection can be nurtured well beyond these few examples by creative scholars and government policies.

A different challenge lies ahead for the collection of gene data. The cost and ease of collecting DNA has been greatly improved over the past decade, and it can be envisioned that personalized genotyping will become common among the current generation before it grows old. However, the collection of DNA for research purposes remains a political challenge, as the description by Kaufman and Perepletchikova (Chapter 9) vividly describes. Their research has been halted by administrators who fear the political fallout of measuring genes in the context of the study of family violence. The tasks of science policy are tall ones. They will be to educate the public that gene data can be collected and stored securely; protected from outside interference by criminal prosecutors, health insurance detectives, and divorce custody attorneys; remain free from political issues about stereotypes of ethnic groups; and prove useful to scientific discoveries that have practical import.

Data Analyses Should Be Guided by Theory
and the Search for Pivotal Phenotypes

Advocating for enhanced collection of environment data does not imply abandonment of standards of scientific rigor in conducting data analyses. We do not advocate that scholars examine every possible available environment variable through experiment-wise controlled tests, as is now the practice with the testing of genes in GWAS studies. Rather, science must proceed with reciprocal influence between theory and empirical findings. Refined theory should both guide and respond to data collection and analysis. The number of possible G × E tests (let alone gene and environment main effect tests) is so large that atheoretical approaches that are based solely on blind empiricism will require such large sample sizes that they will not move the field forward.

So how should theory match empirical testing of G × E effects on developmental psychopathology? The bridge may be identified in phenotypes that link genotypes with psychiatric outcomes. Because it is highly unlikely that individual genes (or even sets of genes) will directly cause a disorder, it is also unlikely that a specific G × E combination (or a single environment, for that matter) will directly cause a disorder. There is no gene for conduct disorder or depression. More likely, genes (and G × E) will lead to important phenotypes that increase the probability that a particular disorder will ensue. Hariri (Chapter 3) brilliantly identifies amygdala reactivity as a crucial mediating phenotype in the relation between genes and behavior. Meyer-Lindenberg (Chapter 4) has identified abnormality in dorsolateral prefrontal cortex response as an intermediate phenotype in schizophrenia.

HEALTH SERVICES POLICY

The most direct practical implication of the G × E revolution would seem to accrue to the field of personalized medicine. Large individual differences have been observed in responsiveness to both pharmacological and psychological interventions for virtually all forms of psychopathology, and the hope has been that G × E effects can improve the prediction of responsiveness to therapies. In 2004, Francis Collins (Guttmacher, Collins, & Drazen, 2004) presented his vision that personalized medicine would revolutionize medical practice within a decade. He continues to embrace that vision today (Collins, 2010), in spite of limited progress toward this goal. Even advocates of personalized medicine such as Roden and colleagues (2006) have acknowledged that findings have not always replicated, due to false positives from many tests, differences in patient groups, and subtle differences in the definitions of clinical symptoms. After a review across many domains, Nebert, Zhang, and Vesell (2008) concluded, "The continuous discoveries, even today, of new surprises about our genome cause us to question reviews declaring that 'personalized medicine is almost here' or that 'individualized drug therapy will soon be a reality' "(p. 187). One of the problems is that attempts to identify specific genes that account for risk for pathology have proven challenging. For example, even though cardiovascular disease has a significant family history association, the risk for a cardiovascular event associated with the aggregate of the supposed major genes is negligible (Paynter et al., 2010). Even though commercial vendors are ready to sell genotyping to any paying consumer who wants to know what drug will work uniquely for him or her, the incremental value of this kind of personalized pharmacogenetics seems questionable at this time.

Although Collins's claim was wildly overstated, research in personalized medicine has marched forward, revealing important discoveries about the process of development of psychopathology. Uher (Chapter 8) presents a cogent case that G × E interaction effects are important and complicated. They imply causal heterogeneity for some disorders, such as depressive disorder. Furthermore, different genes and environments may be implicated at different points in the life course of depression, from initial onset of symptoms to disorder to treatment receptivity and to recidivism. He sets forth the intriguing hypothesis that long-term memory traces from early life experiences such as maltreatment mediate the impact of experience on adult depression through epigenetic changes, and that both pharmacological and psychosocial interventions might counteract such changes. The matching of intervention to an individual's genes and environmental history could prove crucial in successful treatment. If so, future classification systems might subtype depressive disorder according to distinct causal pathways, different effects of genes and environments on various points in the course of disorder, and, plausibly, distinct responsiveness to different pharmacotherapies based on robust findings of G × E.

As a prime example, Uher (Chapter 8) summarizes findings that a polymorphism of the serotonin transporter gene (5-HTTLPR) has been associated with poor response to the serotonin reuptake inhibiting antidepressants (SSRIs), for which the serotonin transporter is the molecular target, at least among adults of European origin. Likewise, an environmental history of early maltreatment appears to predict relatively poor response to pharmacotherapy but relatively good response to psychological intervention. Uher concludes that G × E interaction effects are very important to identify and to understand, primarily because they inform the nature of how psychopathology develops and changes over the lifecourse. In turn, once we understand how a disorder develops and changes through interaction between genes and environments, we can design treatments that apply to subsegments of the population based on genes and life experiences. However, the magnitude of interaction effects that have been identified to date has not been strong enough to alter clinical practice significantly, and the hope of personalized medicine has not yet been fully realized.

Personalized prevention is also a plausible idea gaining momentum. Recent studies by Brody, Beach, Philibert, Chen, & Murry, (2009) and Bakermans-Kranenburg, van IJzendoorn, Pijlman, Mesman, and Juffer (2008) indicate that genetic variation moderates (i.e., exacerbates or limits) the effects of preventive interventions on children. In a randomized controlled trial of a family intervention designed to prevent risky behaviors in rural African American early adolescents, Brody and colleagues found that the intervention was effective, but only for children with a specific allele of 5-HTTLPR. The evidence suggested that levels of involved-supportive parenting that were enhanced by intervention decreased youths' opportunities to engage in risk behavior. In a second randomized controlled trial, Bakermans-Kranenburg and colleagues found that a parent-training program designed to increase rates of sensitive discipline in parents of 1- to 3-year-old children reduced subsequent externalizing behavior, but only in the subgroup of children with a particular preexisting G × E pattern, that is, those children who had a form of the dopamine DRD4 receptor gene and previously had been exposed to the highest levels of sensitive parental discipline. These studies suggest that clinical therapies and preventive interventions might be most effective if targeted to subgroups who meet particular G × E criteria.

Before we jump to intervention policies, however, Kaufman and Perepletchikova (Chapter 9) have shown that replicated G × E interaction effects may themselves be moderated by significant three-way interactions. In their case, a polymorphism in the brain-derived neurotrophic factor (BDNF) genotype moderated the previously reported interaction effect between 5-HTTLPR and maltreatment history in predicting depression. In turn, this triple interaction effect was moderated (muted) by social supports in the child's environment. This G × G × E × E interaction effect indicates that we do not yet know with high precision which combination of genes and environments will be most responsive to particular treatments for depressive disorder.

Should our goal still be to identify empirically robust G × E effects in order to tailor interventions? In concept, this idea has strong merit, if the G × E effect is theoretically sensible, empirically robust, has a strong effect size, and applies to a large enough subsegment of the population to make tailored interventions cost-effective. We expect that some such G × E effects, and therefore such interventions, will soon be identified. However, we suggest that if tailored clinical behavioral interventions are based solely

on atheoretical, empirically discovered interaction effects, they will ultimately prove ineffective. Is there a wiser strategy for the future of clinical
medicine? We suggest that coupled with this empirical approach must be
the push to understand basic principles and mechanisms of human behavior
and then to use these principles to identify ways to shape that behavior.

This theory-guided, empirically validated approach to clinical intervention policy is similar to the search for pivotal phenotypes described
above. Rather than search solely for interventions that alter a psychiatric
disorder outcome, a more fruitful strategy may be to identify interventions
that shape important "environmental phenotypes." Consider an analogy
to the prevention of myocardial infarction. We know that blood pressure
is such a strong predictor and mechanism for long-term heart attack risk
(as well as other morbidities) that now we try to identify ways to shape
blood pressure through pharmacotherapies, exercise, diet, and stress reduction. These environmental interventions indirectly lower the risk of a heart
attack by more directly altering a mediating process. Are there such pivotal
interventions in developmental psychopathology? Reiss and Neiderhiser
(Chapter 6) suggest that parenting practices, especially in fostering warm
parent–child relationships, may be one candidate. They also point out that
important phenotypes might be discovered in unexpected domains, such as
the act of getting married. Their work indicates that this outcome can be
predicted with modest precision from a $G \times E$ effect.

As personalized medicine and prevention based on $G \times E$ evolve in
practice, the field must reconcile several crucial issues that will otherwise
hinder this movement. First, the public must be educated about genetic
tests. Horrible histories of eugenics and unwitting participation of African
Americans in genetic studies have led to public skepticism and misinforma-
tion about what a genetic result does and does not confer. Policymakers
should be urged to promote public education because the future is clear
that consumption of genetic testing will grow whether or not the science
catches up. We daresay that virtually every Western-culture baby born
today will undergo genetic testing for at least one disorder prior to reaching
adulthood. Scientists and health educators alike must become more aware
of the ancillary effects of $G \times E$ testing on consumers. Consumers are likely
to respond to testing results with momentous actions. Furthermore, testing
completed for one disorder might inadvertently confer information about a
second disorder, and so the consequences reverberate. With the discovery
of $G \times E$, public education is even more complicated.

Knowing the momentous impact of their findings on public actions,
scientists have an ethical responsibility to report their $G \times E$ findings accurately and with an appropriate degree of enthusiasm/caution. Public health
educators must learn what $G \times E$ actually implies about the probabilities,
causes, and prevention of disorders. It will be important to resolve issues of

informed consent for testing, secure storage of data, and protection of privacy (or not) from legal and public health officials interested in the broader safety of society.

Engineering Populations
through Environmental Manipulations

Costello (Chapter 10) has documented the large, apparently real, changes that have evolved in Western population-level intelligence, height, and psychopathology over the past century. Intelligence, height, and forms of psychopathology have all increased, and the gap between high and low socioeconomic status groups is growing wider. Although these characteristics have a high heritability, Costello suggests that environmental factors are responsible for these rapid shifts in outcomes. Cook-Deegan (Chapter 12) goes further in arguing that heritability does not imply immutability. He suggests that advocates of eugenics, such as Herrnstein and Murray (1996), mistakenly assume that the environment offers little hope for engineering change, thus elevating their call for genetic engineering as the only hope for population-level progress. He calls on scientists to fulfill their responsibility to get the science right.

The possibility that science could identify environmental causal factors in secular changes suggests that public policy might be able to engineer population-level changes for future generations. One of the most vexing questions for public policy that is raised by G × E discoveries is whether we should genetically and environmentally engineer populations. If certain G × E groups seem to fare best, should governments support the extinction of "bad" genes and "bad" environments? There is obvious backlash against doing so, just as there has been backlash against cloning and stem-cell research. The most ardent supporter of population engineering is the influential philosopher Savulescu (2001; Savulescu & Kahane, 2009), who argues in favor of procreative beneficence, the concept that parents and society at large have a moral responsibility to select the best next generation of offspring that they can, through enhanced use of *in vitro* fertilization and preimplantation genetic diagnoses (PGD) to determine the intelligence and risk of disorder for the fetus. He unabashedly states, "I will argue that we have a moral obligation to test for genetic contribution to non-disease states such as intelligence and to use this information in reproductive decision-making" (p. 414). He goes on, "I will argue that Procreative Beneficence implies couples should employ genetic tests for non-disease traits in selecting which child to bring into existence" (p. 415).

We do not disagree with the moral goals guiding Savulescu's plea; however, the current case against genetic engineering goes well beyond moral conservatism. It starts with a requirement to get the science right. Not only does the science not yet provide a clear picture of which genes are "best," it suggests that supposedly "bad" genes might well have adaptive functions under certain environmental conditions. The very concept of "good" and "bad" genes is mistaken. Most genes have pleiotropic effects that depend on environmental circumstances. Recent G × E discoveries suggest that we do not yet know all of the effects of specific genes in all contexts and that the effects of genes might be surprising. Polymorphisms of genes such as *MAOA* have been found to increase risk for violent behavior and disordered outcomes in some environments, suggesting that they might be candidates for selective extinction in Savulescu's world. However, this risk is obliterated in other environmental contexts, indicating that prevention of the disordered outcome might be achieved by means other than genetic engineering. Furthermore, these polymorphisms might prove to be adaptive in other environments, and if we extinguish these genes we may obliterate the beneficial effects for the species.

A related question is whether we should engineer environments. Obviously toxic environments, such as sexually and physically abusive experiences, have no apparent adaptive value and can be condemned outright. Other rearing environments are more ambiguous, however, and recent G × E findings render caution. Environments that confer risk for disorder have been found to yield no such risk in certain genetic contexts. It might be found, just as with so-called high-risk genes, that "high-risk" environments for some individuals turn out to be health-promoting environments for other individuals. Does this interaction absolve environmental engineers from altering toxic environments because not all individuals will be adversely affected? We are not so Luddite as to advocate fatalism. Rather, we suggest that scientific knowledge in the developmental psychopathology of some disorders is currently too crude to be able to engineer outcomes responsibly. The task for scientists is to understand the adaptation value of G × E combinations so as to craft interventions and policies that optimize outcomes.

Two kinds of G × E findings illuminate this issue. First, many G × E effects have been identified in genes for which the current population base rate is well above 10%. The rate for the "risky" polymorphism in *MAOA* has been reported to be 33–40% (Caspi et al., *www.ncbi.nlm.nih.gov/ omim*; Edwards et al., 2010). The rate for the "risky" short-allele polymorphism in *5-HTTLPR* is 43% (Online Mendelian Inheritance in Man, *www.ncbi.nlm.nih.gov/omim*), and the base rate for the "risky" polymorphism in *avpr1* reported by Reiss and Neiderhiser (Chapter 6) is 40%. How could such "bad" genes survive at such a high base rate unless they serve some survival value? Genes with a base rate over 10% probably have adaptation value for the species, at least under some environmental conditions. Artificially engineering their extinction might threaten the species under as-yet unknown conditions.

The second relevant G × E finding is that some genes may carry risk for susceptibility to environmental influence, in both positive and negative directions. Initial G × E hypotheses had been framed as "diathesis–stress" models for which the risky gene would lead to bad outcomes under stressful environments and, at best, average outcomes under ordinary or extraordinary environments. Belsky (Belsky et al., 2009) has proposed, instead, the vulnerability hypothesis that the very same individuals who are at highest risk for psychopathology under adverse circumstances are the most likely to display exceptionally positive outcomes under other circumstances. They are the so-called orchids living in a world of dandelions (Ellis & Boyce, 2008).

Recent evidence suggests that the susceptibility-to-environments hypothesis might have empirical support and implications for preventive intervention policy. Bakermans-Kranenburg and colleagues (2008) hypothesized that toddlers with the dopamine-processing *DRD4* risk allele for ADHD and externalizing behaviors (population base rate of 33%) would actually be *more* responsive to preventive intervention than would toddlers without the risk allele. Their intervention involved using videorecords of parent–toddler interaction to show parents how they might become more contingently responsive to their toddler's behaviors, in order to promote healthy development. The toddlers with the risk allele decreased their externalizing scores by almost 27%, whereas the protective-allele toddlers decreased externalizing behaviors by just 12% (a negligible difference with the 11% decrease among the protective-allele population in the randomly assigned control group). The hypothesis that the highest risk children will be the most responsive to intervention has been supported in other randomized controlled trials as well (Conduct Problems Prevention Research Group, 2007).

Ellis and Boyce (2008) argue even further that the very same children who are at highest risk for psychopathology might also be at highest probability for excelling. Genetic engineering to extinguish these genes from the population could extinguish chances for extremely positive outcomes. The difference in outcomes for these children depends on the environment.

This work suggests the importance of practices and policies that shape environments, especially for highest risk groups. Reiss and Niederhiser (Chapter 6) take this concept one step further by reporting a study by Hicks, South, DiRago, Iacono, and McGue (2010) which shows that inheritance and environmental risk for externalizing problems in late adolescence are positively correlated such that the highest genetically at-risk adolescents reside in the highest environmentally at-risk contexts. Also, environmental risk is higher in high genetically at-risk individuals, and vice versa. Costello (Chapter 10) suggests a similar argument to explain rapid secular changes in intelligence that might be explained by "multiplier effects" of individuals with particular genetic patterns selecting particular environments that nurture or hinder their development. So it becomes extremely important for policy to intervene in high environmental-risk contexts, both because the environmental risk is high and because the genetically vulnerable individuals are likely to reside there. The major caution here is not about the potential value of intervention; rather, the caution is that we, as a field, do not yet know how to change environments effectively.

JUDICIAL POLICY

A final set of issues concerns the implications of recent $G \times E$ findings for judicial policy, individual culpability for illegal actions, criminal sentencing, and juvenile justice.

Morse (Chapter 11) argues the case for holding individuals responsible and culpable for their crimes, without any exceptions based on $G \times E$ findings. No matter what the genetic or environmental circumstance, he maintains that individuals act out of choice, that they deserve the fate that justice might impose, and that society at large is well served by this seemingly harsh policy. Morse's premise is that choice and free will should be the contemporary bases for judicial policy. He does not distinguish between the guilt–innocence decision and the decision about sanctions (i.e., sentencing and rehabilitation). An alternative perspective is that, although declaration of guilt or innocence might well be based on whether an individual acted with volition to commit an illegal act, sanctions and forced interventions should take into account the developmental processes that underlie behavior and that suggest targets for rehabilitation.

It makes sense that the recent $G \times E$ findings should not change judicial policy in a radical way; however, Morse's initial premise is that choice and free will are contemporary bases for judicial policy, not with regard to declaration of guilt or innocence, but in imposing sanctions and forced interventions on perpetrators.

Two recent important legal cases provide context for these issues. In the first case (Feresin, 2009), an Italian court reduced by 1 year the sentence that had been applied to a convicted murderer, based on evidence presented by his attorney that he has a variant of the *MAOA* gene linked to violent behavior coupled with a life history of physical abuse with which *MAOA* interacts. Abdelmalek Bayout admitted in 2007 to stabbing and killing Walter Perez. According to Bayout, Perez had insulted him over the kohl eye makeup he was wearing for Islamic religious reasons. Bayout was convicted and sentenced to several years in prison. At an appeal hearing, Pietro Pietrini, a molecular neuroscientist, testified, "There's increasing evidence that some genes together with a particular environmental insult may predispose people to certain behavior." Using Bayout's DNA, Pietrini and a colleague found a polymorphism in the gene encoding the

neurotransmitter-metabolizing enzyme *MAOA*. They concluded that Bayout's genes would make him more prone to behaving violently if provoked,
and apparently the victim had provoked him. On the basis of this report,
the judge reduced Bayout's sentence by 1 year, arguing that the defendant's
genes "would make him particularly aggressive in stressful situations."
Giving his verdict, Judge Reinotti said he had found the *MAOA* evidence
particularly compelling.

Like Morse, we would disagree with this direction taken by the court,
but not for the reasons that Morse argues. Morse argues that individuals
must be held accountable for their actions no matter what their genes–
environment configuration has been. We agree that there seems little question that the defendant engaged in the criminal action and is guilty. With
regard to sanctions, however, we do not endorse the decision to adjust a
sentence because a possible cause (even a complicated G × E cause) has been
identified for the action. One problem is that the science at this point is
probabilistic rather than conclusive in this particular case. A second problem is that one task of science is to account for variance in outcomes, and
if science becomes successful, close to 100% of the variance in criminal
outcomes will be accounted for by future studies. Multiple genes will be
identified in interaction with multiple environments and causal pathways.
If we come to that point, would that state of science then render *every*
criminal behavior worthy of reduction in sentencing?

It seems that the merit in considering sentencing modification comes
not from merely identifying a cause for a criminal behavior, but from a
broader understanding of the causal context, the societal function served
by sentences, and the individual's future outcomes from various sentences.
Every behavior has a cause in scientific inquiry. No contemporary scientific study attributes the cause of a behavior to free will. Therefore, every
criminal action is "caused" by a configuration of genes and environments
in current context. There is nothing special in this regard about the case of
Abdelmalek Bayout.

The legal strategy by attorneys for Bayout is not unique and will
undoubtedly be followed by many similar cases in the near future. A recent
review (Feresin, 2009) indicates that in the past 5 years alone attorneys
have presented genetic evidence to support the defendant's predisposition
to criminal behavior in at least 200 cases.

Although we do not endorse alteration of sentencing based solely on
identifying a genetic or environmental cause of criminal behavior, we disagree with Morse that these and other factors should carry no weight in
considering sanctions for the defendant. Emerging judicial practice across
the world considers the age, intellectual competence, and mental status of
the defendant, as well as circumstances of the criminal event, including
provocation, in determining the appropriate sentence. The basis for sentenc-

ing is becoming less and less retribution and revenge and more and more societal deterrence and individual rehabilitation. Science can contribute to knowledge about deterrent value, and the consideration of retribution is one of legal precedent and values. More pertinent to the present discussion is the impact of sentencing on the defendant's rehabilitation. Here, a second recent important legal case is enlightening.

In the case of *Graham v. Florida*, the U.S. Supreme Court (May 2010) ruled that minors cannot be sentenced to life in prison without chance of parole. Terrance Graham was a 17-year-old adolescent who had committed armed robbery and then violated probation and had been sentenced to life in prison without any chance for parole. His attorneys argued successfully that such a sentence should never be levied against a juvenile under age 18, noting that the United States is one of the very few nations still imposing such sentences on minors. A previous case, *Roper v. Simmons*, in 2005, had established that juveniles could not be sentenced to death. The judges in the new case reasoned that "juveniles have lessened culpability (and) are less deserving of the most severe punishments." As compared to adults, juveniles have a "lack of maturity and an underdeveloped sense of responsibility"; they "are more vulnerable or susceptible to negative influences and outside pressures, including peer pressure" (p. 17); and their characters are "not as well formed" (p. 17). Accordingly, "juvenile offenders cannot with reliability be classified among the worst offenders" (p. 17). A juvenile is not absolved of responsibility for his or her actions, but his or her transgression "is not as morally reprehensible as that of an adult" (p. 17). Furthermore, "As petitioner's *amici* point out, developments in psychology and brain science continue to show fundamental differences between juvenile and adult minds" (p. 17). "For juvenile offenders, who are most in need of and receptive to rehabilitation (see Brief for J. Lawrence Aber et al. as *Amici Curiae*), the absence of rehabilitative opportunities or treatment makes the disproportionality of the sentence all the more evident" (p. 23). Finally, "The Eighth Amendment does forbid States from making the judgment at the outset that (juvenile) offenders never will be fit to reenter society" (p. 24). "An offender's age is relevant to the Eighth Amendment, and criminal procedure laws that fail to take defendants' youthfulness into account at all would be flawed" (p. 25).

With this ruling, the Supreme Court acknowledged that adolescents' brains are still developing, that desistance from criminal behavior may occur even without external treatment, and that some interventions have been successful at treating some receptive juvenile offenders. Thus, reduced sentencing, or a different kind of sanction, makes sense for a particular class of individuals. Morse's arguments would not seem to allow for such exceptions, but we view them as highly appropriate. The Supreme Court's ruling even goes beyond age in identifying features that might appropriately alter the sentence that a judge should impose. Even the highly conservative chief justice, John Roberts, wrote in a separate opinion that, Graham's "lack of prior criminal convictions, his youth and immaturity, and the difficult circumstances of his upbringing noted by the majority, *ante*, at 1, all suggest that he was markedly less culpable than a typical adult who commits the same offenses" (p. 8). Thus, the Court acknowledges that upbringing is relevant in understanding the circumstances of one's criminal behavior and in imposing sanctions. The intent of reducing sanctions is not to reduce guilt but to acknowledge the likelihood of developmental maturing and change through intervention. This is the basis for our disagreement with Morse.

CONCLUSION

No doubt, emergent G × E effects in developmental psychopathology have implications for scientific practice. They highlight the need for better measurement of the environment, better sampling in studies, and better theory of processes in development. Their implications for clinical practice policy, public policy, and legal policy are less clear. Although these findings have led policymakers to raise issues for personalized medicine, genetic and environmental engineering, and legal sanctions against criminals, the state of science seems premature to make binding decisions that may have unintended ramifications. We argue that caution is necessary until findings, and theory, become clearer. Nevertheless, it is already clear from the findings on gene–environment interdependence that we need to think in new ways with respect to numerous policy issues. It is very unusual for science findings to lead directly to policy change (see British Academy Working Group Report, 2009) but soundly based policy decisions need to pay full and proper attention to relevant scientific findings. The chapters in this volume provide examples of how the first steps can and should be taken.

ACKNOWLEDGMENT

We thank Zoe Dodge for editing.

REFERENCES

Bakermans-Kranenburg, J. M., van IJzendoorn, M. H., Pijlman, F. T. A., Mesman, J., & Juffer, F. (2008). Experimental evidence for differential susceptibility: Dopamine D4 receptorpolymorphism (DRD4 VNTR) moderates intervention effects on toddlers' externalizing behavior in a randomized controlled trial. *Developmental Psychology, 44,* 293–300.

Belsky, J., Jonassaint, C., Pluess, M., Stanton, M., Brummett, B., & Williams, R. (2009). Vulnerability genes or plasticity genes? *Molecular Psychiatry, 14*(8), 746–754.

British Academy Working Group Report. (2009). *Social science and family policies.* London: Author.

Brody, G. H., Beach, S. R. H., Philibert, R. A., Chen, Y., & Murry, V. M. (2009). Prevention effects moderate the association of 5-HTTLPR and youth risk behavior initiation: Gene × environment hypotheses tested via a randomized prevention design. *Child Development, 80,* 645–661.

Brown, G. W., & Harris, T. O. (1978). *Social origins of depression: A study of psychiatric disorder in women.* New York: Free Press.

Caspi, A., Sugden, K., Moffitt, T. E., Taylor, A., Craig, I. W., Harrington, H., et al. (2003). Influence of life stress on depression: Moderation by a polymorphism in the *5-HTT* gene. *Science, 301,* 386–389.

Collins, F. S. (2010). *The language of life: DNA and the revolution in personalized medicine.* New York: Harper.

Conduct Problems Prevention Research Group. (2007). The Fast Track randomized controlled trial to prevent externalizing psychiatric disorders: Findings from grades 3 to 9. *Journal of the American Academy of Child and Adolescent Psychiatry, 46,* 1250–1262.

Dodge, K. A., Bates, J. E., & Pettit, G. S. (1990). Mechanisms in the cycle of violence. *Science, 250,* 1678–1683.

Edwards, A. C., Dodge, K. A., Latendresse, S. J., Lansford, J. E., Bates, J. E., Pettit, G. S., et al. (2010). MAOA-uVNTR and early physical discipline interact to influence delinquent behavior. *Journal of Child Psychology and Psychiatry, 51*(6), 679–687.

Ellis, B., & Boyce, T. (2008). Biological sensitivity to context. *Current Directions in Psychological Science, 17,* 183–187.

Feresin, E. (2009, October 30). Lighter sentence for murderer with "bad genes": Italian court reduces jail term after tests identify genes linked to violent behaviour. *Nature News.* Available at *nature.com/news/2009/091030/full/neas.2009.1050.html.*

Graham v. Florida. 56 U.S. (2010).

Guttmacher, A. E., Collins, F. S., & Drazen, J. M. (Eds.). (2004). *Genomic medicine: Articles from the New England Journal of Medicine.* Baltimore: Johns Hopkins University Press.

Herrnstein, R. J., & Murray, C. (1994). *The bell curve: Intelligence and class structure in American life.* New York: Free Press.

Hicks, B. M., South, S. C., DiRago, A. C., Iacono, W. G., & McGue, M. (2009). Environmental adversity and increasing genetic risk for externalizing disorders. *Archives of General Psychiatry, 66*(6), 640–648.

Lansford, J. E., Chang, L., Dodge, K. A., Malone, P. S., Oburu, P., Palmerus, K., et al. (2005). Physical discipline and children's adjustment: Cultural normativeness as a moderator. *Child Development, 76*(6), 1234–1246.

Monroe, S. M., & Reid, M. W. (2008). Gene–environment interactions in depression research. *Psychological Science, 19,* 947—956.

Nebert, D. W., Zhang, G., & Vesell, E. S. (2008). From human genetics and genomics to pharmacogenetics and pharmacogenomics: Past lessons, future directions. *Drug Metabolism Review, 40,* 187–224.

Paynter, N. P., Chasman, D. I., Paré, G., Buring, J. E., Cook, N. R., Miletich, J. P., et al. (2010). Association between a literature-based genetic risk score and cardiovascular events in women. *Journal of the American Medical Association, 303*(7), 631–637.

Risch, N., Herrell, R., Lehner, T., Liang, K. Y., Eaves, L., Hoh, J., et al. (2009). Interaction between the serotonin transporter gene (5-HTTLPR), stressful life events, and risk of depression: A meta-analysis. *Journal of the American Medical Association, 301,* 2462–2471.

Roden, D. M., Altman, R. B., Benowitz, N. L., Flockhart, D. A., Giacomini, K., Johnson, J. A., et al. (2006). Pharmacogenomics: Challenges and opportunities. *Annals of Internal Medicine, 145,* 749–758.

Roper v. Simmons. (2005). 541 U.S. 1040.

Rutter, M. (1985). Resilience in the face of adversity. Protective factors and resistance to psychiatric disorder. *British Journal of Psychiatry, 147,* 598–611.

Rutter, M., Maughan, B., Mortimore, P., & Ouston, J. (1979). *Fifteen thousand hours: Secondary schools and their effects on children.* Cambridge, MA: Harvard University Press.

Savulescu, J. (2001). Procreative beneficence: Why we should select the best children. *Bioethics, 15*(5), 413–426.

Savulescu, J., & Kahane, G. (2009). The moral obligation to create children with the best chance of the best life. *Bioethics, 23*(5), 274–290.

Index

Page numbers followed by *f* indicate figure, *t* indicate table